THE HEALTHY BODY HANDBOOK

The Healthy Body Handbook

A Total Guide to the Prevention
and Treatment of Sports Injuries

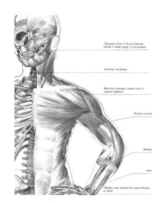

David C. Saidoff, P.T.
and Stuart C. Apfel, M.D.

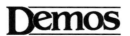

Demos Medical Publishing, 386 Park Avenue South, New York, NY 10016

Visit our website at www.demosmedpub.com

Although a great deal of care has been taken to provide accurate and current information, the ideas, suggestions, general principles, and conclusions presented in this text are subject to your personal health and sound medical advice. Not every possibility is represented, nor do we presume that all possibilities relate to your situation. This book should not be used as a substitute for recognized medical treatment modalities. Always consult your health care practitioner for medical advice.

Library of Congress Cataloging-in-Publication Data

Saidoff, David C.
 The healthy body handbook : a total guide to the prevention and treatment of sports injuries / David C. Saidoff and Stuart C. Apfel.– 1st ed.
     p. cm.
 Includes index.
 ISBN 1-932603-04-2 (pbk. : alk. paper)
 1. Sports injuries–Prevention. 2. Sports injuries–Treatment. 3. Wounds and injuries–Prevention. 4. Wounds and injuries–Treatment. I. Apfel, Stuart C. II. Title.
 RD97.S255 2004
 617.1'027–dc22

                                    2004015563

To: Debby, Elisha, Yishai, and Barak
David C. Saidoff, P.T.

To: Sari, Chaim, Avi, Shira, Ariella, and Rivka
Stuart C. Apfel, M.D.

Acknowledgments

Many thanks are offered to Dr. Diana M. Schneider and her team at Demos Medical Publishing for making this book a reality. Many thanks to my family for the time spent away from them while preparing this book. Above all, thanks to Debby, my wife and best friend.

David C. Saidoff, P.T.

Contents

Preface

A HEALTHY, STRONG BODY is essential to the enjoyment of life. We have written *The Healthy Body Handbook* is about learning to be proactive and keeping our bodies is top condition. It deals with the many conditions that affect individuals of all ages, from overdoing an exercise routine or simply rushing into sport activity after a period of inactivity, which can result in overuse and injury. Today the emphasis in sports is on taking the time to learn how to care for ourselves and prevent injury. A key concept is to pace yourself, learn to warm up, stretch before and after exercising, and not throw yourself headlong into exercise. This is as essential to wellbeing as it is to strength and stamina building. This handbook teaches about the dangers of the mind pushing the body beyond its limits. It educates you on exercising the "right way" and learning to avoid injuries and overuse through knowledge, patience with oneself, and appropriate exercise.

The Healthy Body Handbook will help you understand the basic structure and function of the musculoskeletal system of the human body. This knowledge is essential to the prevention of many health problems. It is written in a straightforward and readable format and is generously illustrated. Some chapters discuss specific areas of the body; others discuss conditions that affect the whole body; and the last chapter offers instructions for staying fit. There is also a detailed chapter that discusses a variety of strategies for pain relief. The information in this book will empower you to be proactive about your health, make positive lifestyle choices, prevent injuries, and participate fully in the healing of injuries—especially those that are sports-related.

The body sends out many warning signals of impending overuse and the resultant potential for injury. With the *Handbook* you will learn to listen to these signals, evaluate them, and make healthy decisions. It also includes information about the remedies and procedures your doctor is likely to recommend if you have been injured or have an illness. All of the chapters are self-contained; you can read any chapter independent of the others if you are interested in a specific condition, or read the book from cover to cover in order to become fully informed as to everything you can do to stay healthy and avoid injury.

The primary theme of this book is the lifelong necessity of exercise—without overdoing it! To this end, we have included detailed advice regarding various exercises and the appropriate regimen for stretching and strengthening, both of which are essential to warding off age-related problems. A healthy body also supports a healthy intellectual and emotional life. As the great American naturalist and philosopher Henry David Thoreau said, "Methinks that the moment my legs begin to move, my thoughts begin to flow."

Daily life in modern society can be overwhelming. There is just too much to do and there are too many demands requiring our attention. The Healthy Body Handbook stresses the importance of slowing down! Exercise should be fun. Do not push your body beyond its biomechanical limits. Respect your body and make time to give it the rest it needs. Take the middle ground and always seek balance.

Investing in your health is as essential as investing in your financial portfolio, so be proactive, take good care of yourself, and live a long and prosperous life.

David C. Saidoff, P.T.
Stuart Apfel, M.D.

1 The Musculoskeletal System

■ THE BASICS

THE MUSCULOSKELETAL SYSTEM is a marvel of balance and symmetry. More than 650 muscles are connected to the 206 bones of the skeleton. Together with the joints, tendons, and ligaments, the muscles and bones in the body comprise a *musculoskeletal system* that functions like a system of struts and levers. This system allows us to move and function within our environment.

Our bodies are designed using engineering principles that make us appear flawed when compared to other life forms. If a person could drive his legs as quickly as an ant, he would be able to run at speeds close to 100 miles per hour. However, at this speed his bones would break and his muscles would be torn to shreds! An engineer cannot increase power output by simply designing a larger model of the same machine. Although the human body is only about 25% efficient (about 75% of the energy we generate is lost), it still works efficiently when compared to man-made machines. When we reach our physical limits, we simply build machines such as bulldozers, cranes, and automobiles to compensate for our limited strength and stamina.

■ MUSCLES

The skeletal muscles are located beneath the skin, and they convert chemical energy into mechanical movement. Muscles exist in two states: contraction and relaxation. When muscles contract, they create movement; when they relax, they do not. A muscle cannot push, it can only pull. During contraction, muscles shorten by almost one-half, bringing their points of attachment closer together. This pulling force is first exerted on a tendon, which in turn pulls on a bone. By attaching to bones, muscles are arranged to act like levers.

There are about 6 trillion muscle fibers in the body—about two-thirds more muscles than bones—which provide a muscular, contoured surface to our figure. Each fiber is thinner than a hair and can support up to 1,000 times its own weight. Muscles thrive on exercise, and resting them too much causes them to shrink. It is for this reason that the limb will be thinner when a cast is removed from an arm or leg. The unused muscles have become *atrophied*, or shrunken.

■ INTERESTING FACTS ABOUT MUSCLE

Breasts are composed of *adipose tissue*—another word for fat—and no amount of exercise will make a woman's breasts larger. Unlike muscle, fatty tissue does not have the ability to contract and, therefore, it cannot not be exercised and enlarged. However, exercising the large pectoralis muscles located beneath the breasts may make the bosom appear to be somewhat more pronounced.

The muscle bearing the longest name is the *levator labii superioris alaeque nasi*. Contraction of this

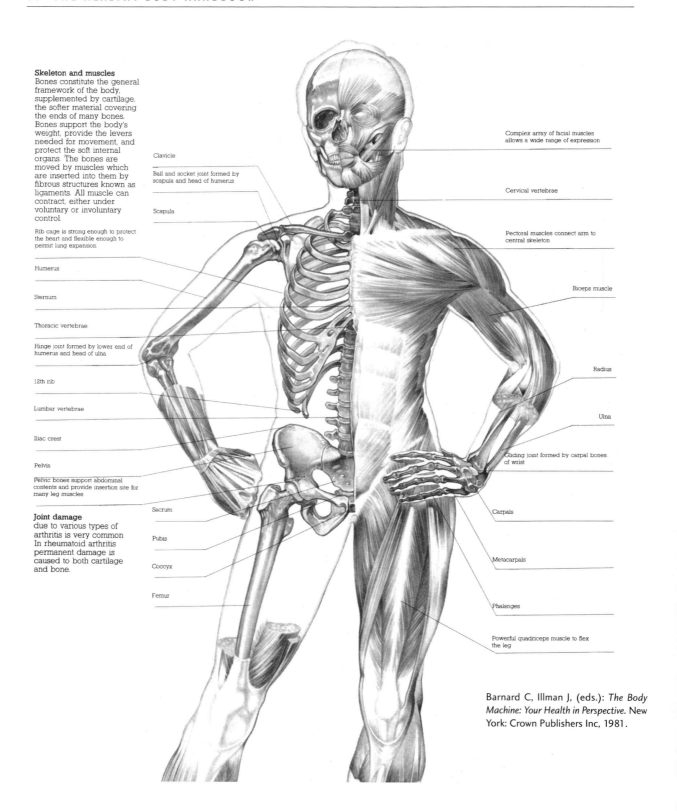

Skeleton and muscles

Bones constitute the general framework of the body, supplemented by cartilage, the softer material covering the ends of many bones. Bones support the body's weight, provide the levers needed for movement, and protect the soft internal organs. The bones are moved by muscles which are inserted into them by fibrous structures known as ligaments. All muscle can contract, either under voluntary or involuntary control.

Rib cage is strong enough to protect the heart and flexible enough to permit lung expansion

Humerus

Sternum

Thoracic vertebrae

Hinge joint formed by lower end of humerus and head of ulna

12th rib

Lumbar vertebrae

Iliac crest

Pelvis

Pelvic bones support abdominal contents and provide insertion site for many leg muscles

Joint damage

due to various types of arthritis is very common. In rheumatoid arthritis permanent damage is caused to both cartilage and bone.

Clavicle

Ball and socket joint formed by scapula and head of humerus

Scapula

Sacrum

Pubis

Coccyx

Femur

Complex array of facial muscles allows a wide range of expression

Cervical vertebrae

Pectoral muscles connect arm to central skeleton

Biceps muscle

Radius

Ulna

Gliding joint formed by carpal bones of wrist

Carpals

Metacarpals

Phalanges

Powerful quadriceps muscle to flex the leg

Barnard C, Illman J, (eds.): *The Body Machine: Your Health in Perspective.* New York: Crown Publishers Inc, 1981.

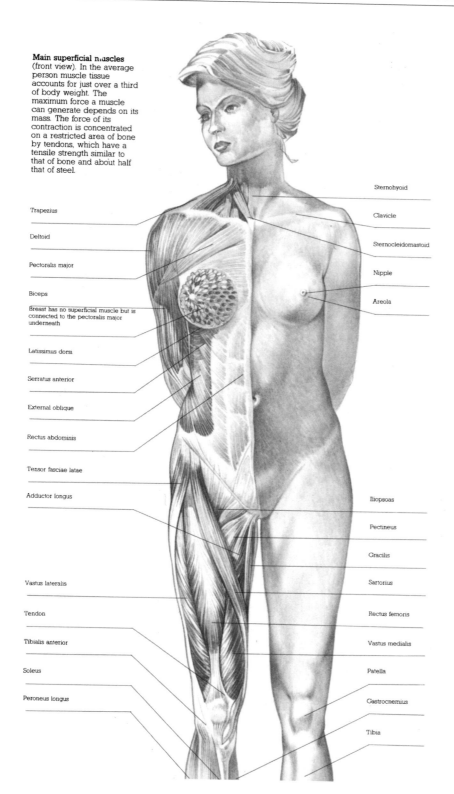

Main superficial muscles (front view). In the average person muscle tissue accounts for just over a third of body weight. The maximum force a muscle can generate depends on its mass. The force of its contraction is concentrated on a restricted area of bone by tendons, which have a tensile strength similar to that of bone and about half that of steel.

Trapezius

Deltoid

Pectoralis major

Biceps

Breast has no superficial muscle but is connected to the pectoralis major underneath

Latissimus dorsi

Serratus anterior

External oblique

Rectus abdominis

Tensor fasciae latae

Adductor longus

Vastus lateralis

Tendon

Tibialis anterior

Soleus

Peroneus longus

Sternohyoid

Clavicle

Sternocleidomastoid

Nipple

Areola

Iliopsoas

Pectineus

Gracilis

Sartorius

Rectus femoris

Vastus medialis

Patella

Gastrocnemius

Tibia

Barnard C, Illman J, (eds.): *The Body Machine: Your Health in Perspective.* New York: Crown Publishers Inc, 1981.

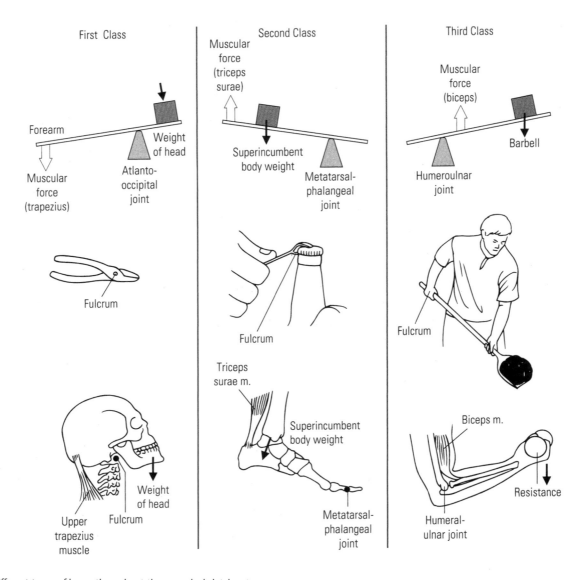

Different types of levers throughout the musculoskeletal system.
Saidoff DC, McDonough AL: *Critical Pathways in Therapeutic Intervention: Extremities and Spine,* St. Louis: Mosby, 2002.

facial muscle, which connects your upper lip to your nostril, results in an "Elvis Presley" lip curl. The *sartorius,* your longest muscle, extends from the knee to the waist, while your *latissimus dorsi* ("lats" for short) covers the largest area. It spreads, wing-like, across your upper back. The sit muscle—the *gluteus maximus*—is strong enough to help us climb stairs,

and the *masseter* muscles, which are located on the sides of the jaw, can generate a biting force of up to 150 lbs. The eye muscles have the fastest reaction time.

The smallest muscle in the body is the *stapedius*. It is about 1/20 of an inch in length and thinner than a dime; it is attached to the stapes bone, which is the smallest bone in the body. The stapes bone is located in the middle ear, where it sends vibrations through the eardrum. Another interesting fact: when you frown you use 43 muscles, but when you smile you only use 17. Moral: Be happy and save energy!

TENDONS

A *tendon,* known as a *sinew,* is a flexible, strong cord that attaches the end of a muscle to a bone. Tendons are an intermediate form of tissue that links muscle to bone and, like strings on a marionette, they make motion possible. By blending with the surface fibers of the bone (the *periosteum*), tendons carry the pulling force from the muscles to the bone, allowing the bone to move. A tendon cannot stretch for, if it did, the muscular force would be lost. While many tendons are short, others, like those belonging to the forearm muscles, are quite long. They pass through the wrist and allow movement of the hand and fingers. As a result, tendons often permit control from a distance. Tendons are enveloped in a delicate membrane known as a *synovial sheath* that protects them and provides nutrients.

The most familiar tendon is the *Achilles tendon,* which connects the calf muscles to the heel bone. This muscle-tendon-bone complex enables us stand on our toes: when the calf muscle contracts, it pulls upward on the heel by way of the Achilles tendon.

The *hamstring tendons* are the great tendons of the thigh muscles. They may be felt on either side of the back of the knee. Athletes often "pull a tendon." This refers to a stretch or tear of tendon fibers that results in a painful and disabling condition.

BONES

Most people think of bones as dead material but, in fact, they are like trees. They are quite alive and without their support we would collapse into a blob of jelly. Bones provide a rigid framework that supports the body, and they also provide the surface where muscles are anchored. In this way, bones provide the levers needed for movement. Acting as a chassis, the skeleton allows us to twist and bend through a wide range of movement unequalled by any man-made machine. Bone has the equivalent strength of steel-reinforced concrete, although it only accounts for 14% of body weight. Steel bars of comparable strength would weigh about 4 to 5 times that much! Bones also protect our vulnerable internal organs.

Bones are anything but dead and inert. In fact, bone is one of the most biologically active tissues, a living organ with a host of responsibilities beyond supporting and protecting the body. Bone is made up of one-third water and contains virtually all of the body's mineral supply. It is responsible for moving calcium, phosphorus, and other essential trace elements to wherever they are needed. In addition, the soft core of bone—known as the *marrow*—manufactures blood cells. Every minute, about 180 million red blood cells die, and most of the new ones are created in the bone marrow, along with the white blood cells that protect the body from infection.

Like a well-organized factory, a division of labor occurs within bone that is shared between its different types of cells. *Osteoblasts* create more bone by creating a protein-like substance known as *osteoid* that traps calcium, which is then mineralized; *osteoclasts* remove or remodel bone by secreting enzymes that dissolve bone; and *osteocytes* govern bone metabolism.

Bones disappear as we grow to adulthood. We start off with 350 bones at birth, but many of them fuse as we mature, reducing the number to 206 in the full-grown adult. Bones come in all sizes and shapes. The largest bone is the thighbone, or femur. It is a myth that women have an extra rib.

LIGAMENTS

Ligaments (from the Latin *ligare*, "to bind") are tough, fibrous bands that are found where bones meet at joints. They bind the two connecting bones together. Ligaments act as tie-pieces between bones by fastening around or across bone ends in bands— for example, the ribs or the bones of the forearm. In this way, ligaments guide the movement of joints and prevent excessive motion, which can cause injury. In activities such as gymnastics, which involve remarkable agility and often astounding suppleness, the joints are regularly moved in ways they were not intended to be moved. While beautiful to watch, these activities eventually undermine the protective function of the ligaments and cause joint problems in later years.

JOINTS

Getting around on Earth requires living things to have joints. Whether your means of locomotion is hopping forward like a kangaroo or rabbit, scuttling sideways like a crab, moving on all fours, or walking around like we humans do, living bodies must have joints. Otherwise, our only means of getting around would be to roll, log-like, in different directions— and that would not work well at all!

A joint is a connection between two or more

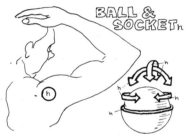

The ball-like head of one bone fits into the socket-like head of another, permitting all movements. Examples: shoulder and hip joints.

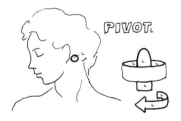

The C-shaped surface of one bone swings about the rounded surface of another. Movement is limited to flexion/extension. Examples: elbow, ankle, interphalangeal joints.

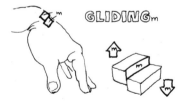

The concave surfaces of two bones articulate with one another. All movements are possible, but rotation is limited. Example: carpometacarpal joint of thumb.

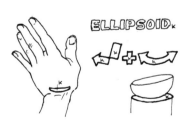

This is a reduced ball and socket configuration in which rotation is not permitted. Example: radiocarpal (wrist) joint.

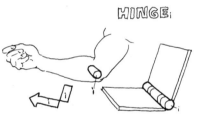

A ring of bone rotates about a process of bone. Movement is limited to rotation. Example: skull on its atlas (1st cervical vertebra) rotates about the odontoid process of the 2nd cervical vertebra.

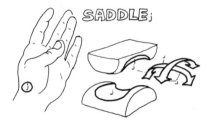

Two opposed flat surfaces of bone glide across one another. Movement is limited to gliding. Examples: intercarpal joints.

Kapit W, Elson LM: *The Anatomy Coloring Book*. New York: Harper & Row, 1977.

bones such as the knees or elbows. Some joints, such as those in the spine, have a limited range of movement. Others, such as those making up the hips, knees, elbows, wrists, fingers, ankles, and toes, allow for a good deal of movement. The body has several types of joints, classified according to how much movement they allow. For example:

- *Fixed joints* occur as seams between the pieces of bone making up the skull.

- The joints at the knees and fingers move back and forth in one direction only, or open and close like hinges on a door. These are called hi*nge joints*.

- The joint between the two topmost vertebrae (bones in the spine) is considered a *pivot joint* because it allows the highest bone to pivot on the lower one so that the head can turn from side-to-side.

- The very flexible joint that connects the thumb to the hand is called a *saddle joint* because of the saddle-like shape of its two ends. This joint allows the thumb to move in two directions: from side-to-side and from back to front.

- The shoulder and hip joints are called *ball-and-socket joints* because the bulbous head of one bone is round and fits into a hollow depression on the other bone.

A joint is endowed with the type of movement necessary for its particular function. Relatively little movement is needed in the back because the spine needs protection. In contrast, our hands would be little better than claws without the unique shape of a saddle joint—imagine trying to pick up a cup of coffee without your thumb! The opposable thumb allows us to pick up small items such as needles or tiny screws. On the other hand, it is a real advantage to have a wide range of movement at the hip or shoulder joints. Ball-and-socket joints allow for a very wide range of motion and are used for just getting around and much more. With almost 360-degree movement capability, the shoulder has different uses for different creatures. Gibbons use their shoulders to swing from tree to tree; moles use them for digging; birds use them to fly; antelopes use them to run; and human shoulders enable the hand to be placed in virtually any position—something extremely valuable when we are holding and using tools.

The weight of our bodies, our relationship to gravity, and simply moving around cause the ends of the bones to rub against each other. Eventually, this friction can be destructive to the joint. All movable joints, whether man-made (such as a door hinge) or biological, are prone to wear and tear. Automobiles and other man-made machines often wear out for this very reason. Unlike biologic systems, they do not have the ability to go to sleep and wake up refreshed. On the other hand, because we are alive, we have the capacity to heal, and any minor wear can be compensated for. For example, the body has evolved a special strategy to protect the joints from friction by covering the ends of the bones with *cartilage*—a smooth, springy, and spongy material that limits friction by acting like a shock absorber.

The space between the bones is called the *joint cavity*, which is enclosed by a *joint capsule*, a sac that covers both ends of the joint.Lining the inner capsule is a special layer of tissue called the *synovial membrane*, which releases a slippery lubricating fluid that keeps the bone ends from rubbing against each other. Synovial fluid provides nutrition to the cartilage and is essential for keeping it healthy. Because of cartilage and synovial fluid, friction within a joint is kept so low—even less than two pieces of wet ice rubbing against each other—that it beats the best low-friction materials designed by engineers! How-

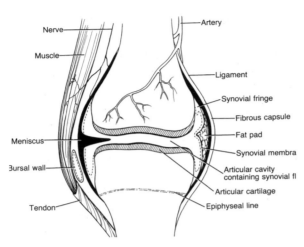

Anatomy of a typical joint.
Gould JA, Ed.: *Orthopaedic and Sports Physical Therapy*, 2nd Edition.

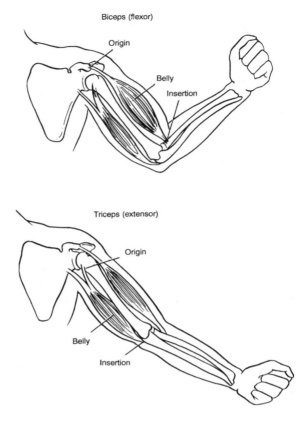

Antagonist and agonist in the upper arm. The biceps flexes upward, while the triceps extends downward.
Siegel Irwin M: *All About Muscle: A User's Guide.*
New York: Demos, 2000.

ever, this friction-reducing strategy eventually gives out with increasing age because the tissues that maintain it age. This wear and tear of the cartilage is the cause of osteoarthritis.

The tough ligaments that protectively wrap the joint comprise the outer capsule and keep it stable when it is moving. Ligaments also narrowly restrict movement of the joint so that only those portions of the joint ideally suited to take on wear are exposed to friction. Continuous stretching damages these ligaments and allows portions of the joint that were never meant to be in contact rub against each other. This frequently occurs in athletes.

■ MUSCLE BALANCE —
AGONIST AND ANTAGONIST

The muscles that make up the musculoskeletal system are paired, so that when one contracts, the other relaxes. For example, when you make a muscle in your arm, your biceps bunch up in the center of your upper arm. At the same time, the triceps muscle on the back portion of the arm relaxes as it stretches and becomes elongated. The muscle that contracts (the biceps) is the prime mover and is therefore called the *agonist*, while the muscle that is relaxed and elongating (the triceps) is called the *antagonist*. However, when the elbow is straightened, the triceps becomes the agonist and the elongating biceps assume the role of antoagonist.

There is a constant interplay between muscles during ordinary motion. The agonist and antagonist muscles on either side of a joint must be in proper balance for the joint to work properly. Both muscles must be able to stretch and contract, in turn. Like other types of soft tissue, muscles easily adapt to the changing positions of the adjacent joints. While this enables us to move, favoring one joint position over another will bias one muscle group over its opposite. If a position is held too long, one muscle will become permanently bunched up and the other will become excessively elongated.

The normal balance between them will be affected when one muscle gets stronger than its paired opposite. For example, an executive who spends lots of time in the sitting position will develop tight hamstring muscles because the sitting position favors shortening of the hamstring muscles and lengthening of the opposite muscles, the quadriceps group in the front of the thigh. This muscle imbalance between the muscles in front of and behind the thigh may cause problems and it will become difficult to straighten her legs. The executive will feel a stretching pain behind her knee because the hamstring muscle has become less flexible. This condition is called "tight hamstrings," and it can be corrected by regular stretching. Without regular stretching, these muscles will become more or less permanently tight in what is called a *contracture*.

Contractures of the hamstrings can be a major problem because they affect the nearby joints such as the knee, hip, and pelvis. Because they are large, long muscles, they attach on the pelvis and, if they are overly tight, they will pull too hard on the pelvis. This, in turn, upsets the pelvic posture and may strain the lower back and cause pain. Typically, as we grow older, paired muscles become excessively tight on one side and weaker on the other side.

It is essential that muscles have the right amount of contraction as well as flexibility in order to maintain healthy muscles and the joints they surround. Maintaining this balance between paired muscles is accomplished by both strengthening and stretching. Because muscle balance and good posture are so important, it is essential to perform regular stretching exercises.

▨ YOU HAVE LOTS OF NERVE!

A *neuron,* also called a *nerve cell,* communicates by transmitting electric signals between the brain or spinal cord and the entire body, much like a tele-

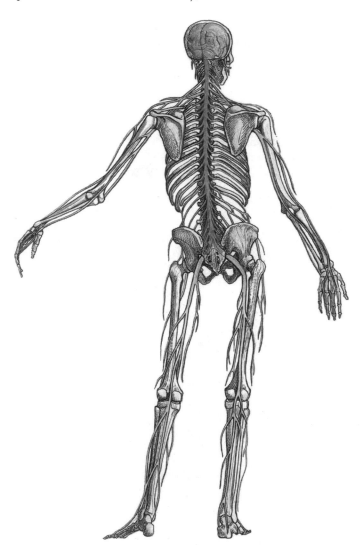

The central nervous system (dark) is made up of the brain and spinal cord, whereas as the peripheral nervous system extends from the spinal cord and reaches out to the limbs.
Bloom FE, Lazerson A, Hofstadter: *Brain, Mind, and Behavior.* New York: W.H. Freeman and Company, 1985.

phone system. This vast communication network is known as the *nervous system,* and it involves approximately 28 billion nerve cells, each of which is connected to thousands of others. It is similar to using a telephone system; when you dial a telephone number, you generate a series of impulses that travel along the telephone wire to an exchange that automatically connects the call to the number dialed.

The nervous system has two main components: (1) nerves that make up the brain and spinal cord, which form the *central nervous system* (CNS), and (2) those that link the central system to the rest of the body, which form the *peripheral nervous system* (PNS). The peripheral nervous system is made up of cells that perform certain functions according to instructions from the CNS, and others that provide information that is relayed back to the central system. The CNS houses all of the controls that allow information to be gathered and processed.

Afferent nerves carry information, such as the feeling of stepping on a thumbtack, back to the brain and spinal cord, whereas *efferent* nerves are sent from the brain and spinal cord to the legs to make them jump away from the thumbtack. A typical nerve cell consists of a cell body with many *dendrites* that receive information from other cells in the form of impulses. A long filament called the *axon,* which originates in the center of the nerve cell, sends out messages to other nerve cells. A *motor*

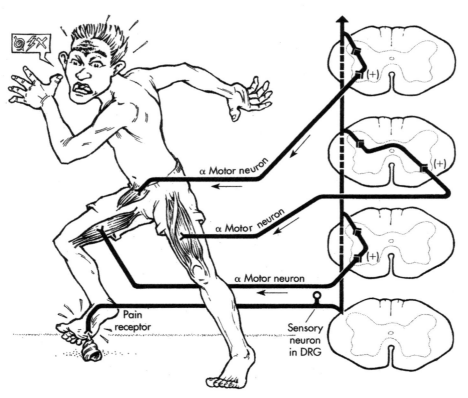

The sensation of stepping on a sharp object is carried to the central nervous system (brain and spinal cord) by a sensory neuron, and the excited withdrawal reflex reaction occurs through a motor neuron.
Leonard CT: *The Neuroscience of Human Movement.* St. Louis: Mosby, 1998.

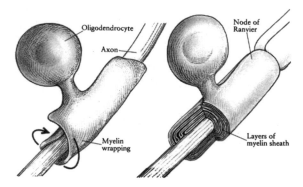

Myelin surrounds the nerves and serves as insulation to speed up the rate of electrical transmission. It is made up of fatty cholesterol. Bloom FE, Lazerson A, Hofstadter: *Brain, Mind, and Behavior*. New York: W.H. Freeman and Company, 1985.

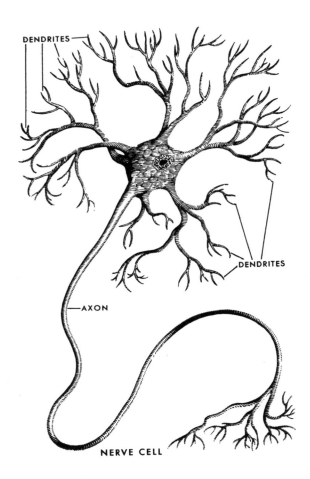

Typical nerve cell.
Asimov I: *The Human Brain: Its Capacities and Functions*.
New American Library, 1965.

insulation conduct impulses at a speed of 1½ miles (2.4 km) per hour, whereas those with thick myelin sheathing conduct impulses of nearly 325 miles (523 km) per hour. One reason that newborn babies cannot walk is because they have not yet developed the insulating myelin sheath around the nerves leading to their legs. In diseases such as multiple sclerosis, the myelin sheath degenerates and normal function is impaired.

Nerves transmit electrical impulses that are passed along in a "spark-gap" manner and are therefore not continuous. At the end of each nerve is a *synapse* that connects it to another nerve or to a muscle. When a nerve impulse reaches the end of an axon, it triggers the release of chemicals known as *neurotransmitters* that travel across the tiny gap that lies between two nerve cells—the *synaptic junction*. Each nerve cell chemically communicates with surrounding cells via these neurotransmitters. For example, if a neighboring cell is a muscle fiber, that muscle will contract. There are many types of chemical neurotransmitters: acetylcholine, norepinephrine (known as *noradrenaline*), serotonin, and dopamine. Excessive dopamine in the brain is associated with schizophrenia, while dopamine deficiency is associated with Parkinson's disease, in

nerve sends axons out from the brain and spinal cord to muscles that move the skeleton, whereas *sensory nerves* such as those involved in sight, hearing, taste, smell, or touch send information about experience and the environment to the brain and spinal cord for processing.

The speed with which information is sent depends on how much insulation covers the nerve fiber. Nerve fibers have an insulating sheath called *myelin* that wraps around the nerve fibers and speeds up the rate of electrical impulse. The thicker the sheath, the faster the impulse. Fibers lacking

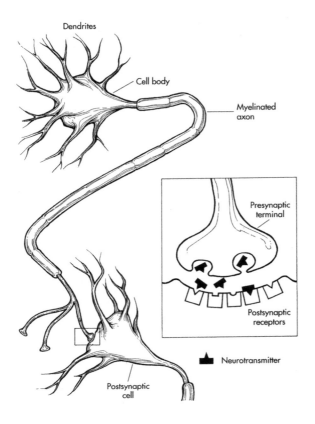

The tiny space (synapse) between the two nerve cells is where they communicate via chemical release of neurotransmitters.
Leonard CT: *The Neuroscience of Human Movement*. St. Louis: Mosby, 1998.

other words, the illness produced depends on which neurotransmitters are involved.

■ NERVE CELLS ARE SPECIALISTS

Neurons are highly specialized cells that are quite vulnerable to many types of injuries and disease. Nerve cells are more sensitive to poisoning by alcohol and drugs because they are specialized and the damage is often permanent and irreversible. Nerve cells are less tolerant than other types of cells to oxygen deprivation and will die within a few minutes if they are deprived of the oxygen and nutrients delivered via the blood. This deprivation can occur as the result of a stroke in the brain or spinal cord. The same thing occurs in *carpal tunnel syndrome* at the wrist. The nerves in the brain and spinal cord (the CNS) are incapable of repair if damaged, although nerves of the arms and legs (the PNS) are capable of some repair. If a nerve is cut at the wrist or compressed as in carpal tunnel syndrome, it can heal and normal function may return.

The peripheral nerves wind down through the arms and legs, around bones, under muscles, behind tendons and ligaments, and beneath skin and fascia. Fortunately, they can elongate and bend during our body movements. The downside is that they may become entrapped, inflamed, or injured. If we break a bone, a sharp shard may tear a nerve. If we hold our wrists in one position and use our fingers for long periods of time—as we do when typing or playing the piano—fluid buildup can compress the nerves and prevent the delivery of sufficient oxygen and nutrients. When the wrist tendons are overworked and swell, the median nerve passing between them into the hand is compressed, resulting in carpal tunnel syndrome. (See chapter 24)

Another problem that occurs as we grow older is that without proper stretching of our arms and legs, the soft tissue surrounding our peripheral nerves may become accustomed to poor posture and become taut. This excessive soft tissue tautness is experienced as inflexibility, which may press on the nerves within the arms and legs. This may cause painful compression of the nerve at various sites throughout the body (known as *fibrosseous tunnels*) in which the nerve is pressed between soft (fibrous) and osseous (hard bony) tissue. This may result in pain, weakness, and wasting in the muscles con-

trolled by that nerve. When no symptoms occur, the nerve becomes stressed and is more likely to develop problems if it is compressed at another point along its length. For example, if the median nerve is compressed or pinched near the neck, it will become stressed along its entire length and be more likely to succumb to carpal tunnel syndrome at the wrist. This is known as a "double crush" (see chapter 24) and may be avoided by regular stretching exercises that keep the spine, legs, and arms flexible.

2 Soft and Hard Tissue Injuries

■ MUSCLE AND TENDON INJURIES

INJURIES to muscles are common, especially during sporting activities. One of the most common problems is muscle cramps that occur during or after intense or prolonged exercise. This type of cramp is called a "charley horse" because the seventeenth century policemen in the service of King Charles often had aching legs from patrolling on horseback.

By drawing on stored sugars, muscles attempt to generate more power for a lot of activity or during activities such as sprinting that require brief, intense, bursts of energy. All activities utilize oxygen, but intense bursts of energy require more power than normally available, and so muscles work anaerobically—meaning "without oxygen." This process is less efficient in the long run and, although it allows for increased power, it generates the waste product *lactic acid*, which builds up in the muscles and causes them to cramp. It is this buildup of waste material and its slow removal that causes discomfort to be felt for several days after intense or prolonged activities.

■ STRAINS

Muscles and tendons work by contracting and relaxing in much the same way as sliding doors open and close. They may become stretched, frayed, or torn if they are overworked. When muscles and tendons are injured without a direct bruise or cut, we say they are *strained*. A *muscle strain* occurs from overexertion and may either result in a *stretch* or *tear* of the muscle fibers. Common types of muscle strains include a pulled hamstring or groin pull injury, both of which occur in sprinters from muscle overload.

When a muscle tear occurs, the torn space is not filled in by new muscle tissue. Instead, a poorer quality *scar tissue* fills the gap. Undamaged muscle tissue consists of fibers that run parallel with each other. This distributes force evenly throughout the muscle. The fibers making up scar tissue are randomly oriented, and they not able to contract; they form a weak site that is prone to failure. Because scar tissue is not as strong or capable as muscle, the muscle is weakened and more prone to re-injury.

Strains are classified according to how much disruption occurs in the muscle and tendon fibers. A *mild muscle strain* (1st degree strain) occurs from overstretching or minor tearing of a muscle or tendon and often heals without treatment. A *moderate strain* (2nd degree strain) involves tearing of more muscle fibers and must be treated with care so that it will heal to its pre-injury level. With a *partial muscle tear*, the muscle can still contract, although weakly and painfully. A moderate strain may lead to *total muscle rupture* (3rd degree strain) if untreated. A complete muscle tear can be felt as a gap in the muscle, and any attempt to contract the muscle will be useless.

Muscular *hematoma* refers to an isolated internal bruise from a blunt hard blow. The resulting bleed-

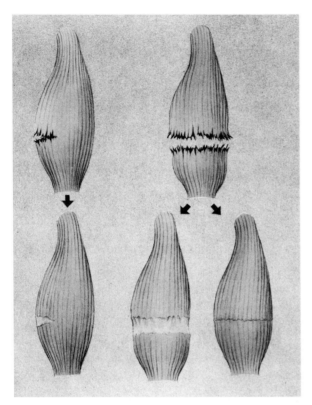

Partial and total muscle ruptures and the results of healing. Left: Partial rupture that has not been operated on fills with scar tissue. Right: A full rupture that has both been operated on (right) and which has filled in with scar tissue (left) because no operation occurred.
Peterson L, Renstrom P: *Sports injuries: Their Prevention and Treatment.* Chicago: Yearbook Medical Publishers, 1986.

ing within the muscle may simply go away or may develop into a serious problem. Because of this, a significant bruise to any muscle should be brought to the attention of a doctor.

■ TENDON DISEASES

Many tendons have a poor blood supply and are enveloped in a supportive *synovial sheath* of tissue that provides them with nutrients. Many of the tendons in the body may take a long time to heal after becoming injured because they lack their own

blood supply. Excessive use of the tendons causes the tendon to slide up and down within its synovial sheath. At some point, the friction imparted to the delicate synovial sheath will injure the sheath and provoke inflammation, which is known as *tenosynovitis* ("itis" means inflammation) or inflammation of the synovial sheath.

Tendons without sheaths, such as the Achilles tendon, may also become inflamed from excessive overuse of the calf muscles. The tendon may pull on the heel bone very hard and repetitively in a person with a normal foot, causing the tendon insertion on the bone to become inflamed. In a foot that has an arch that is either too flat or too high, the tendon may move to the right or to the left with each step, causing it to become inflamed at its insertion point on the heel bone. With either source of inflammation, the tendon becomes stressed from overuse and the resulting inflammation is called *tendonitis*. (See Chapter 5 for information regarding pain and inflammation.)

■ LIGAMENT SPRAINS

In general, ligaments are not capable of stretching. Therefore, they are able to bind the two ends of a joint securely together, like taut Scotch tape. A torn ligament is called a *sprain* and results in a less stable joint. Ligament injuries occur quite often, especially in the ankle and knee joints, and they are very painful. A mild sprain (grade I sprain) involves a tear of only a few ligament fibers, while a moderate sprain (grade II sprain) involves a tear of less than one-half of the fibers making up that ligament. A complete sprain (grade III sprain) involves a rupture of all of the fibers in the ligament. Aside from pain, a ligament sprain involves bleeding that causes the neighboring joint to swell up after the injury. The affected joint will usually turn blue or purple the next day.

Ligaments are so strong—stronger even than bone—that they will occasionally pull away a bit of bone from the area where they attach, rather than tear. Sprains may occur anywhere in the musculoskeletal system, but they most often occur in the wrist, elbow, shoulder, ankle, and knee.

The torn space is not filled in by new ligament tissue when a ligament tear occurs. Like muscle, poorer quality *scar tissue* fills the gap. This distributes force unevenly throughout the ligament and represents a weak site that is prone to failure with excessive joint motion. Because scar tissue is not as strong or capable as the ligament, it is weakened and more likely to be re-injured in the future.

■ BURSAE

A *bursa* is a fluid-filled bag (*purse* in Latin) reflecting its shape. The bursa itself is made up of synovial membrane, the same material that lines the inside of many joints. Compare a bursa to a balloon filled with water that is placed between two wooden boards moving in different directions. The balloon makes sure that the surfaces of the two boards do not touch, but it allows them to move while being very close to each other. Bursae work in the body just like water balloons. They are present at sites of high friction to minimize the friction from moving parts, especially at large joints such as the shoulder, hip, and knee. They help fine-tune motion at these joints. The walls of the bursa may wear down if motion is excessive at a joint, and this may result in inflammation of the synovial walls that make up the bursa. This is the body's way of telling us to slow down and rest. If we do not slow down, the inflamed bursa may swell and develop into a painful condition known as *bursitis*. Bursitis may also occur from infection if bacteria get into a bursa. Additionally, infection will trigger an immune response that releases pus and makes the bursa swell. This sort of

bursitis is known as *septic bursitis,* and it must be treated by a doctor immediately to prevent the spread of infection.

■ CARTILAGE WEAR – OSTEOARTHRITIS

As described in Chapter 1, the constant wear and tear of joints causes the cartilage that caps the bone ends to wear down to bare bone. Imagine the human knee tolerating the pounding that occurs with each step taken. The weight of the body pushes downward at the knee joint, and the upward push from the ground meets this equal but opposite force at the knee. These forces collide at the knee and wear down the cartilage, over time. The body attempts to limit the wearing down of the joints by various mechanisms, including the lubrication of the synovial fluid and the smooth surface of the cartilage. Tissues such as the *menisci*—which act as a washer at the knee joint—also absorb some of these colliding forces. Whatever damage occurs, for example from running a long distance or performing heavy work, the body often has the ability to heal itself when resting. However, due to increasing age or excessive wear, the body eventually begins to lose its ability to repair cartilage and it degenerates. This process of cartilage degeneration in large body joints is called *degenerative joint disease* or *osteoarthritis.* Osteoarthritis occurs most commonly in women and diabetics; it is worsened by obesity; and it is uncommon in people of Asian descent. (See chapter 33.)

■ SUBLUXATIONS/DISLOCATIONS

Many joints are wrapped by a joint capsule and ligaments for protection. However, despite the protection offered to joints, some injuries and forces applied to the body are so strong that they pull the joint out of alignment. A *subluxation* occurs when the outside force is strong enough to alter the perfect alignment of the two bones that make up a joint. This happens because the capsule and surrounding ligaments absorb the force of the injury and tear. In doing so, the protective ligaments make sure that the two bone surfaces remain in contact. However, with still greater force, contact between the two opposing bones making up the joint is lost and a *dislocation* occurs. This happens more easily in some joints than others, including the knee, shoulder, and finger, because these joints are very shallow.

Subluxations usually affect the knee cap, ankle, and *acromioclavicular* joint of the shoulder, while dislocations usually affect the shoulder, elbow, and finger joints. Subluxated joints often return to their original positions on their own and remain stable with healing of the capsule and ligaments. Dislocations require immediate medical attention, including x-rays, to make sure that no bones have been broken; the doctor must return the joint back to normal very quickly, or this may become impossible without surgery.

Bone Bruises

Bones may be injured by banging into something hard—for example, when you accidentally hit your elbow against a hard surface. The inner, soft core making up bone is supplied by blood vessels, and the hard outer core acts as a lever to protect the bone from forces that would damage the delicate blood vessels that run through it. Because of this, the outer portion of bone has a unique glove-like covering (the *periosteum*) that makes up for the lack of surface blood vessels. A nasty bump from a fall can cause this bone covering to bruise. This type of bone bruise is aptly named *perostitis* (inflammation of the "bone-skin"), and a bump swells at the site of impact. This bump occurs because the resulting inflammation causes fluid to accumulate between the periosteum and bone in an attempt to protect and heal the bruised bone.

When Bones Break - Fractures

Bones can bend just like a tree branch or trunk in a strong wind. Unfortunately, just as a wooden branch can snap and break off, a bone can break, given enough force. This results in a *fracture*. How exactly does this happen?

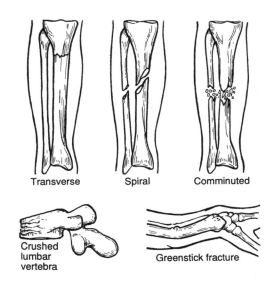

Different types of fracture patterns, meaning a *break* in Latin. From left: transverse fracture, spiral fracture, and comminuted fracture. Dandy DJ: Essential *Orthopaedics and Trauma*. Churchill Livingstone. Edinburgh, 1989.

Bones are similar in hardness to many rocks because they are primarily made of calcium and other mineral salts. About one-third of bone is made up of a tough elastic protein fiber called *collagen* (from the Greek words *kolla* meaning "glue" and *gen* meaning "forming"). Mineral will be removed from the bone if a chicken bone is placed in vinegar for several days because of the acetic acid contained in vinegar. The submerged bone will become so pliable that it may be tied in a knot. Collagen provides the framework for calcium and other salts to be deposited within the bone. Calcium provides hardness and rigidity, and collagen allows bone to momentarily become as flexible as rubber, which enables it to withstand tension. It is this remarkable ability to withstand both compression and tension forces that makes bone similar to the modern building material of choice: reinforced concrete. Calcium withstands compression very well, and collagen withstands tensile forces—much like concrete and steel beams.

With every step we take, the world we live in is constantly bumping into us, or we are bumping into it. The ability of bones to withstand *compression* and *tension* allows it to stand up to enormous forces. However, in the same way that buildings will collapse from excessive force during an earthquake or explosion, our bones also have a limit beyond which they cannot tolerate force. When this limit is reached, the bone will fail and break. The good news is that, unlike a broken tree branch that falls off, bones can heal!

Bones have a poor ability to withstand shear and torsion forces, which impart simultaneous equal and opposite forces. This is especially true in older people, whose bones are more porous from osteoporosis and contain less calcium. Many older women who break their hips do so even before they fall. It is not hitting the ground that causes the hip to fracture. Typically, they may have suddenly turned at the waist, leaving their feet planted on the ground in front of them. This causes a twisting of the delicate, thin portion of the femur bone known as the femoral neck, causing it to snap.

Another category of bone fracture is a *stress fracture*, which most often affects the leg and foot. A good analogy for the kind of stress your foot and leg undergoes with each step is to take a baseball bat and whack it hard against the floor several times. Vibrations will pass up through the bat into your hands, and the tip of the bat will soon become marred and scratched. Similarly, you place incredible amounts of pressure on your feet every time you walk. A person weighing only 135 lbs. absorbs a pressure of over 2.5 million pounds in the soles, heels, and toes during a typical day of walking. The large upward forces from the ground are absorbed by the muscles, which act like cushions to minimize the jarring impact to the bones in the foot and leg. However, if you push yourself too far and too hard, the muscles will fatigue and work less efficiently, and the bones will have to absorb more and more stress. At some point, the bones will become unable to tolerate this stress and they will fatigue and break. For this reason, a stress fracture is also called a *fatigue fracture*.

An *open fracture* occurs when the broken ends of bone pierce the skin. Bone splinters into many pieces in a *comminuted fracture*. Similar to a freshly cut wood sapling that can be broken on one side and only bent on the other side, children commonly suffer *greenstick fractures* because their bones are so springy. Fortunately, fractures begin to heal soon after they occur.

3 Fatigue and Injury

DESPITE ITS ABILITY to regenerate, the musculoskeletal system is governed by the same principles of wear and tear that apply to other mechanical systems. Whether the material we are considering is steel, concrete, bone, muscle, tendon, or ligament, each has its own breaking point beyond which it ceases to function and injury may occur. The likelihood of injury is increased by *fatigue*. The body can be pushed only so far before it starts to fatigue. Once this happens, you are more likely to develop what has been alternately called *overuse syndrome* or *repetitive stress injury*.

The term *fatigue* may be used to describe the tendency of a material to break or fail under stress. Fatigue also refers to weariness or exhaustion from labor, especially if any body part is worked to the point of injury. Overuse can lead to tissue failure. Knowledge is power, and understanding the physical limits of the musculoskeletal system will allow you to pay attention to your body and avoid overuse to the point of fatigue.

Getting hit with a baseball bat by accident or having someone attack you may certainly cause injury. However, fatigue is the most common cause of musculoskeletal injury. Bone and muscle work together, hand-in-hand, to ward off the effects of fatigue and the likelihood of sustaining an overuse syndrome or athletic injury.

■ MUSCLE FATIGUE

Many different types of muscles in the body may be categorized into either *voluntary* muscles such as those that move the skeleton, or *involuntary* muscles such as those of the heart and other internal organs. The latter group rarely tires; your heart can beat continuously without stopping or undergoing fatigue for an entire lifetime. In contrast, skeletal muscles can become fatigued. Why these muscles fatigue depends upon the way they burn energy. The biceps muscle in your arm can generate a quick, short burst of energy at the expense of quickly building up a waste product referred to as *lactic acid*. Lactic acid buildup causes the muscle to gradually become inefficient, and rest is required to give the body a chance to rid itself of the lactic acid. We certainly could not walk very far on our hands because the muscles of our arms and hands would tire quickly. However, our legs can walk mile after mile without tiring to the point of having to stop. This is because the muscles of our legs are composed of a different kind of fiber that does not easily fatigue.

By virtue of their sheer bulk and number, muscles play an important role in absorbing much of the stress and force delivered to and through the musculoskeletal system from the weight of the body and its relationship to gravity (the ground reaction forces moving upward from the floor through your feet) and injurious forces such as when you bump into something. These forces can cause bones to break, muscles to strain, tendons to tear, and ligaments to sprain. To be able to ward off injury, muscles should be in top form, not fatigued. Even leg muscles, which are fatigue-resistant, may fail to protect the adjacent bone from injury.

BONE-SPLINTING MUSCLES

Imagine skiing downhill and suddenly getting your ski boot caught in a snowdrift. Your body above the ski boot—whose upper edge abuts against the front of your shinbone—continues moving at least 15 to 20 miles per hour, depending on how fast you are going. Because your foot is stuck in one place, your shin bone will be momentarily bent forward, due to experiencing too much tension and compression in a very short time. If you multiply your body weight (100 to 200 lbs.) by the speed at which this happens, the forces generated are very strong and can easily break the shinbone. Yet this does not always happen. Why not? Breaks such as this can be prevented by a large, powerful, and very important muscle group called the *triceps surae*. (See chapter 8.) This muscle group is comprised of the *gastrocnemius* and *soleus* muscles (as well as the Achilles tendon). It suddenly and reflexively contracts in response to sudden stretching in order to provide a counterforce behind the shin. This counterforce cancels the tension exerted in the front of the leg. This bone-sparing strategy is an example of how muscles and bones work together to protect each other throughout the musculoskeletal system.

BONE STRESS AND FRACTURE

Bones are the strong, internal structure of the body. When engineers build a modern building, they utilize both concrete and steel beams. They do this because concrete withstands compressive forces, while steel withstands bending or tensile forces.

That is why concrete with steel beams within it is called steel-reinforced concrete. Bone is so resistant to compression forces that you can jump from a considerable height and your skeleton can, to a large extent, prevent a break. On the other hand, bending bone subjects it to tensile forces, which can overcome the cement holding the bone cells (*osteons*) together.

If you try to bend a long chicken leg into a bow, it will break on the convex side. Bending a bone converts it from a straight rod into a bow with a concave and convex side. The concave side undergoes compressive forces while the convex side undergoes tensile forces.

Bending a thigh bone can occur if you are headed down the ski slope and one leg is abruptly stopped by becoming stuck in a snow bank. The thighbone, which is loaded with your body weight, undergoes momentary bending, causing tension force (arrows moving apart) on the convex side and compressive forces (arrows moving toward each other) on the concave side. Gould JA (ed.) *Orthopaedic and Sports Physical Therapy*, 2nd Edition. St. Louis: Mosby, 1990.

Because bone handles tension poorly, the fracture will occur on the convex side, causing a *transverse fracture* (known as a *cross-wise fracture*). The bony break will occur across the length of the bone. As in the skier analogy above, a transverse fracture can be avoided if the *triceps surae* can quickly generate enough force to counter the tensile forces in the tibia bone.

If you load or overload bone quickly, you may subject it to so much compressive force that it will break, despite the fact that bone is resistant to compressive forces. If you jump out of a two- or three-story building and land on your feet, you are very likely to break either your heel bone or one or more of the vertebrae in your spine. This can also happen if you slip on ice and land hard on your buttocks, especially if your bones are brittle due to osteoporosis or some other degenerative condition. The bone virtually collapses in on itself and becomes short and squat, as can be seen on x-ray. This is called a *compression fracture*.

■ SHEAR AND TORSION

The body can recover quite well from either tensile or compressive forces. Shear and torsion are two destructive forces on bones. Shear forces occur when two forces act on a bone in opposite directions. When this occurs, the bone can shear off in different directions, causing an oblique distortion of the bone. If the force is greater than the adjacent muscle, a *shear fracture* will occur because the frac-

ture line passes obliquely through the bone. The ability of the adult skeleton to heal itself by remodeling bone with this type of fracture is compromised when shear forces cause an oblique fracture, because the magnitude of disruption to the bone is so severe that healing is not likely to restore it to its original strength. Children can recover nicely if they break a bone before puberty because they have better recuperative abilities.

Torsion forces applied to the body have the worst effect. *Torsion* occurs when two forces are applied to bone in such a way that one force rotates it one way, and the another force rotates it in the opposite direction. This causes a *spiral fracture*. When this happens, the skeletal system of either an adult or a child cannot remodel the bone well enough over time to compensate for the injury. If the injury caused the bone to bend more than 20 degrees, only traction or surgical intervention can correct the problem.

■ HOW BONES HEAL

When a fracture occurs, blood from broken vessels within the bone form a mass of blood clots (hematomas) around the site of breakage. This has the effect of splinting the two bone ends together so that they will not move very far apart. The surrounding muscles go into a spasm in order to help this splinting. Blood is a versatile substance that is converted into other substances according to the body's needs. For example, a woman's breast converts blood into milk in order to nurture an infant. With a bone fracture, the blood clot surrounds the two broken bone ends like a glove and serves as a framework for calcium deposition. The hematoma, working as a framework, is called an *osteoid*.

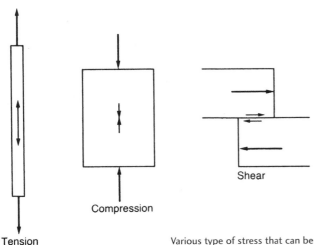

Tension   Compression   Shear

Various type of stress that can be applied to bone that will cause a fracture (with the exception of a break of the heel bone). Gould JA (ed.). *Orthopaedic and Sports Physical Therapy*, 2nd Edition. St. Louis: Mosby, 1990.

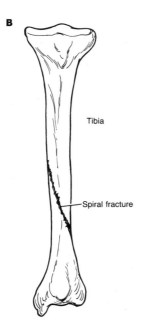

B

Tibia

Spiral fracture

Torque applied to the ski tip is transferred to the shinbone, resulting in a spiral fracture. Gould JA (ed.). *Orthopaedic and Sports Physical Therapy,* 2nd Edition. St. Louis: Mosby, 1990.

It gradually becomes impregnated with calcium crystals that are brought into the tissue by blood vessels growing into the osteoid. Once enough calcium is deposited, the red-colored, soft, osteoid become white and hard and is called a *callus.* This callus is eventually chiseled into the bone's original shape by a process known as *bone remodeling.*

THE ECCENTRIC MUSCLE

Strenuous exercise, activity, or trauma can cause injury to the musculoskeletal system. Muscles that become fatigued generate less tension and are poor protectors of bones and other tissues. The same can happen if a muscle is too weak. Keeping muscles in optimal shape in terms of proper strength and flexibility is essential to warding off injury.

Muscles work in several ways. An *isometric* con-

traction occurs when muscles contract in such a way that the limb and joint do not move. An *isotonic* contraction occurs when muscles contract in such a way that the joints and limbs do move. There are two types of isotonic contraction. When you pick up a gallon of milk, your biceps contract *concentrically*— meaning that the muscle fibers bunch up together. Alternatively, after you have poured milk in your coffee and you are lowering that heavy gallon back down to the table, you are still using your biceps, but now the muscle fibers are working by doing the opposite of contracting; they are *distracting,* which means that the fibers are slowly moving apart instead of closer together, allowing the milk to be placed on the surface in a gradual, controlled manner. This type of muscle work is known as *eccentric* work. (Referring to eccentric muscle activity, "contraction" is a misnomer because the fibers are distracting rather than contracting. It is for this reason that this type of muscle activity is called "eccentric," referring to its odd and peculiar nature.)

One way to appreciate the value of an eccentric contraction is to consider the crumple zones developed by the automobile industry. In the event of a crash, this strategy allows the brunt of an automobile crash to be absorbed by the metal body of the car crumpling, accordion-like, so as to spare the passengers occupying the car from the force of the impact. Eccentric contraction is extremely important for the body because it also absorbs energy. In the example above, the biceps muscle eccentrically absorbed the downward force of gravity on the gallon of milk. In the case of the skier whose foot got caught in a snow bank, the counter-tensile force generated by her calf muscles was eccentric and absorbed the tensile force in the bent bone, thereby sparing the shinbone from breaking. An essential part of rehabilitation when fractures occur is to exercise the affected muscles eccentrically, because this sort of contraction will counter the tendency toward re-injury. Eccentric exercises are also valu-

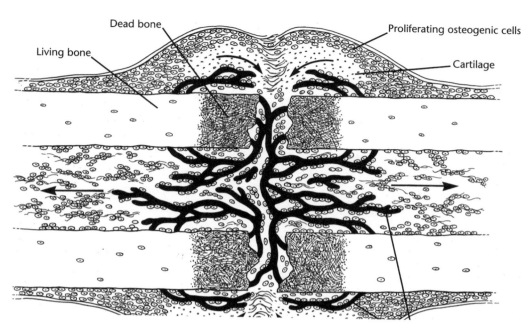

Callus formation and healing around a fracture site of a long bone.
Greenstein GM: *Clinical Assessment of Neuromusculoskeletal Disorders*. St. Louis: Mosby, 1997.

able in protecting other tissues such as tendons and ligaments from injury. An eccentric exercise program designed by a physical therapist or exercise trainer can be part of an overall exercise program for remaining strong and healthy.

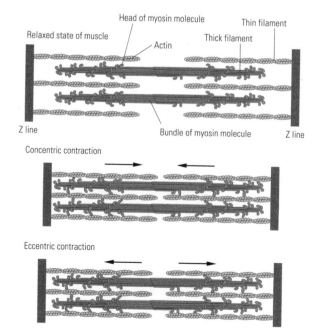

Top: Relaxed state of muscle. Middle: Concentric contraction occurs when the muscle filaments move together, similar to when you lift a gallon of milk by bending your elbow. Bottom: Eccentric contraction occurs when the muscle filaments move apart, similar to when you lower a gallon of milk by straightening your elbow slowly.
Saidoff DC, McDonough AL: *Critical Pathways in Therapeutic Intervention: Upper Extremities*. St. Louis: Mosby, 1997.

4 Pain and Inflammation

ALL OF US experience acute pain in the course of our daily lives. We might experience it as a stubbed toe, pinprick, upset stomach, headache, or other manifestation of trauma or disease. Pain is an unavoidable consequence of being alive. About 80 million Americans suffer from chronic pain and spend more than $90 billion each year on pain relief. As many as 600 million workdays are lost each year, with headaches alone being responsible for the majority of those sick days, followed by joint pain, stomach pain, backaches, muscle pain, premenstrual pain, and dental pain. Pain is strongly related to a person's psychological state, and this may explain why people who experience high degrees of stress experience greater pain. There are currently more than 1,000 pain clinics in the United States.

■ WHAT IS PAIN?

A judge was asked during a famous court proceeding to define pornography for the purpose of deciding a legal case. He responded that although he was unable to define it, he knew it when he saw it. Pain is perhaps the most fundamental human experience, and virtually all human beings experience it many times during their lives. We can easily recognize pain when it occurs, yet experts have wrestled with giving it a precise definition. The International Association for the Study of Pain offers the following formal definition: "Pain is an unpleasant sensory and emotional experience associated with actual or potential tissue damage, or described in terms of such damage." Another way of looking at it is that commonly experienced pain may be characterized as a warning mechanism that protects a person by encouraging the avoidance of potentially harmful experiences.

Careful examination of this definition reveals several useful facts:

1) Most types of pain have two major components: a *sensory component* and an *emotional component*. The sensory component refers to what is actually felt by the individual. This is the result of information being carried by the nerves to the brain; it generally reflects some type of physical disturbance at the site where the pain is felt. The emotional component describes how our perception of pain may be colored by factors that are unrelated to any physical injury. These factors influence how we react to pain and how intensely the pain is felt.

2) Pain may be associated with physical injury, but physical injury is not a prerequisite for pain. The fact that no physical injury can be identified does not make many types of pain any less real or severe than when tissue injury is readily apparent.

3) Sometimes the pain associated with anticipation of injury is far worse than the pain associated with the actual injury. For example, fear of the dentist often exacerbates what would otherwise be a moderate level of discomfort. People who over-

come this fear are often able to tolerate most dental procedures with minimal or no pain medication.

WHAT GOOD IS PAIN?

Pain cries for immediate relief, and we may think that all pain is bad. However, the truth is that pain is often *good* for us. People with some types of congenital conditions are insensitive to pain, and they usually do not reach adulthood without unintentionally breaking many of their bones, scarring large parts of their bodies, or biting their tongues and the inside of their mouths. Most importantly, pain is *protective*. It protects by teaching us—through negative reinforcement—not to damage ourselves.

Pain serves as an early warning system by causing a reflexive withdrawal from any source of potential injury. For example, if you are walking barefoot on the beach and feel something sharp under your foot, the pain will cause you to quickly draw your foot upwards. This minimizes the penetration of the object, which might cause a cut or bruise. Your heart rate will go up at the same time in preparation for running away, just in case you accidentally stepped on a beehive or jellyfish and need to get out of there in a hurry!

Some parts of the body feel no pain. For example, the brain has no sensory nerves, even though it is ultimately the organ where all pain is perceived. It is possible to operate on the brain of a person who is awake and he will feel no pain. However, the brain is surrounded by tissue called the *meninges* that does have pain-sensitive nerves. Stretching or irritation of this tissue can be quite painful—for example, during bleeding into the brain. Other soft tissues that feel no pain include the lining of the lungs and liver. The absence of pain-sensitive nerves in these tissues allows local diseases such as tumors or cirrhosis to progress to an advanced state without the

person being aware of it. The absence of pain is harmful in such circumstances because early detection of disease might result in more successful treatment.

The positive aspect of pain is often overlooked when an individual is experiencing it. People with advanced neuropathy—a condition in which the peripheral nerves degenerate over time—may no longer be able to feel painful stimuli in their feet, and they may injure them without being aware of it. As a result, minor cuts or bruises can easily become chronic, infected ulcers that can ultimately lead to gangrene and amputation. Some people with this condition may walk around for weeks with foreign objects such as shards of glass stuck in their feet without being aware of it. They must be cautioned to visually inspect their feet at least twice every day.

TYPES OF PAIN

There are several different types of pain, each having different origins, different underlying mechanisms, and different approaches to treatment. This results in various—albeit incomplete—classifications of pain. Apart from the commonly used word "pain," there are other less familiar terms that warrant definition. Each describes a sensation with its own particular characteristics and associated conditions:

- **ALLODYNIA** is pain provoked by a mechanical or hot or cold stimulus that would not normally be painful. For example, individuals with a condition called *reflex sympathetic dystrophy* may be extremely sensitive at the site of a previous injury, even if the injury itself was minor. (See Chapter 32.) The touch of a blanket, clothing, or someone gently brushing against the affected area may produce severe pain.

- **HYPERALGESIA** refers to a condition characterized by excessive sensitivity to pain (a lowered pain threshold). For example, even a mild touch or lukewarm water may be perceived as painful if you have local inflammation.

- **HYPERPATHIA** describes a condition where there is a normal pain threshold, but the pain is perceived as being much more severe than it actually is because of abnormal processing of information in the brain.

CLASSIFICATION OF PAIN

The subdivision of pain into specific categories is perhaps of greater importance than an overall definition, and a number of classification schemes have been proposed—most of them are useful to some degree—but none are complete in and of themselves. For example, pain may be classified according to its duration:

- **TRANSIENT PAIN** is brief pain elicited by the activation of pain-sensitive nerves without any accompanying tissue injury or persistent disease-like state. This type of pain is self-limited and there is no need to consider therapy—for example, stepping on a sharp object. The pain may be intense at first but it will subside once the object is removed.

- **ACUTE PAIN** is of recent onset and usually associated with a noxious stimulus such as an injury, disease process, or other abnormal functioning. This type of pain will be felt after spraining an ankle, developing an abscessed tooth, angina, or playing a rigorous game of touch football after spending 20 years as a couch potato. Childbirth may also fall into this category, although some parents may think of it as a more chronic type of pain that persists until the child finally moves out of the house. Acute pain will usually respond to correction of the underlying disease process or injury, or to pain-relieving (analgesic) medications.

- **CHRONIC PAIN** often begins with an acute injury and then takes on a life of its own over the course of time. It is persistent and can last from several months to years, typically well beyond the time of the original injury. It is often associated with altered behavior resulting from the ongoing experience of pain, and it can intensify. Chronic pain dramatically affects many aspects of a person's life and should be considered a disease state of the nervous system, not simply prolonged acute pain associated with some other condition. Medication or simple medical management is rarely adequate to control chronic pain. Behavioral therapy as well as some re-education is often necessary.

Pain may also be classified according to its underlying source: either *nociceptive* (from the Latin root word *noci-*, meaning capable of being harmful) or *neuropathic*:

- **NOCICEPTIVE PAIN:** This type of pain is caused by an external stimulus that irritates pain-sensitive nerves. This may include a transient irritation such as stepping on a tack or touching a hot object. It also includes any type of tissue injury or disease process that irritates nerve endings.

- **NEUROPATHIC PAIN:** This type of pain is caused by a problem in the nerve itself and does not reflect true tissue injury. People with peripheral neuropathy experience this type of pain; although they might not feel a piece of glass embedded in their foot, they may frequently experience severe burning or sharp shooting pains in their feet without any external stimulus because the nerves that normally relay sensory information are not functioning normally. Similarly, people who have had limb amputations, yet continue to feel pain in the missing limbs, may experience neuropathic pain. This is referred to as *phantom pain* (see below). Unlike nociceptive pain, which is an important defense mechanism against injury, neuropathic pain provides absolutely no benefit to the person who suffers from it. Unfortunately, it is often a very difficult type of pain to treat effectively.

- **REFERRED PAIN:** Pain is not always helpful in letting you know the location of the problem. Sometimes pain is felt in one part of the body but it is actually caused by an injury or illness in another part of the body. This is *referred pain*. For example, the pain associated with angina or a heart attack may be felt in the left arm, even though the heart is in the chest. An ulcer or other irritation of the diaphragm may be perceived as pain in the shoulder. This is because during fetal development the nerves that attach to different organs come out of the spinal cord at levels close to where those organs are located in the fetus. However, when the organs migrate to new positions as the fetus grows, the attachments that lead from the spinal cord stay in the same place. As a result, we feel pain as if the affected organs are still located where they were at early stages of embryonic development.

- **PHANTOM PAIN:** This type of pain is experienced by an individual with an amputated limb; it is an extreme example of misperception as to the location of pain. This type of pain is perceived as coming from the missing limb, even though the limb is no longer present. The amputee might complain of peculiar sensations and even severe pain. The cause of phantom pain is still not fully understood, although it is believed to be caused by a reorganization of connections among neurons in the brain following loss of normal input from the missing limb.

HOW PAIN IS FELT

Sensory nerves have specialized nerve endings that convey information such as touch, vibration, pressure, and injury. These nociceptive pain receptors are simple branches of nerves located in the superficial layers of skin, muscle, bone surface, and other parts of the body. Pain receptors may be excited by three types of stimuli: mechanical (pressure or a cut), thermal (heat or cold), and chemical.

PAIN PATHWAYS

There are two different phases of pain. The first is an immediate, intense pain of short duration. The second phase begins just as the first subsides and is represented by a dull, vague, throbbing, and persistent sensation. We experience acute pain in two waves because there are two different types of pain receptors made up of two different types of fibers:

- **FAST PATHWAY:** A-delta fibers are thin and have a small fatty sheath around them called *myelin* that serves as insulation to help nerves conduct electrical signals. These fibers transmit information about well-localized heat and mechanical pain, which may be felt immediately as sharp and prickling. They transmit this information slowly compared to other types of sensory nerves, but much faster than type C pain fibers do. The first wave of pain mediated by A-delta fibers is known as the *fast pathway* because of its quick transmission.

- **SLOW PATHWAY:** Type C fibers are thinner and lack the fatty insulation that aids in the conduction of electrical signals. They are the *slow pathway* because they transmit impulses more slowly than A-delta fibers. They typically convey the poorly localized, diffuse, burning pain that may arise from mechanical, thermal, or chemical stimuli.

Pain impulses from both pathways enter the gray matter of the spinal cord and relay information to the CNS by way of the neurotransmitter *substance P*. Once pain messages reach the spinal cord, they travel up to the brainstem and the thalamus by way of two separate routes: the spinoreticular and spinothalamic tracts. The *thalamus* is located in the center of the brain and serves as a relay station for information received from the senses such as pain, touch, temperature, vision, vibration, hearing, and the position of limbs. It organizes the information and sends it to the cortex—the conscious, reasoning part of the brain.

▪ THE INFLAMMATORY PROCESS

A series of vascular and cellular events known as the *inflammatory response* is set in motion whenever cells are injured or destroyed. The inflammatory response is positive because it walls-off or destroys invading germs and paves the way for cellular restoration. The inflammatory response may be compared to the response of emergency personnel in an urban disaster such as the sudden collapse of a building. Within minutes, police, firefighters, and ambulances rush to the scene, each with a specific task. They clear the area, control onlookers, search for survivors, extricate those who are trapped, administer emergency aid to the wounded, carry them in ambulances to the hospital, examine structures still standing to see if there is danger of additional collapse, and put out fires. Similarly, at the site of an injury there are specialized cells that per-

form specific functions. For example, in a bacterial infection the sequence of events in the inflammatory process begins with the release of chemical signals that cause the small blood vessels to dilate (vasodilatation) and leak. This increases blood flow to the injured area and allows fluid and additional inflammatory cells to accumulate. At the same time, clear fluid leaks out of vessels into the injured area and dilutes the effect of harmful substances. Once this happens, white blood cells flow out of the vessels and begin attacking the bacteria that have infected the site of injury. White blood cells also begin to destroy the damaged tissue—literally eating it and recycling any material that is still useful. This process is known as *phagocytosis*. The dead bacteria, cellular debris, and white blood cells create a mixture known as *pus*.

The major signs of inflammation are redness and increased warmth, swelling from accumulated fluid, and pain. *Inflammatory pain* is the most common type of pain and occurs whenever there is an injury or infection. The affected cells release a variety of different chemicals during the inflammatory process that either directly stimulate pain fibers to signal pain or enhance the sensitivity of nociceptors, making local nerve endings hypersensitive. Chemicals that excite pain receptors include bradykinin, histamine, prostaglandin, serotonin, potassium, and nerve growth factor. Inflammatory pain is an important response to injury because it forces us to slow down and immobilize the injured part of our body, preventing further injury and allowing us to heal. Acute inflammation from a skin cut lasts only a few days, while chronic inflammation can last much longer.

A coward dies a thousand deaths,
but a brave person dies but once.

This common folk wisdom suggests that fear of pain heightens its intensity. The experience of pain differs significantly between different people because our perception of pain is shaped by many factors, including childhood experiences, genetic make-up, gender, and cultural attitudes. Learned behavior strongly influences the way people respond to pain. For example, women in many societies are conditioned to expect terrible pain during childbirth and, thus, this fear may be realized. Childbirth is not dreaded in other societies and women go back to work a short time after their babies are born. The basic premise of the Lamaze method of training for natural childbirth is that women in most Western cultures are conditioned to expect and fear the pain of childbearing. This fear increases pain by producing changes in muscle tone and breathing patterns that hamper the birthing process.

Most Westerners believe that pain is an evil to be avoided whenever possible. In contrast, male Australian aborigines are brought up in a society that considers stoic indifference to pain to be a sign of manliness; their initiation rites include ritualistic circumcision, chest scarring, and extraction of the upper two teeth, all while showing no reaction. Self-flagellation with knives by men during the Muslim festival of Muharram in Pakistan, as well as face and tongue piercing by females, is performed ecstatically in religious ceremonies. (Muharram is a festival commemorating the escape of the Israelites from Egypt *and* the day Noah's ark touched ground after the flood.) Some Hindu fakirs pierce their cheeks with pins or rest on beds of nails with utter disregard to pain.

THE MIND CAN MAGNIFY DISTRESS

Our anticipation of pain may be far worse than the actual pain experienced. For example, fear of the dentist may exacerbate what would otherwise be a relatively moderate level of discomfort. People who overcome this fear are often able to tolerate most dental procedures with minimal or no pain medication. Those who are not able to overcome their fear may have a more painful experience because their perception of pain is worsened by anxiety. The lesson to be learned is that the more you focus your attention on pain, the worse it will be.

Evidence of how our state of mind relates to our perception of pain may be understood when we consider the conditions under which pain occurs. When battle-wounded soldiers in World War II were compared with civilians who suffered similar injuries, it was discovered that the majority of soldiers did not need pain relief for injuries of similar severity. The soldiers may have had a higher threshold for pain because being wounded was not unexpected. Being injured was a positive event, in one sense, because they were temporarily spared from more combat.

PAIN RELIEF

Although about 40% of all people get some pain relief from placebos (medicine that contains no active ingredient) many people need various types of pain relief. While most seek relief from medical doctors or dentists, many people go to chiropractors, pharmacists, nutritionists, acupuncturists, spiritual counselors, and even faith healers. Non-drug treatment methods to effectively control pain include acupuncture, biofeedback, hypnosis, and electrical stimulation. (See Chapter 36 for more information on remedies for pain relief.)

GATEWAY TO PAIN RELIEF

Pain signals may be modified many times by interactions with other parts of the nervous system while they are being transmitted from the stimulated pain receptor to the cortex. Modification of the signal can begin even in the peripheral nervous system. Researchers Patrick Wall and Ronald Melzack noticed, in the early 1960s, that the stimulation of large diameter peripheral sensory nerve fibers, which are not normally involved in pain sensation, decreased the responsiveness of spinal cord neurons to signals coming from pain-sensitive nociceptor neurons. Spinal cord neurons responded more intensely to pain signals coming from nociceptors if the activity of these other sensory neurons was blocked. As discussed in Chapter 36, this led to the "Gate Control Theory of Pain Perception, which maintains that pain perception may depend upon a balance between the activity of the pain-sensitive nociceptor neurons and the other larger diameter, better insulated sensory neurons. Pain sensation is heightened when activity is high in nociceptor neurons and low in the large fiber neurons; it is diminished when the opposite is true.

The practical outcome of this theory is that it supplies a rationale for other non-medicinal approaches to pain management. For example, the Gate Control Theory may explain why vigorous rubbing of the skin at the site of a minor, painful injury often helps relieve pain, in that it stimulates the large diameter sensory fibers. It also explains the rationale underlying a popular method of pain control called *Transcutaneous Electrical Nerve Stimulation* (TENS), which uses a device that stimulates the large diameter sensory fibers electrically. This stimulation suppresses the response of *dorsal horn neurons* to nociceptor signals.

ADDICTS AND JOGGERS

Luckily for us, our bodies produce pain-suppressing chemicals, not just chemicals that enhance pain. These natural painkillers inhibit the transmission of pain sensations to the brain. They are similar to opium, an ancient analgesic that comes from the dried juice of the opium poppy. Another commonly known narcotic (*numb* in Greek) is hashish. Others include codeine, heroin, and morphine. When addicts take these drugs to get high, they are using *exogenous* (produced outside the body) *morphine*. These chemicals interfere with pain impulse transmission by precisely fitting into receptors in the brain in exactly the same way that a key fits into a lock.

The discovery that the brain contains receptors that can attach to opiates led scientists to wonder whether there are naturally occurring chemicals in the brain that behave exactly like morphine and other narcotics. Why else would our brain have receptors for these chemicals? Research revealed many such chemicals, which are known as *endogenous* (produced within the body) *morphine*, or *endorphins*. These chemical analgesics are one hundred times more potent than plant-derived morphine and share with them an identical short sequence structure of amino-acids. This sequence comprises a unique geometrical template that gives these molecules their specificity.

During extreme circumstances such as combat or athletic competition, stress and excitement cause the release of a relatively large amount of endorphins within the brain that serve to mask injuries until the stressful situation has ended. They allow us to accomplish whatever is necessary to escape without being handicapped by pain. A dramatic demonstration of this phenomenon occurred during the 1996 Summer Olympics in Atlanta, Georgia when gymnast Kerri Strug performed a near perfect vault despite spraining her ankle and her team won the gold medal.

A classic and often quoted description of this phenomenon comes from David Livingstone, a Scottish missionary and explorer of Africa. He reported that he was suddenly attacked by a lion while searching for the source of the Nile River.

Livingston described the event in his memoirs as follows:

"... I heard a shout. Starting, and looking half round, I saw the lion just in the act of springing upon me. I was upon a little height; he caught my shoulder as he sprang, and we both came to the ground below together. Growling horribly close to my ear, he shook me as a terrier does a rat. The shock produced a stupor similar to that which seems to be felt by a mouse after the first shake of the cat. It caused a sort of dreaminess in which there was no sense of pain or feeling of terror, though quite conscious of all that was happening. It was like what people partially under the influence of chloroform describe, who see all the operation, but feel not the knife.... The shake annihilated fear, and allowed no sense of horror in looking round at the beast. This peculiar state is probably produced in all animals killed by the carnivora; and if so, it is a merciful provision by our benevolent creator for lessening the pain of death."

David Livingstone,
Missionary Travels, 1857

5 As We Get Older

THE QUEST for immortality is one of the most cherished dreams of mankind. The legendary knights of King Arthur searched for the Holy Grail and Don Quixote searched in vain for the fountain of youth and the imagined El Dorado. The Bristlecone Pine tree can live up to 4,900 years, the Sierra Redwood up to 2,300 years, and the English Oak for about 1,500 years. The Galapagos tortoise lives to more than 100 years, a swan lives for as many as 70 years, and an elephant for as many as 50 years. In ancient Greece (700 B.C.) the average life expectancy was 17 years, which increased to 26 years in Rome (50 B.C.). Life expectancy was 33 years in England in 1500, and this figure had risen to 33.5 years in the United States by 1790. King David of the Psalms supposedly lived four score and ten (70) years. According to the Bible, Methuselah lived to an ancient 969 years.

In recent times, the oldest person in the world was Shigechiyo Izumi of Japan, who was 120 when he died in 1986. The oldest American was Mrs. Fannie Thomas, who was almost 114 years old when she died in 1981. Life expectancy at birth in most developing countries increased from between 35 to 40 years in 1950 to 61 years by 1990, mostly due to the use of insecticides, vaccines, antibiotics, and the high-yielding varieties of seeds produced since the 1950s. Today, with the advent of successful genetic cloning, living far beyond this seems to be a possibility.

The average life expectancy for most Americans is about 75 years, almost twice what it was in the early twentieth century. More people are now living into their 90s and more – about sixty thousand Americans are 100 or older. Today, approximately 13% of the population – about 34 million Americans, are 65 or older.

An Aging World

In the past several decades, the elderly population in the United States has grown more than twice as fast as the rest of the population. A baby born in 1900 might expect to live an average of about 47 years, while a baby born in 1985 may expect to live almost 75 years. Only 4% of the U.S. population was older than 65 years of age in the year 1900. By 2050 (when people born in 1985 turn 65), almost one in four Americans will be 65 or older.

American women outlive their male counterparts by an average of 7 to 8 years. Today in the United States, people over age 75 comprise the fastest growing age group in the country. Tens of thousands of centenarians currently live in the U.S., and more are expected over the next 50 years. Luckily, because of modern medicine and changes in the workplace, many people are living longer, productive, and enjoyable lives. This chapter is about living longer and healthier by taking better care of ourselves.

The Aging Musculoskeletal System

No two people age in exactly the same way or at the same rate. However, age-related changes occur in just about every single body system, including the heart, lungs, skin, hair, brain, kidneys, and the senses such as sight, hearing, and taste. As the body ages, we become shorter. This occurs because the discs between the vertebrae that make up the spinal column gradually lose fluid, causing overall height to shrink by several inches. The arches of the feet become less pronounced, which also contributes—albeit slightly—to a loss in height. The body joints become stiff and less flexible, and arthritis may develop. In addition, muscles and bones are affected in a number of ways.

Muscle strength is at its maximum between ages 20 to 30, after which lean body mass begins to diminish as muscle fibers gradually shrink and are replaced by fat. A steady decline in stamina and muscle tone begins around age 40, especially in sedentary people. Middle-aged people are more likely to experience muscle strains from excessive exercise. Muscle weakness contributes to fatigue, weakness, and reduced exercise tolerance. By age 65, muscle strength is diminished by as much as 80%, and about half of the body's entire muscle mass is lost by age 80.

Bone mass reaches its peak at approximately age 35 and then starts to decrease. Loss of bone mass following menopause in women can make bone so brittle (a condition known as *osteoporosis*) that fractures are a common injury. Hip fractures start to rise in frequency in the 40s and double thereafter every 6 years.

THEORIES OF AGING

Aging is an irreversible, inevitable change that occurs in all body organs over time. While no one knows exactly why we age, all of the cells in the body experience changes with aging that render them less able to divide and reproduce. Cells have difficulty getting oxygen and nutrients, and they also accumulate waste as the body becomes increasingly less efficient in ridding itself of carbon dioxide and metabolic by-products. Connective tissue becomes increasingly stiff and less resilient. A number of theories have been proposed to explain why these processes occur, and it may be that several or all of them contribute to the aging process:

- **WEAR AND TEAR THEORY:** The human body progressively wears out with each advancing year; this is the "wear" part. "Tear" refers to the fact that inadequate nutrition, disease, stress, and accumulated exposure to pollution and sunlight wear down our bodies. Just the simple act of living causes wear and tear to accumulate to the point that the body cannot cope, and it eventually gives out. Two examples of this are the need for dentures in old age and skin cancer resulting from prolonged exposure to the sun.

- **CELLULAR ACCIDENT THEORY:** We are all exposed to a lifetime of toxic substances, pollutants, and radiation that are present in the air we breathe, the water we drink, and the food we eat. We are at the top of the food chain and we often eat other top food chain predators. For example, tuna is a carnivorous fish that some researchers estimate to contain significant amounts of heavy metals (e.g., mercury), and we ingest these heavy metals every time we enjoy a tuna sandwich. This is only one example of how pollution causes mutations within the DNA of our cells, causing the newly reproduced cells to be imperfect. As more cells become affected, progressively more cells are less able to work efficiently, causing a decline in function and eventual death.

- **FREE RADICAL THEORY:** Free radicals are the by-products of normal metabolism. They are the molecules generated by normal chemical reactions in the cells of the body as we metabolize food and turn it into energy. Free radicals contain an unpaired electron—a chemical situation that is very unstable—that causes them to easily react with other molecules in a process called *oxidation*. When these free radicals bond with the fats contained in the cell membrane, they damage the ability of that cell to function properly. To prevent this, our bodies produce scavenger enzymes known as *antioxidants* that roam the body in search of free radicals. Antioxidants such as Vitamin E combine with free radicals and neutralize them—hopefully before any significant damage occurs. The number of free radicals eventually outpaces the antioxidants, causing progressive dysfunction and eventual cell death. Free radicals are thought to exacerbate—or even cause—diseases such as stroke, heart attacks, and diabetes. The problem is that our bodies produce fewer of these antioxidants as we age, which is why eating right and taking supplemental vitamins is so important. Foods such as blueberries, for example, have a high content of antioxidants.

- **PROGRAMMED AGING THEORY:** This theory proposes that the rate at which a species grows old is predetermined by its genes, which determine how long cells will live. Until the 1960s, cells were thought to have an unlimited ability to replicate. Cells have a fixed reproduction limit, which means that aging and death are built into the blueprint of our genes. Research shows that specific DNA-protein sequences at the end of chromosomes (*telomeres*) are responsible for maintaining other chromosomes and may play a role in both aging and cancer. Telomeres set a finite limit as to how many times a cell can replicate. By the same token, cancer cells are considered immortal because, unlike the normal cells in the body, they continue to replicate. Cancer cells avoid damage from telomeres by activating an enzyme called *telomerase*, which deactivates the telomeres and allows for unlimited growth. This is an exciting area of research.

Aging is a complex process that is influenced by heredity, environment, cultural influences, diet, exercise, leisure, past illnesses, and many other factors. The most important factor to keep in mind is that there are things you can do to keep yourself youthful and healthy, despite the passing years.

FACTORS THAT AFFECT LIFE EXPECTANCY

Avoid cigarettes. Smoking can lower your life expectancy by as much as 12 years! Obesity lowers life expectancy by 1 year for every 10% over normal body weight. Pollution of the air, water, and food may occur from many sources, including food additives, pesticides, and weed-killers. These pollutants contaminate our environment and may account for a wide range of diseases that includes leukemia and other forms of cancer.

DECONDITIONING AND DISUSE

Sitting around being a couch potato is not very healthy. Lying in bed because of illness is even worse, although necessary, because at least you are trying to get better. Excessive bed rest negatively affects every system in the body and has the overall effect of weakening the body. This is especially true for older people who may have trouble getting out of bed after coming down with the flu or a cold. They may feel weak, dizzy, unbalanced, and unsure of themselves. Their muscles were not used during the time they were sick in bed, and they may have became atrophied (a condition known as *disuse atrophy*), which makes the simple activities of daily living difficult. The musculoskeletal system must experience regular conditioning in order to remain strong and healthy. This means that it must have the regular exercise that accompanies everyday life, at the very least, such as getting out of bed, preparing meals, performing housekeeping, and negotiating stairs. In the absence of these basic exercises that many take for granted, the body becomes out of condition or *deconditioned*. In this state, flu or other illness can cause major problems. A good way to prevent deconditioning is to engage in regular exercise in the years *before* your sixth decade. This time and exercise investment is as important as regularly setting aside investments in a financial portfolio. What good is setting aside money for your retirement if you are not going to be healthy enough to enjoy it? Be mindful. Take care of yourself today— invest in tomorrow!

STRESS

Stress is both a good and bad thing. In a way, *stress* is the revved up energy we harness to meet the demands of life. It can be the deepest source of our vitality and joy in life, provided we can meet those demands. On the other hand, *distress* can be either physical or mental. Mental stress often happens because of the gap we encounter between our expectations and our inability to fulfill those expectations. Physical stress can occur from pushing the body over and above its tolerance level. Too much of either kind of stress results in our immune system becoming less capable of warding off the attack of organisms such as the viruses and bacteria that are all around us, rendering us more susceptible to illness.

Virtually every body system is affected by stress. The hectic pace of urban life is especially stressful. Our cell phones, beepers, portable computers, e-mail, personal digital assistants, and telephones with call-waiting options seem to have imprisoned us more than they have helped us. We are busier than ever. Americans work harder and longer than their counterparts in other first-world countries, and the preoccupation with more and bigger everything places enormous stresses on individuals, families, and communities. More and more people are choosing to opt out of the fast lane in exchange for simpler lives, making less money, and moving away from urbanized areas.

How long can the mind and body cope with physical and mental stress? Some theorize that people have a certain amount of "adaptation energy," a reserve of internal energy or drive that allows us to adapt to changing and perhaps difficult environments. This inherited adaptation energy, which varies from person to person, is like inherited wealth. However, although we can draw upon it during our lives, we may never add to it. We can recoup some of it—for example, after a good night's sleep following a hard day's work. Taking a much-needed vacation serves the same purpose. We can never recoup it entirely, however, and if we continue to experience high levels of stress during our lives, we may lose our ability to adapt just like a spendthrift heir who squanders his inheritance. It is essential to pace yourself, take breaks and naps, eat well, and generally live in moderation.

PERSONALITY TYPE AND STRESS

Certain personality types handle stress in different ways and, consequently, react to its effects differently as well. People are often said to have one of the following three types of personality:

- **TYPE A:** People with this personality type typically eat fast, move and walk quickly, speak in quick bursts with loud, jarring voices, hold a tense posture or facial expression, do two or more things simultaneously whenever possible, interrupt others or finish their sentences, schedule too many activities in too little time, play nearly every game to win, drum their fingers or jiggle their knees, get annoyed and angry by delays, and feel guilty when spending time doing nothing. The combination of these behaviors describes an individual with excessive hostility, cynical mistrust of the motives of other people, anger, and impatience, who can work himself up to having a heart attack and is five times more at risk for doing so when compared to the general population.

- **TYPE B:** This type of person is more relaxed and easily satisfied, unhurried, and capable of choosing from a spectrum of coping mechanisms without having to resort to competitive hostility.

- **TYPE C:** These individuals tend to suppress their true feelings in the face of stress and are at a higher risk for developing diseases such as cancer. Other characteristics of this group include a tendency to have one valued person as their emotional focus and a tendency to become depressed if they experience disagreement, a quarrel, or separation from that person. Breast cancer is almost six times as likely to recur in a woman who is experiencing severe stress such as a life-impacting event with long term consequences: divorce, a breakdown of family relationships, or the death of a loved one.

THE MIND-BODY CONNECTION

In one study, doctors performing cervical biopsies on women with abnormal Pap smears were able to accurately predict—before getting the biopsy results—which women were most likely to have cancer based on the feelings of hopelessness expressed by these women. This underlines the importance of the will to live. A positive attitude goes a long way in maintaining good health and longevity. Often, people with cancer and other catastrophic illnesses are buoyed up by an optimistic outlook. How this affects the immune system is unknown, but there is so much circumstantial evidence for this that it merits attention. In contrast, people who give up and express indifference or hopelessness often succumb to disease. Keeping a positive outlook on life is not something you hope for, but rather something you work toward every single day. This state of mind is helped by regularly taking good care of your body.

HEALTHY STRATEGIES

The following strategies can help you live a longer and healthier life:

- **AVOID SMOKING:** Do not smoke; cigarettes cause cancer, heart disease, emphysema, stroke, and other diseases.

- **EAT WELL:** Eat a balanced diet and maintain a desirable weight. Avoid junk food, cut down on carbohydrates, reduce fat intake to 30% or less of calories. Saturated fat intake should be less than 10% of ingested calories, and cholesterol intake should be less than 300 milligrams per day. Eat lots of salad and fiber. Watch your sugar and salt intake, and do not eat too much. Studies have shown that eating less may prolong life. Too much food seems to overload the system; eating a lighter diet, at the very least, protects against kidney and heart disease.

- **EXERCISE REGULARLY:** Exercise may help delay the effects of aging, including reduced muscle mass and lower aerobic capacity. Regular exercise increases your health, maintains flexibility, and increases resistance to disease.

- **MODERATE ALCOHOL CONSUMPTION:** Studies have shown that drinking a glass of white or red wine each day actually helps fight heart disease. Avoid other forms of alcohol and drink responsibly when it is unavoidable. Avoid beer—the calories go straight to your waistline. Heavy drinking has been linked to all kinds of problems, including strokes and malnutrition.

- **VISIT YOUR DOCTOR REGULARLY:** Having regular medical checkups is necessary. Women should be regularly checked for breast and other forms of cancer, and men should undergo annual checks for testicular cancer. Everyone should be checked for colon cancer after middle age, especially if they have a positive family history.

- **SLEEP WELL:** Get enough sleep each night, but do not sleep too much. Mortality rates increase for people who sleep too little and for those who sleep more than ten hours nightly. People who take a nap during the day not only feel refreshed afterwards, they also live longer.

- **BE SAFE:** Practice good safety habits wherever you are, be it in the home, car, or elsewhere.

- **STAY MARRIED:** Married people have lower mortality rates than those who are divorced, widowed, or who never married.

- **HAVE PETS:** Regular contact with pets—especially dogs and cats—can reduce heart rate, blood pressure, and levels of stress. In addition to providing companionship, pets are a source of constancy in an ever-changing world. They make us feel safe and needed, comfort us with touch, stimulate us to exercise, and engage us in play.

- **CARE FOR YOUR TEETH:** Recent studies have demonstrated a link between the plaque buildup in your teeth and plaque buildup in the coronary arteries. People with gum disease have a significantly higher incidence of stroke and heart disease. Have regular dental check-ups and cleaning, and brush and floss your teeth daily.

- **GET YOUR FLU SHOT:** Disease-fighting proteins known as *antibodies* may be reduced by as much as 30% by age eighty-five. As a result, a bout of flu that might result only in a high fever for a few days in a younger person may be fatal to an older one. It is important to be vaccinated against both the flu and pneumonia.

- **AVOID OVEREXPOSURE:** As people grow older, they do not handle temperature variations as well as they did when they were younger. Because of this it is important to avoid overexposure to heat and cold.

- **STAY INVOLVED:** Maintain positive relationships with friends, family, and co-workers.

- **POSITIVE OUTLOOK:** Keeping your chin up is something not to be taken for granted—work on it every day. A good attitude is extremely important in determining the quality and duration of life. Take pleasure in enjoying yourself. This satisfaction can help contribute to a long life. Try to surround yourself with positive experiences and other positive people.

- **EASE UP:** Be good to yourself—you deserve it! The old adage "no pain—no gain" should be set aside whenever possible. Do not let your mind push your body beyond its limits. Know when to quit and do not be too hard on yourself. Do not ignore one of the most important relationships in your life—your relationship with *yourself.* Set aside downtime when you are not required to be productive: just put your feet up and relax with a good book or whatever your heart desires. Do not feel guilty about it! Take care of yourself and your body will take care of you.

Foot, Ankle, and Leg

THE FOOT CONTAINS one quarter of all the bones in the human body, 107 ligaments, 30 joints, and 19 muscles, which is an incredible number of biomechanical parts that must work together to get us where we want to go. The full force of the body weight comes to bear on the foot with each step, making proper care of the feet essential in preventing injuries. The ankle is a hinge joint that links the bones of the lower leg to the topmost bones of the foot and is especially vulnerable to sprains and fractures. The lower leg is also susceptible to an overuse injury known as "shin splints."

6 Your Feet

T HE FOOT IS BOTH an architectural nightmare and anatomic wonder. Leonardo da Vinci claimed that feet were "a masterpiece of engineering and a work of art." A single foot contains 28 bones—one quarter of all the bones in the human body—107 ligaments, 30 joints, and 19 muscles. That is an incredible number of components that work together in a complex way to get us to where we want to go. The average person spends approximately four hours on his or her feet every day, taking between eight to ten thousand steps. This is the equivalent of about 2,000 miles per year. Each of us covers enough distance in a single lifetime to have circled the globe about four times! The full force of the body weight comes to bear on the foot with each step, and anyone who is overweight increases this force. Proper care of the feet is essential in preventing overuse injuries and other problems.

■ THE "FEAT" OF WALKING

Try walking on two pogo sticks. The bottom of each pogo stick is considerably smaller than the soles of our feet, so this gives you an idea of what is involved in balancing our full body weight. Walking consists of repeatedly throwing ourselves off balance by leaning forward with one leg and catching ourselves before falling by moving the other foot ahead into a new forward position. This is done in cooperation with the contraction and relaxation of many muscles of the foot, leg, hip and pelvis, rotation of the trunk, and swinging our arms. Essentially, the supporting leg acts as an advancing base that vaults the body forward over the foot.

The foot would soon be pulverized if it were to hit the ground flatly with each step forward. That is what happens to wooden stilts—the wood eventu-

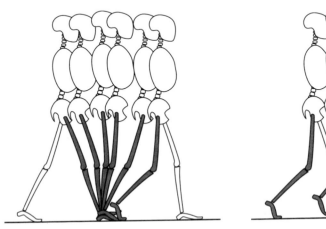

During stance —that portion of gait in which one foot is in contact with the ground.
From: Perry J: Gait analysis: normal and pathological function, SLACK, Thorofare, NJ, 1992. p. 23, fig. 3.4.

ally wears away. The foot meets the ground in a special, three-sequence way designed to minimize stress. The initial shock is absorbed by the fat cushion covering the heel bone. This *heel strike* absorbs the initial impact and transmits the force along the five metatarsal bones that fan out toward the ball of the foot. The foot literally rolls forward into the *foot-flat* phase and the foot ligaments absorb the energy of impact like a spring as the foot unlocks. The foot continues to roll forward toward the toes and the ligaments lock the foot into a solid support that catapults the body forward as the heel rises and the big toe thrusts back during the *toe-off* phase.

We perform this *gait sequence* over and over without thinking about it. Constant communication between the feet and brain enables us to walk by constantly readjusting muscle contraction, muscle tone, speed, and balance.

■ INTERESTING FACTS ABOUT FEET

No two feet are similar—not even your own—because one is usually larger than the other. Feet are always changing. If you gain weight, feet widen; if you lose weight, they slim down. Size can vary by 5% daily, depending on whether you are standing, walking, or sitting. Although most feet stop growing by age 20, they continue to elongate as foot muscles lose tone and broaden as one approaches middle age. The weather causes feet to contract in cold weather and expand in hot weather. The foot becomes more susceptible to malady and injury with increasing age because of the thinning of the protective fat pad cushioning the skin and bone on the bottom of your feet. Speaking of shoe size, the 16-inch footprint of the semi-mythological creature known as the Abominable Snowman (or Bigfoot) wandering the North American wilderness would require an incredible size 25 shoe—presumably extra wide!

■ A GLUTTON FOR PUNISHMENT

Feet sustain an incredible amount of pressure. For example, the sole, heel, and toes of an average individual weighing only 135 pounds and taking an average of 18,000 steps per day translates into a cumulative pressure of more than 2.5 million pounds during a typical day! It is no wonder that the number one foot complaint people have is sore,

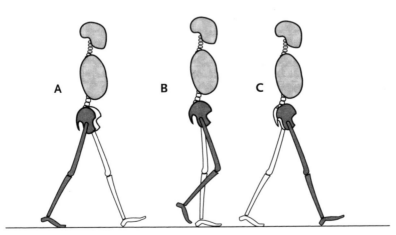

Three basic phases of stance during walking involve (view the non-shaded leg): A. heel strike; B. foot flat; and C. heel rise.
From: Perry J: Gait analysis: normal and pathological function, SLACK, Thorofare, NJ, 1992. p. 23, fig. 3.6.

aching feet; about three out of every four Americans have problems with their feet at some time during their lives, although the vast majority of them are over age 50. Most men suffer from athlete's foot, injuries, and odor; females are more likely to develop blisters, corns, painful bunions, calluses, and ingrown toenails. Very active children may experience heel pain between the ages of 8 and 13 because high-impact exercise may irritate the growth center of the heel. Adults who engage in high-impact sports such as jogging, aerobics, or racquet sports are more prone to developing foot problems.

■ CIVILIZATION AND FEET

Foot problems are often a result of civilization because shoes contribute to as much as 80% of foot-related problems. The approximately 1 billion people in the world who walk shoeless have fewer foot problems than those who wear shoes, although these people do not live as long as those in Western society and do not travel as much. Shoes protect feet from injury, but they also unnaturally imprison feet in leather or man-made materials. Consider the fact that about one-fifth of all men and almost one-half of all women in the United Stated admit that they are willing to wear shoes that hurt in order to be more fashionable. Poorly fitting shoes and high-heeled shoes cause most foot problems..

The American Indians either walked barefoot or wrapped their feet in animal skins and walked on yielding, uneven terrain. This is the finest possible exercise for feet. Most people relish the idea of kicking off their shoes and walking barefoot on grass. The onset of civilization brought shoes and flat, hard surfaces such as cement sidewalks and hard floors—all of which are not very good for the long-term health of your feet.

The feet of girls in China were traditionally bound tightly to prevent growth. This painful practice made women who could squeeze their small feet into tiny shoes more sexually desirable. Pointy-toed shoes were popular in post-medieval Europe as protection against witchcraft—remember the shoes of the Wicked Witch of the West in the *Wizard of Oz*? In the fifteenth century, aristocratic women in Italy wore platform heels 10+ inches high. This caused so many accidents that a law was passed to prohibit pregnant women from wearing them because it placed their unborn children's lives at risk!

The feet of newborns are best compared to little packs of soft jelly with lots of fat obliterating any visible arch and bones, which are soft and rubbery. Unfortunately, many well-intending parents tuck crib sheets around their babies tightly enough to produce mild foot deformities and force their children's feet much too early into socks and shoes in an attempt to civilize the feet.

■ PRONATION VERSUS SUPINATION

Your foot hits the ground with one-half of the weight of your body, multiplying the force by the speed that your leg moves forward. This is Newton's second law: Force = mass x acceleration. The ground pushes back with equal force. This is Newton's third law. These forces meet at the foot and can cause problems, if not for two protective strategies: *pronation* and *supination*.

The term *pronation* means "the act of assuming the prone position," such as when lying face down on your stomach. *Supination* means "the act of assuming the supine position," such as when lying face up on your back. These positions are referred to in biomechanics as angular, rotating motions. This is what occurs in the forearm when the radius bone twists around the ulna so that the palm faces downwards in pronation or upwards in supination.

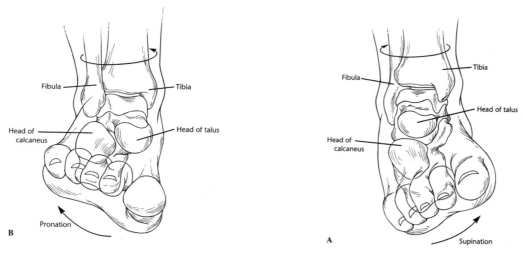

Pronation and supination positions in foot biomechanics that occur constantly throughout the gait cycle.
From: Greenstein GM: Clinical assessment of neuromusculoskeletal disorders, Mosby, St. Louis,, 1997, p. 197, fig. 6-9.

Pronation and supination of the foot refers to a sequence of joint movements that are accompanied by rotation of the shinbone in one or the other direction throughout the gait.

Our pelvis, thighbones, shins, spine, and shoulders all rotate when we walk. These rotations are known as torsion, and they occur throughout our musculoskeletal system; they are an evolutionary strategy that dissipates the many injurious forces we meet as we move around.

LOOSE BAG OF BONES VS. RIGID ARCH

The first thing someone learning to parachute out of an airplane learns is how to fall properly. A parachutist who keeps her body rigid when landing would probably break a bone or two, or worse. The parachutist is taught how to sequentially expose the body to the force of landing by rolling *into* the landing. This distributes the impact throughout the

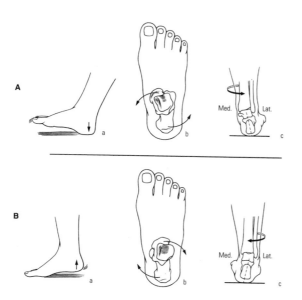

A. The foot crumples into pronation during heel strike as a strategy to dissipate forces. This is accomplished by inward rotation of the talus bone within the foot and inward rotation of the shin bone in the leg and thigh bone in the thigh.

B. During heel rise, the opposite occurs —the foot is reconverted in supination into a rigid base to propel the body forward. This is accompanied by outward rotation of the talus, shinbone, and thigh bones. These rotations are enormously helpful in dampening the enormous forces passing through the foot.
From: Saidoff DC, McDonough AL: Critical pathways in therapeutic intervention: Extremities and Spine, Mosby, St. Louis, 2002, p. 377. fig. 30-14.

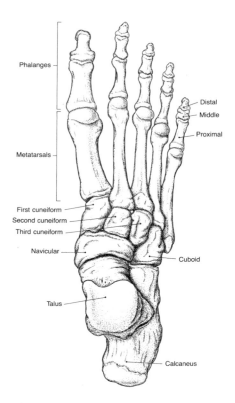

Phalanges

Distal
Middle
Proximal

Metatarsals

First cuneiform
Second cuneiform
Third cuneiform
Navicular

Cuboid

Talus

Calcaneus

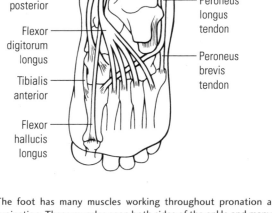

Tibialis posterior

Flexor digitorum longus

Tibialis anterior

Flexor hallucis longus

Peroneus longus tendon

Peroneus brevis tendon

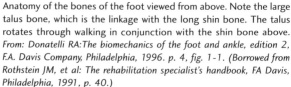

Anatomy of the bones of the foot viewed from above. Note the large talus bone, which is the linkage with the long shin bone. The talus rotates through walking in conjunction with the shin bone above. *From: Donatelli RA:The biomechanics of the foot and ankle, edition 2, F.A. Davis Company, Philadelphia, 1996. p. 4, fig. 1-1. (Borrowed from Rothstein JM, et al: The rehabilitation specialist's handbook, FA Davis, Philadelphia, 1991, p. 40.)*

The foot has many muscles working throughout pronation and supination. These muscles span both sides of the ankle and many of them attach underneath the foot. *From: Saidoff DC, McDonough AL: Critical pathways in therapeutic intervention: extremities and spine, Mosby, St. Louis, 2002, p. 418, fig. 32-5.*

body, not to just one area. Similarly, every time the foot meets the ground during walking the impact is evenly distributed.

The foot recoils into a spring that absorbs the brunt of impact when it first hits the ground. The keystone of the foot (the *talus*) is designed like an arch that rotates inwardly and disengages the foot out of its locked arch. The arch collapses slowly as the sole fully contacts the ground, aided by the muscles of the leg that attach to the arch of the foot. These muscles contract *eccentrically* (meaning they lengthen during contraction) and relatively slowly. This allows them to absorb many of the forces sus-

tained during impact. This process of unlocking the arch is pronation, and it allows the foot to come down on its inner margin. Incidentally, this also helps your balance by getting the maximum amount of your foot onto the ground.

The foot prepares to push off and propel the body forward after the foot-flat phase and *must* be converted into a rigid lever in order to successfully do this. Imagine trying to row a boat with cloth oars instead of wooden ones. You would go nowhere fast! It is the same with the foot. This process of being converted from a loose "bag of bones" into a rigid arch is supination.

This sequence of pronation and supination occurs with each step. However, no two people have the same feet. In the ideal foot, pronation and supination occur at precise times during the gait cycle. Deviations from the ideal foot are extremely common: too much pronation or too much supination. The foot with too much pronation is soft and unlocked during a time when it needs to be rigid in order to push off. This exposes the foot to undesirable stress. In contrast, the foot with too much supination is locked into a rigid arch that does not properly absorb the impact of heel strike causing injurious force to the foot. Both overpronation and oversupination lead to every type of foot ailment known. These problems typically do not show up in youth; they usually occur as middle age approaches.

FOOT TYPES

It is estimated that about three-fourths of all foot problems may be inherited. Your genes dictate a characteristic foot shape anywhere along the spectrum between flat feet to highly arched feet. You may be predisposed to problems that are aggravated by poor care or ill-fitting shoes. A good way to prevent these problems is to have a prescribed *orthoses* or *orthotic* fitted specially for your foot from a cast taken of the sole. Known as *shoe cookies*, orthoses fit into shoes and help realign the foot in relation to the ground in order to provide a more ideal alignment.

On one end of the spectrum of foot deformities are flat feet (known as *pes planus*) in which the foot is postured in perpetual pronation because of a collapsed arch. Many people are born with an inherited tendency to have poor arches. This used to be cause for dismissal from the United States armed services during World War I and II, but it is no longer considered a disqualifying disability. Many people get through life rather well with flat feet. Interestingly, there may be a positive relationship between flat feet and stress incontinence in females. The flat foot lacks the ability to absorb energy and may transmit forces up the leg into the pelvis that jar the muscles supporting the pelvic floor, causing

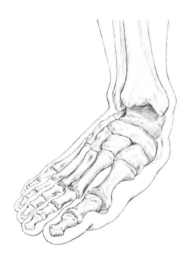

Flat feet lack the ability to become rigid during heel rise and do not efficiently propel the body forward—note how the arch sags inwardly. *From: Peterson L, Renstrom P: Sports injuries: their prevention and treatment, Yearbook Medical Publishers, Chicago, 1986.p. 356.*

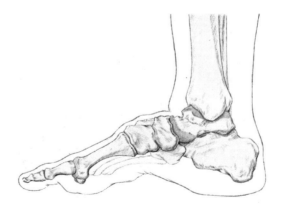

A foot with a high instep is too rigid and does not easily absorb the forces during walking. *From: Peterson L, Renstrom P: Sports injuries: their prevention and treatment, Yearbook Medical Publishers, Chicago, 1986.p. 358.*

urinary leakage. Many babies are born with what looks like flat feet because of the fat obscuring the arch of the foot.

At the other end of the spectrum are people who have high arches (known as *pes cavus*), also known as a hollow foot, claw foot, or high instep. Interestingly, foot studies of Army recruits show that people with high arches have a greater likelihood of injuring their feet and legs than those with flat feet.

HIGH HEELS

Narrow shoes with pointed toes and high heels were first introduced to Western women by Catherine de Medici of France (1519-1589), and many women continue to place the vogue of fashion above what is best for their feet, despite persistent pain and deformity. Four times as many women as men have foot problems. High-heeled shoes pitch body weight forward, shorten calf muscles, and throw the spine off balance. This accomplishes a forward protruding bosom, prominent buttocks, and outlined calves—desirable sexual attributes that can also cause short and long-term injury to the feet. It is no wonder that many woman kick off their shoes at every opportunity. They would do better to simply throw them away. The cumulative effect of wearing such shoes results in severe foot pain in many older women. Pumps may even lead to arthritis of the knee.

■ THINGS THAT CAN GO WRONG

There are many things that can commonly go wrong with feet:

• **CALLUSES** are thick flat pads of dead, hard skin found anywhere along the sole from the heel to the ball of the foot. The skin on the sole of the foot is about forty times thicker than anywhere on the body, and a callus can double this normal thickness. Calluses occur in certain patterns in accordance with the shape of the foot due to friction between the shoe and foot. The body reacts protectively to excessive friction by building layers of skin in an attempt to protect the foot from too much pressure. This is especially helpful as people get older and the fat pad along the bottom of the foot thins out. Removing a callus during a pedicure session may make your foot more attractive, but it deprives it of a natural shock protector. The best management of calluses is to wear properly fitting shoes with a cushioned insole such as moleskin to protect the foot. Keeping the foot well lubricated or powdered helps diminish friction to the skin of the foot. Callus pads cushion the ball of the foot and help prevent thickening of the skin. Several soothing foot creams rich in various fruit acids such as alpha hydroxy acid (known as *glycolic acid*) can help soften calluses and eliminate the layers of dead skin. Look for products that contain at least 10% alpha hydroxy acid in a 70% solution.

■ **CORNS** are very common. They are most likely result from wearing shoes that create a pressure spot on the skin, often around the toe joints or the sole of the feet. Corns are usually less than a ½ inch in diameter and occur when the skin responds to friction by building up protective tissue made up of dead skin cells. Over time, the patch of thick, hardened skin develops into a knobby, hard core that grows larger and larger to the point of causing painful pressure. Corns develop on toe joints (usually the little toe) but they can also develop between the toes. Wearing shoes that are too small, pointed, or so rigid that they squeeze the toes contributes to the development of corns. People with hammertoes or bunions are at increased risk for developing corns because of the increased friction owing to the abnormal shape of their toes. These problems can be prevented by wearing shoes that fit correctly and do not rub or squeeze the toes together. Avoiding tight hosiery is also helpful. Cutting a corn or using an acid corn remover may lead to infection. Remove the layers of the corn with a pumice stone carefully, layer by layer. Protect the corn with a moleskin plaster or petroleum jelly and cover it with a band-aid. Then buy shoes that fit. Corns may also be protected with small, dough-nut-shaped pads known as "corn pads." Placing lamb's wool between the toes may act as a cush-ion and reduce perspiration. Contact your podia-trist if these suggestions do not give you relief.

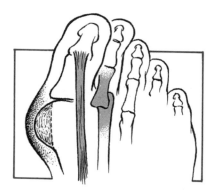

The big toe lies in valgus (outwardly) while the second toe rides beneath it or may overlap it, causing the joint of the second toe to dislocate. The outer side of the big toe develops an inflammation of the bursa known as a bunion. *From: Dandy, DJ: Essential orthopaedics and trauma, Churchill Livingstone, Edinburgh, 1989, p. 405, fig. 25.11.*

■ **BUNIONS** are gradually enlarging bumps on the side of the big toe that are accompanied by an inward tilt of the big toe toward the second toe. Sometimes, the big toe will overlap the second toe by folding above or underneath it, or push-ing it outward in what is known as *hallux valgus.* Some people are genetically predisposed to developing bunions. However, they are more likely to develop in females because of high-heeled shoes. Wearing shoes that are not wide or

roomy enough may also be a cause. When the metatarsal bone juts outward and rubs against the inner side of the shoe, the underlying soft tissue become inflamed and a painful, red, bump devel-ops. The underlying bone reacts to this stress by building up additional bone as a bulwark against pressure. Wearing good shoes or a specially designed splint for use inside the shoe may help prevent bunions from getting worse, although there is no fully effective means of prevention. Treatment involves wearing low-heeled shoes with a large rounded toe box. Wearing sandals is also helpful. In some cases, an orthoses may take pres-sure off the bunion by redistributing weight. Ice may be applied to painful bunions, followed by a soak in warm water. Taking non-steroidal anti-inflammatory medications may also relieve pain. Bunions can be surgically removed, although they tend to come back because the underlying problem—the structure of the foot—has not changed. The best way to prevent bunions, including recurrence following surgery, is to use a custom-made foot orthotic worn inside the shoe. Typically, a mold is taken of the foot and orthotics are designed based on the mold. They align the biomechanics of the foot in such a way as to minimize the forces that create bunions.

■ **BLISTERS** are accumulations of fluid cushions that form when the outermost layer of skin is damaged by pressure or friction from shoes or socks, or because the skin is either too dry or too sweaty. Blisters are a very common, minor injury. Covering a blister with an adhesive bandage is helpful, and shoes and socks that fit well are essential. Apply moisturizer if feet are too dry. Sprinkle talcum powder or cornstarch into shoes and socks if feet are too sweaty. Small blisters may simply be covered so they will not interfere with walking and they can heal. If the blister is very painful and prevents you from walking, puncture and drain it using a sterile needle along its base, followed by an application of antibiotic ointment and covering with a protective pad. Hands should be washed with soap and water before and after this procedure.

■ **ATHLETE'S FOOT** occurs when fungi that live on the skin enter a moist crack or crevice where they can develop and multiply, usually between the toes. It may cause itching, burning, cracking, and blistering of the toes. Athlete's foot is prevented by keeping feet clean and dry, and wearing absorbent socks and shoes made of breathable materials. Some people can resist fungi better than others, but it is possible to contract athlete's foot from someone else, especially if you are walking around a locker room in your bare feet. It is important to keep the feet and toes dry, and wear protective bath slippers when swimming and showering at a pool. This is not an easy task when we consider that the sole of the foot has more sweat glands than anywhere in the body except for the palms of the hands. Non-prescription and prescription anti-fungal medications are helpful in ridding oneself of athlete's foot. If this does not work, newer prescription-strength medications such as terbinafine (Lamisil®) and naftifine (Naftin®) have fewer side effects than older generation drugs and clear up athlete's foot in four to six weeks by gradually building up compounds that are toxic to the fungi.

■ **INGROWN TOENAILS** occur when nails are trimmed too short or curved, allowing the side of the growing nail to grow painfully under the skin. Ingrown toenails most commonly occur in the big toe and can lead to inflammation and infection. This condition is made worse by wearing tight shoes that compress the toes. Ingrown toenails can be prevented by cutting nails straight across. The recommended treatment for an ingrown toe-

nail is soaking the foot in warm water with one tablespoon of salt per quart for about 20 minutes, twice per day. Tuck a wisp of cotton with a small amount of antibiotic ointment under the nail to hold the nail edge away from the skin after soaking. Change the cotton once daily until the nail grows out beyond the corner. Wearing open-toed shoes or sandals is also helpful. If no infection has occurred, and the toenail is only mildly ingrown, making a V-shaped notch in the center of the nail will redirect the growth of the nail toward the center and away from the painful hard edge of the nail. If this does not help, see your podiatrist. Some ingrown toenails are caused by fungal infections, so simply fixing the ingrown toenail without also treating the fungal infection will not help in the long run.

■ **HAMMERTOES** commonly occur in the toe next to the big toe, causing both toe joints to become clenched like a claw, similar to a hammer that strikes the strings in a piano. This condition is sometimes accompanied by painful corns. Although there may be an inherited tendency to develop hammertoes, improperly fitted, tight shoes are a common cause because the toes are pushed forward and do not have room to lie flat in the shoe. Crowding from a bunion increases the risk of hammertoes. Hammertoes can harden into fixed deformities if they are ignored. They can make it impossible to walk normally without pain and contribute to disability. Hammertoes can be prevented by wearing shoes with a wide toe box. Pain may be relieved by placing an over-the-counter toe pad into the shoe. Using splints or shoe inserts (known as *orthotics*) may help redistribute weight and ease the position of the toe. Surgery may be the best option in some cases.

■ **PLANTAR WARTS** are spongy, flat warts that occur on the soles of the feet. They are caused by a highly contagious virus. They are most common in children and young adults because of their immature immune systems. Plantar warts can make walking painful because they may eventually press on underlying tissue and nerves. They have the appearance of circular craters consisting of small black dots. This condition can be prevented by keeping the feet dry and wearing thongs or pool shoes at the beach or health club. Plantar warts are best dealt with by a podiatrist rather than by over-the-counter treatment.

■ **POOR CIRCULATION** to the feet is common in older people because plaque buildup in the arteries prevents blood from reaching those areas farthest from the heart, possibly resulting in coldness or numbness. This condition is progressive and often relentless, however, some studies suggest that walking progressively longer distances over months or years improves circulation and may cause new vessels to grow into the feet in a process known as *collateral circulation*. Taking tepid baths helps dilate blood vessels and improves circulation. Propping your feet up on an ottoman also helps, especially if you move your ankles back and forth repeatedly. This type of condition needs careful medical management because clots may form and be released into the blood stream. Many people with this condition wear elastic stockings to help push the blood back up the leg toward the heart. Surgical intervention may be recommended.

■ **STRESS FRACTURES** occur when one of the long, slender metatarsal bones fractures due to high-impact aerobics, jogging, or walking for long periods of time. This type of break in the bone is known as a *march fracture* or *fatigue fracture* because it results from overuse and fatigue. Stress fractures occur most often in the second or third metatarsals. This type of fracture will heal over time without intervention.

■ **SESAMOIDITIS** is injury to the tiny, free-floating sesamoid bones embedded within the tendons under the base of the big toe. The sesamoid points act as a pulley for the tendons by helping the big toe thrust forward during late stance. High-impact activities such as aerobic exercise, jogging, or ballet dancing may injure these bones or the surrounding tendons.

■ **PUMP BUMPS** are technically known as *Haglund's deformity*. They are bony growths on the back of the heel bone that develops as the result of wearing high-heeled shoes (also called "pumps"). Often these shoes have a rigid leather edge that rubs the back of the heel, aggravating the tissue and turning it red. The underlying bone reacts by trying to protect the area by growing a bony bump as a cushion.

■ TAKING CARE OF YOUR FEET

Many older people experience painful feet due to years of neglect and misuse, and spend much of their time sitting in rocking chairs and on park benches when they could be healthy and more active. It pays to take care of your feet.

Toenails should be trimmed short and straight across. A cotton swab may be used to clean under the nail. Filing is best performed straight across with a single movement, lifting the file before the next stroke rather than sawing back and forth. A loofah sponge and pumice stone can help get rid of dead skin, but keep in mind calluses act to protect the foot and will simply grow back if removed. Skin creams can help keep the skin soft and pliable, and talcum powder absorbs perspiration and odor. It may even prevent the painful blisters that occur with hiking or wearing new shoes. Wearing flat, cushioned inserts made of cork or other shock absorbing material may be helpful in reducing shock and supporting heels and arches. Soaking your feet in a warm-to-hot bath not only feels great but also is good for your feet, especially when followed by a foot massage. Kick off your shoes, wriggle your toes, and walk barefoot around the garden or house as often as possible, but make sure that the walking surface is clean and free of anything that might cause an injury. Walking barefoot, especially on uneven terrain, is probably the best exercise for feet.

Foot care is a major task for people with diabetes and requires the utmost attention daily. The diabetic often has poor blood flow to the feet and is less capable of healing in response to a cut or injury. Some diabetics can step on a piece of glass and not even feel it because diabetes affects the nerves in the feet in a way that makes them less capable of sensation! Preventative foot care can reduce the risk of amputation in people with diabetes by one-half to three-quarters. People with diabetes are best referred to their doctor or podiatrist for instruction in the appropriate care of their feet.

■ CHOOSING THE RIGHT SHOES

The first shoes were probably papyrus sandals worn about 5,000 years ago by the ancient Egyptians, or perhaps by the icemen, who bound their feet with fur to stave off the cold. Today, style is the most important factor in determining the type of shoes to buy—not comfort.

The following suggestions can be used as a guide in choosing the right type of shoes:

■ The best time to purchase a new pair of shoes is in the late afternoon when feet are the most swollen. Otherwise, go for a long walk before trying on shoes. Both feet should be measured while standing because most people have one foot larger than the other. Choose the largest size. There should be at least a ½ inch space beyond the length of the longest toe so that there is enough room to move the toes upward within the toe box. Forget about breaking them in; if you are not comfortable with new shoes when you first try them on, do not buy them.

■ Shoes should be light, flexible, and made of natural materials that breathe such as leather or canvas. Heavy shoes may take a heavier pounding and last longer, but they may be penny-wise and pound-foolish because they can fatigue the muscles of your feet more easily. Look for shoes that have a good arch support, feel sturdy, and are flexible at the ball of the foot, where your feet naturally bend. Soles and heels should be replaced as soon as they show noticeable wear.

■ Fancy, expensive shoes with thick spongy soles do not absorb impact any better than less cushioned footwear and they put extra distance between you and the floor surface, possibly causing a fall. People with high arches may need to skip some eyelets during lacing to avoid pain.

■ Pregnant woman may need a larger shoe size for several reasons. Pregnancy causes swelling in the feet and legs, and the ligaments of the feet relax and stretch, causing the foot to flatten and spread more widely. Sturdy, roomy shoes with wide heels (no higher than 1½ inches) that provide good support are recommended.

7 Plantar Fascitis

A 38-year-old female aerobics instructor complains of pain in the sole of her left foot in the vicinity of her heel. She has taught low-impact aerobics part-time over the past several years and has begun to include high-impact aerobics in her lessons. The pain is becoming increasingly severe at the end of her workouts and is intensely felt when she gets out of bed each morning and takes her first few steps. Applying ice to the painful area and taking oral pain medication provides some relief. Bending her big toe upward or her ankle with toes pointed upward are both extremely painful. Her muscle strength is normal. She has flat feet, although her left foot is flatter than her right. This woman has one of the most common athletic injuries of the foot: plantar fascitis.

THE PLANTAR FASCIAE

T HE *plantar fascia* is a thick, fibrous, broad band of tissue running lengthwise along the bottom of the foot. It attaches at the base of the five toes and extends along the bottom of the foot and attaches at the bottom of the heel. It is located just below the skin and subcutaneous fat. *Fascia* is a type of body tissue made of a tough fibrous outer casing that envelopes certain muscles. The term *plantar* refers to the bottom of the foot: that part of the foot that we "plant" on the ground when we walk. *Plantar fascitis* refers to an inflammation of the fascia at the heel bone. The pull generated by the plantar fascia generates stress between the front and back of the foot. The pull of the five toes is stronger and will overcome the singular pull at the back of the foot where the plantar fascia attaches. This causes fraying, tearing, and the painful inflammation at the heel attachment known as plantar fascitis.

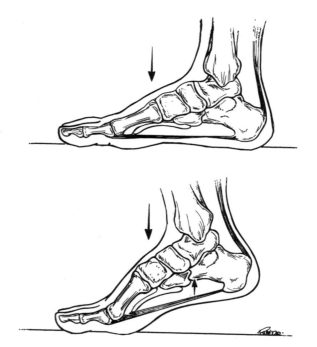

The plantar fascia reaches from the heel bone in the hindfoot to the toes in the forefoot. Acting to tie together the forefoot and hindfoot during quiet standing, it becomes tensed when the heel is lifted. Valmassy RL: *Clinical biomechanics of the lower extremities*, Mosby, St. Louis, 1996. p.23. fig. 1-30. (Modified from Bojsen-Moller R, Lamoreux L: ACTA Orthop Scand 50-411-479, 1979).

THE ARCHED FOOT

The arrangement of the 26 bones and 57 articulations (joints) form an inherent bow shape comprising the arch that spans the *hindfoot* (back of the foot) and the *forefoot* (front of the foot). The foot undergoes enormous *compressive force* when it contacts the ground because of the resistance from the ground pushing against the superincumbent body weight. This follows Newton's Third Law: Every force is matched by an equal and opposite force. Compressive forces occur when something is squeezed together by two different forces pushing in opposite directions. This is exactly what happens at the foot.

An *arch* is a rigid span curving upward between two points of support. The strength of an arch lies in its upper-most link: the crown or *keystone*. The keystone of an arch is wedge-shaped just like the state of Pennsylvania, which is known as the "Keystone State." From an engineering standpoint, the uniqueness of the arch lies in that the stress on it is entirely compressive. The Romans were the first to use the principle of the arch to develop structures on a massive scale. The arch represents an innovative engineering principle that has great advantage over post-and-beam architecture, which is limited by being subject to both compressive *and* tensile forces.

THREE ARCHES IN ONE

Imagine holding up a tall skyscraper! This is similar to what our feet do by holding up the weight of our entire body. The location of the foot at the lowest part of the body means that it must bear the superincumbent body weight of the entire body when standing! Because of the enormous compressive forces which focus on the foot, the bones of the foot assume three different arches. The two *longitudinal arches* of the foot run along the long axis of the foot

and are subdivided into the inner (medial) and outer (lateral) aspects. The longitudinal arch is supported by a post on the back of the foot known as the *heel bone* (calcaneus) and along five posts in the forefoot known as the heads of the five *metatarsals*. A third arch (the *transverse arch*) is located just behind the metatarsal heads and extends from the inner side to the outer side of the front of the foot (*forefoot*.)

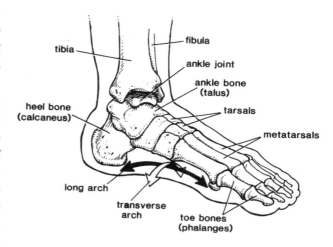

The arches of the foot. Siegel IM: *All About Bone: An owner's manual,* Demos, 1998, p.144, fig.12-1.

TRUSS

A *truss* is created by fastening beams (or bones) together in a triangular configuration. From an engineering perspective, the truss framework distributes the load of the foot in such a way that each bone shares a portion of the load. It is a triangular structure whose lower ends are connected by a *tie-rod* or bar, which keeps the lower ends of a slanted roof truss or arch from spreading outward.

The triangular shape of the truss endows it with structural rigidity capable of withstanding significant compressive and tensile forces. While standing, the forefoot and hindfoot may be likened to the lower ends of a truss, while the plantar fascia (known as the *aponeurosis*) is similar to a tie-rod that ties together the two main beams (the calcaneus and the metatarsals) together. Normally, the effect of weight-bearing on the arches of the foot is to dis-

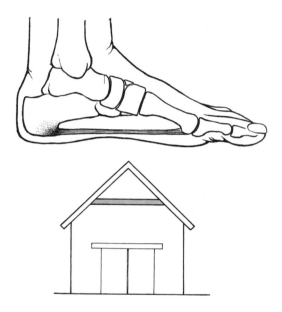

The biomechanics of the foot follow the principles of a truss and tie-rod. Dandy DJ: *Essential Orthopaedics and Trauma*, Churchill Livingstone, Edinburgh, 1989, p.401, fig. 25.4.

tract the front from the back of the foot. This causes increased tension in the plantar fascia, which resists distraction and maintains the shape of the arch. The plantar fascia must be precisely tensioned to function optimally, or it may become inflamed from plantar fascitis.

■ THE COLLAPSING AND RESURRECTED ARCHES

When the foot first contacts the ground during heel strike, the arches sequentially collapse in much the

same way that a compressed spring absorbs the brunt of impact. The talus rotates in an inwardly direction and disengages the foot out of its locked arch as the weight of the body moves over the foot. This process of unlocking the arch is pronation; it is a collapsing strategy that allows the foot to adapt to the impact that occurs with each step.

After the foot-flat phase, during which the sole fully contacts the floor, most of the energy of impact is dissipated. The foot must now prepare to push-off and propel the body forward. The pliable foot converts into a rigid lever so that it can push off the big toe and propel the foot forward. The process of being reconverted into an arch happens because of rotations of the talus and leg. This locking of the arch is supination.

As discussed in Chapter 6, many people have feet that are either excessively pronated or supinated, which stresses the plantar fascia and may result in an increased likelihood of developing plantar fascitis.

■ CONTRIBUTING FACTORS

Plantar fascitis is a classic *repetitive-stress injury* that may develop or worsen for a number of different reasons. While plantar fascitis may affect persons of all ages, factors that increase risk include:

- **AGE:** The plantar fascia becomes less resilient with age due to loss of elasticity, and the fat pad covering the heel bone thins out and is less capable of absorbing the impact of walking, which places more stress on the heel bone and the tissues attached to it.

- **WEIGHT-BEARING ACTIVITIES:** Standing for long periods, walking, jogging, or performing aerobics places added pressure on the feet and may stress the plantar fascia. High-impact aerobics are especially hard on the plantar fascia.

- **OBESITY:** Close to three quarters of the population of the United States is overweight, which is a serious health problem. Extra weight has significant consequences for the foot, and eventually the arches begin to sag under the load, which causes the plantar fascia to be stretched at its weakest point: the inner heel.

- **TIGHT MUSCLES:** The plantar fascia is a direct continuation of the Achilles tendon, which broadens out on each side of the heel and blends into the plantar fascia. Due to this direct linkage, the plantar fascia may act as a quasi-surrogate tendon for the calf muscles (known as the *triceps surae*). This means that tightness of the calf muscles and Achilles tendon is often common in persons with plantar fascitis. The tight calf and Achilles complex pull on the plantar fascia causing strain and predisposing the foot to developing plantar fascitis.

- **FLAT FEET:** This condition is also known as *pes planus*. (See page 57) These are feet where the inner sole of the foot contacts the ground. This has the effect of slowly stretching out the plantar fascia, which eventually pulls on its vulnerable attachment at the inner heel bone. Also, because the plantar fascia becomes less extensible with age due to loss of elasticity, overuse leads to sagging of the longitudinal arches of the foot and may cause the fascia to stretch, resulting in microscopic tears of the fascia at the inner heel bone.

- **HIGHLY-ARCHED FEET:** This condition is also known as *cavus feet*. These are feet that are locked into a rigid arch. This rigid type of foot is not pliant and is less able to absorb the forces of weight-bearing. Highly arched feet absorb much of the concussive forces of impact instead of helping to dilute those stresses because they have poor shock-absorbing capacity. If the foot is subjected to repetitive loading, the attachment of the plantar fascia may undergo micro-tears at its attachment on the heel bone. Furthermore, the person with a cavus posture will have a shortened plantar fascia that will lose extensibility due to the effects of age-related changes over time.

HEEL SPURS

A bony spicule of bone looking very much like a claw will grow out of the place where the planar fascia attaches to the inner heel bone when plantar fascitis becomes chronic. The body grows this extra bone in an effort to heal and stabilize the area and minimize injury. This occurs slowly over a period of time during which calcium is slowly deposited at the attachment of the plantar fascia to the heel. These bony spurs (known as an *exostosis*) are easily detected on x-rays. However, the pain associated with this condition results from micro-tears in the plantar fascia and the resulting inflammatory response rather than the sharp bony spur. While bone spurs may be associated with plantar fascitis, they are not believed to be its cause. Interestingly, many people with plantar fascitis never develop heel spurs. Statistically, 15% of normal feet have heel spurs, whereas 50% of painful heels have no spurs. At times, plantar fascitis may develop in one foot, while the opposite painless foot shows a heel spur on x-ray.

SIGNS AND SYMPTOMS

Plantar fascitis usually develops gradually and is experienced as a nagging discomfort localized in the front, inner part of the heel, along the sole of the foot. The pain tends to be worse when getting out of bed in the morning and the first few steps are the worst. This early morning pain diminishes once the foot limbers up but may recur throughout the day with excessive walking. Standing on tiptoes or climbing stairs may also exacerbate pain. Running is more painful than simply standing or walking. Pain is usually felt immediately when pressing along the inner heel where the plantar fascia attaches on the heel bone.

■ CONDITIONS TO RULE OUT

■ **TARSAL TUNNEL SYNDROME:** This condition results when the *posterior tibial nerve* in the foot is trapped, much like its counterpart at the wrist in carpal tunnel syndrome. The posterior tibial nerve and the artery and vein are located behind the inside anklebone in a tunnel formed by bone (the heel) and a fibrous band (the *flexor retinaculum*) called the *tarsal tunnel.* Tarsal tunnel syndrome may occur after an injury to the foot or ankle and is caused by compression or squeezing of the posterior tibial nerve that provides sensation to the bottom of the foot. Such injuries include ankle sprains, fractures of certain foot bones, or following illnesses such as diabetes or rheumatoid arthritis. Varicose veins in the tarsal tunnel may also compress the nerve. People with flat feet are more prone to developing tarsal tunnel syndrome because over-flattening of the long arch of the foot may also compress or stretch this nerve. A feeling of "pins and needles," burning or numbness, or even shooting pain may often be felt along the inner side of the foot. Certain activities such as standing for long periods or running may worsen symptoms. Wearing tight shoes may also bring on symptoms, which are often worse at night while sleeping. Pain may be felt when the area behind the inside part of the anklebone is pressed.

■ **SEVER'S DISEASE:** This disease is common in children 6 to 10 years old and is characterized by pain, tenderness, and swelling at the Achilles ten-don insertion on the heel bone. Sever's disease occurs in children in one or both heels when the growing part of the heel (the *growth plate*) is injured. The rate of bone growth during puberty often outstrips the growth of the muscles, tendons, and ligaments. They become tight and pull too hard on the soft growth plate, causing the Achilles tendon to pull on and injure the heel. Sever's disease is most common in physically active girls 8 to 10 years old and in physically active boys 10 to 12 years old. Gymnasts and soccer players often develop this condition, although any child performing running or jumping activities may be affected. Sever's disease rarely occurs in older teenagers because the back of the heel has finished growing by the age of 15. Sever's disease typically occurs after a child begins a new sports season or a new sport and may cause the child to walk with a limp and experience increased pain when standing on tip toes. The child's heel may hurt if squeezed on both sides toward the very back. This is called the *squeeze test.* The doctor may also find that the child's heel tendons have become tight. Children with Sever's disease must rest and cut down or stop the activities that produced the heel pain. Applying ice to the injured heel 3 times a day for 25 minutes may help ease the pain. If the child has a high arch, flat feet, or bowed legs, the doctor may recommend orthotics, arch supports, or heel cups. The child should be discouraged from walking barefoot and should wear good quality shoes with firm support and a shock-absorbent sole. Relief is often obtained by elevation of the shoe heel. The child should avoid excessive running on hard surfaces. Non-prescription medications may also relieve pain. Management primarily includes physical therapy and stretching and strengthening exercises. The child should feel better within 2 weeks to 2 months with proper care. The child can start playing sports again only when the heel pain is gone. The doctor will decide when physical activity is safe. Sever's disease may be prevented by maintaining good flexibility of the foot while the child is growing.

- **MORTON'S NEUROMA:** This condition is named for a military doctor who first described it during the Civil War period. It refers to a condition in which a nerve located in the middle of the ball of the foot becomes painfully pinched as the foot widens with the onset of middle age. Morton's Neuroma more commonly occurs in women who wear high-heeled shoes because the nerve is pinched between the bones of the foot that are forced together by the shoes. Wearing good shoes often solves the problem. A podiatrist may recommend wearing an orthoses. Minor surgery may be recommended in persistent cases.

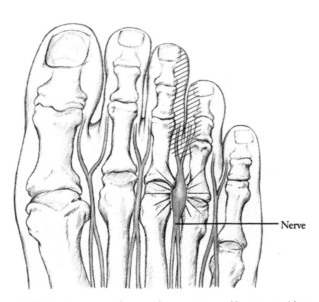

Nerve

In Morton's neuroma, the nerve becomes trapped by an ever-widening and aging foot. The nerve then swells and increasing pressure causes radiating pain and numbness in the shaded area. Peterson L, Renstrom P: *Sports Injuries: Their Prevention and Treatment*, Year Book Medical Publishers INC, Chicago, 1986, p. 372.

■ PREVENTION AND TREATMENT

The goal of treatment is to decrease pain, promote normal walking, heal tears, and decrease inflammation. Patience is often the key to resolution of plantar fasciitis and the majority of cases resolve with conservative management. It is essential to adhere to a conservative management program for as long as pain persists and avoid the temptation to return to vigorous activity prematurely, because doing so may result in relapse and conversion of an acute condition into a chronic disability. The entire process may take from 6 to 12 weeks. The longitudinal arches of the foot are not supported by muscle and a fallen or flattened arch cannot be raised by exercise. An estimated 90% of all cases can be improved by conservative management even though treatment may be frustratingly long in some cases.

- **REST:** The key to effective recovery is rest. Activities such as high-impact aerobics must be temporarily stopped and other activities such as swimming and stationary cycling may be substituted. Lightly stretching and warming the calf muscles is recommended prior to getting out of bed in the morning. The plantar fascia can also be stretched by pointing the toes toward the ceiling and making clockwise and counterclockwise circles with the feet.

- **COLD TREATMENT:** Rubbing an icepack back and forth over the painful area on the sole of the foot is known as an *ice massage* and may be applied up to three times per day to the area of tenderness for 10 to 12 minutes at a time. One technique involves freezing the water in an empty tennis ball and longitudinally rolling your foot over the ball. This will help minimize inflammation and decrease pain.

■ **MEDICATION:** Oral non-steroidal, anti-inflammatory drugs are very helpful in controlling the pain and inflammation associated with plantar fascitis. Non-prescription medications include those containing ibuprofen (Motrin®, Advil®, Nuprin®, and Medipren®) and prescription medications (Naprosyn®, Indocin®, Feldene®, and Relafen®). Some people have found that massaging a topical anti-inflammatory ointment or a 0.025% capsaicin (the active ingredient in hot chili peppers) into the painful area may help relieve pain. All medications should be used under the direction of a doctor because of potential side effects.

■ **SPLINTS:** Wearing splints during sleep initiates healing in an elongated manner and prevents micro-tears caused by stretching and weight-bearing. A plantar fascia splint holds the foot in dorsiflexion (a position wherein the toes are pointed up as much as tolerated) and allows healing to occur with the plantar fascia in a lengthened position, making it less likely to tear.

■ **RANGE OF MOTION:** The pain experienced during the first few steps in the morning can be minimized by performing simple range of motion exercises such as ankle circles and pointing the toes repetitively in different directions before getting out of bed.

■ **STRETCHING:** Stretching of the calf muscles and Achilles tendon complex is a very important part of the management of plantar fascitis. It is also very beneficial to stretch the hamstring muscles because tight hamstrings may indirectly affect the structures of the foot by contributing to tightness of the calf muscles. An excellent method of stretching is using a night splint to stretch the calf muscles and Achilles tendon complex. This approach is beneficial because it stretches the muscle-tendon complex for many hours during sleep. It is also important to stretch the plantar fascia in the following manner: While seated on the floor with the knee and ankle bent (dorsiflexed) toward the chest, pull the toes back toward the ankle and hold for a slow count of ten. This may be repeated up to ten times per session several times throughout the day. Stretching is an excellent way to help prevent onset of plantar fascitis.

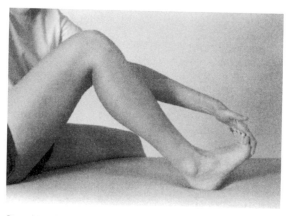

Stretching the plantar fascia.
Brotzman SB, ed: *Clinical Orthopaedic Rehabilitation*, Mosby, St. Louis, 1996, p. 278. fig. 6-40.

■ **CUSHIONED SHOES:** A well-made sneaker or shoe with air cushioning or a gel material will help minimize jarring to the foot. Inserting a longitudinal arch support or heel cushion may also help diminish the forces imparted to the heel.

■ **CUSTOM ORTHOTIC DEVICES:** These devices are appropriate in persons with a foot deformity such as a flattened or excessively high arch. These types of feet may result in poor biomechanics, which places them at increased risk for injury. A custom shoe insert may help compensate for the problem and minimize stress by aligning and thereby distributing pressure more evenly throughout the foot.

- **ULTRASOUND:** Ultrasound involves electricity passed though special crystals, which vibrate at ultrasonic (high) frequencies. This vibration penetrates deep into tissue as heat energy and may provide relief once inflammation passes beyond its acute stage. Ultrasound applied in the pulsed mode may deliver pain-relieving medications to the inflamed extensor tendon.

- **EDUCATION:** Education is a very important part of plantar fascitis management. Avoid exercising and impact sports, such as running, basketball, and high-impact aerobics, on hard surfaces. Performing alternate exercises is important and may include swimming, easy running, and cycling in low gear during the healing process. Prevention should include warm-ups prior to activity, including slow stretching of the calf muscles and the Achilles tendon. Reduction of the intensity, frequency, and duration of workouts is important in the prevention of repetitive stress injuries such as plantar fascitis. Runners should avoid hills and speed work, and long workouts should be broken up into two shorter ones. Wearing the right kind of running shoe is also important in the prevention of plantar fascitis.

- **INJECTIONS**: Steroids injected into the heel may temporarily relieve symptoms but will not address the underlying problem that caused plantar fasci-tis in the first place. Multiple injections are not recommended because they may weaken and eventually cause fraying and even rupture of the plantar fascia. Moreover, steroid shots cause the protective fat pad covering the heel bone to shrink and may increase the likelihood of plantar fascitis and other foot problems over time.

WHEN IS SURGERY NECESSARY?

Surgery should be considered as a last resort, especially for a painful heel spur, because the heel spur is likely to grow back again. This is what forced the retirement of the late, great Joe DiMaggio, whose heel never healed properly after removal of a bony spur. Surgery is appropriate *only* when all other treatments have proven unsuccessful. The surgeon makes a small incision on the inner side of the heel so he can partially release the fascia, remove any bone spur formation, and release any nerve in the area that may have been compressed by the irritated plantar fascia. This process is known as *endoscopic plantar fasciotomy* and is performed on an outpatient basis. It is approximately 85% effective and allows walking within hours after surgery with little or no discomfort. The only exercise recommended during the rehabilitation period following this type of surgery is swimming.

8 Achilles Tendon Injury

An obese 42-year-old housewife followed her doctor's advice to include exercise in her weight reduction program. She began by walking briskly every morning for two and a half hours wearing the worn, soft, comfortable tennis shoes that she normally used for gardening. Three weeks later—and six pounds lighter—she began to feel a burning pain in the back of her right ankle during her daily walk. The pain became less severe as she continued to walk, only to worsen about one hour after she finished. She also felt pain when negotiating steep inclines, climbing stairs, and rising up on her tiptoes. Her symptoms intensified and she began taking ibuprophen twice per day, which provided some relief. About three weeks later, she began to experience early morning pain and stiffness when getting out of bed and taking her first few steps. She has two flat feet and her right long arch appears flatter than the left. Her right Achilles tendon appears slightly red where it attaches to the heel and is warm to the touch. Standing on her right toes or gently stretching her toes upward is painful. Her right hamstrings and calf muscles appear tight. This woman has tendonitis *of her right Achilles tendon.*

THE ACHILLES TENDON

THE *Achilles tendon* is the large tendon connecting the two major calf muscles—the *gastrocnemius* and *soleus*—to the back of the heel bone. The name of this tendon is derived from the mythical Greek warrior Achilles—the greatest of the Greek warriors in the Trojan War. Achilles was the son of the sea nymph Thetis and Peleus, who was the King of the Myrmidons of Thessaly. His mother dipped him into the River Styx when he was a child to make him immortal. The waters made him invulnerable, except for the heel by which his mother held him. As recounted in the Iliad, Achilles led the Greeks to the walls of the city during the ten-year siege of Troy and was killed by Paris, who shot an arrow guided by Apollo into the heel of Achilles—his only weak point. Thus, the tendon that attaches directly to the heel bone is known as the *Achilles tendon.*

The outline of the Achilles tendon is clearly seen as a prominent cord when viewing the leg and foot from behind. It is the thickest and strongest tendon in the body and is capable of withstanding enormous forces. Beginning at the back of the mid-leg, the Achilles tendon is unique in that it is shared by the two major calf muscles. It is therefore considered a *conjoint tendon.* Any understanding of injury to the Achilles tendon is predicated on understanding the role of the muscles attached to it.

TRICEPS SURAE MUSCLES

Triceps surae literally means "three-headed calf muscles." It is actually made up of three muscle bellies that give the posterior leg its rounded, muscular appearance. Comprised of the *soleus* muscle, which lies close to the bone, and the outer *gastrocnemius* muscle, which is actually two muscles called by one name, the triceps surae stands out prominently when you stand on your toes or wear high-heeled shoes. Together, these powerful muscles allow us to stand on our toes by lifting the body onto the heads of the metatarsals. They are also involved when the toes are pointed downwards in *plantar flexion*. The triceps surae helps us jump up or down and, when walking, it pushes the body forward in anticipation of the next step by raising the heel.

Throughout history, soldiers have recognized the value of the Achilles tendon when they captured prisoners and *heel-strung* them, thereby ensuring their inability to escape subjugation and slavery. Today, the savage practice of cutting an enemy's Achilles tendon is outlawed by the Geneva Convention. In addition to playing a major role in helping us walk, the muscles comprising triceps surae play two other very important roles:

- **VASCULAR RETURN FUNCTION:** Contraction of the powerful triceps surae pumps blood from the legs back up to the heart. One of the few reliable signs of summer arriving in London is watching the Queen's guard standing at attention for hours, until inevitably one of them faints and lies on his back for several minutes. During prolonged standing without the benefit of the contraction of the triceps surae during walking, gravity causes excessive venous blood to pool in the feet and legs. This shunts too much oxygen-containing blood away from the brain, and the body's early warning system forces the head to come down to the level of the heart so that the flow of blood to the brain can be restored.

- **BALANCE MAINTENANCE:** The line of gravity falls through our joint axes during quiet standing in such an efficient way that the vertical projection of our center of mass sequentially falls behind our hip joint, in front of our knee joint,

and in front of our ankle joint. This causes the center of gravity to fall slightly in front of the body. and we may topple forward. This natural tendency to lose our balance is prevented by the active contraction of the soleus muscle during quiet standing, because the soleus generates an untiring, constant, counterforce that cancels the tendency to fall forward. Fascinatingly, the soleus

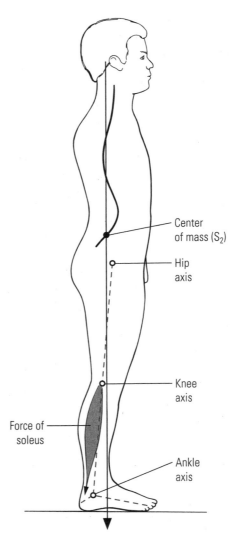

The soleus muscle in the calf is constantly working—even when we are standing still—making sure we do not fall in a forward direction. Saidoff DC, McDonough AL: *Critical Pathways in Therapeutic Intervention: Extremities and Spine.* St. Louis: Mosby, 2002.

can do this for hours on end without succumbing to fatigue!

TONIC VS. PHASIC

Understanding the physiologic difference in the type of muscles comprising the triceps surae is essential to understanding Achilles tendon pathology. Muscles are made up of individual components called *muscle fibers*. While most of the muscles of the musculoskeletal system are comprised of a mosaic of different muscle fiber types known as *tonic, phasic*, or somewhere in between, the gastrocnemius and soleus muscles are unique in that the majority of the fibers they are made of are predominantly one or the other. The energy chemistry of these different types of muscle fibers corresponds to the body's need for either sustained or rapid contraction.

- **TONIC MUSCLE FIBERS:** The word *tonic* derives from the Greek word *tono*, meaning continuous tension. This describes the soleus muscle very well because it allows us to stand for hours without getting tired. The soleus is comprised of 80% *slow-twitch, tonic fibers* that are ideal for continuous low level activity. These tonic muscle fibers are technically known as *Type I*. They are made up of slow acting, intermediate fibers and are red in color because they have a large reservoir of *myoglobin*—an oxygen-carrying molecule found in muscle— that enables them to store oxygen. The small, thin fibers of the soleus muscle experience little or no fatigue because they take turns contracting for brief periods of time. In this way, contraction is continuous. These slow-twitch fibers are designed to sustain the body in an upright position against the continual force of gravity.

- **PHASIC MUSCLE FIBERS:** The term *phasic* derives from the Greek word *phasis*, referring to the cyclic waning and waxing of the stars or moon. This type of muscle is capable of powerful bursts of energy but becomes unable to work after a period of time. Hence, it goes in and out of *phase*. These light-colored, wide-diameter fibers are known as *Type II*. They contain a small amount of blood and are recruited for short duration, intense work—for example, as when running a 40-yard dash or lifting a heavy object. The gastrocnemius muscle propels the body forward during the late stance phase of gait and then rests while the other foot contacts the ground. Phasic muscles accumulate lactic acid quickly and fatigue rapidly, making them incapable of delivering the same initial power output after about 3 minutes of continual activity.

THE BUILDUP OF SHEAR FORCES

Rotation of the pelvis causes the *femur* (thigh bone) and *tibia* (shin bone) to rotate around the long axis of the limb as part of normal gait when walking. Rotations of the thigh and leg usually occur in tandem to synchronize with pronation and supination of the foot. During early stance, when pronation of the long arch of the foot occurs, the thigh and shinbones rotate inwardly. These actions reverse themselves and rotate outwardly during late stance when the arch of the foot re-supinates. However, an individual who excessively pronates will cause her tibia to excessively rotate inwardly at the same time as the femur begins to rotate outwardly. This throws off the synchronous rotation between the shin and thighbones.

The gastrocnemius and soleus muscles both attach to the base of the heel bone, but they originate from different locations. Whereas the gastrocnemius is attached to the femur, the soleus is attached to the shinbones, tibia, and *fibula*.

Shear force typically refers to opposing forces

acting on the body, but it may also develop between the gastrocnemius and soleus muscles in the event that misalignment of the foot causes the shin and thigh bones to rotate asynchronously. This causes shear to be transmitted to the most vulnerable portion of the Achilles tendon: its vascular watershed. In this instance, the term *watershed* refers to an area of tissue that is more vulnerable to remaining injured because of a lack of blood vessels providing nourishment. The Achilles tendon contains such an area at approximately its mid-substance, and shear forces to this area are likely cause degeneration.

CRITICAL ZONE

Like many other tendons in the body that are nurtured by a protective sheath, the Achilles tendon is actually enveloped by an inner and outer sheath. The inner sheath has many nutrient-rich blood vessels that course up and down the length of the Achilles tendon. Unfortunately, a spot exists along the length of the tendon that has no blood vessels. This watershed area is known as the *critical zone* of the Achilles tendon because excessive activity is likely to result in problems at this location. This portion of the tendon is located about ⅓ inch before the attachment at the heel and is nurtured by passive diffusion. It is an anatomically weak spot where trouble is likely to begin.

A SAW-LIKE WHIPPING EFFECT

As discussed in Chapter 6, a repetitive sequence of movements known as pronation and supination that occurs within the foot allows us to walk. Both pronation and supination involve various motions of the bones within the foot, and both involve movement of the *calcaneus* (heel). Because the Achilles tendon attaches to the calcaneus, it is subjected to a whip-

ping, back-and-forth motion when walking that wrings out that area of the tendon that has the most minimal blood supply—the *critical zone*—and hence receives the smallest amount of oxygen and nutrients. This insult to the tendon may be magnified by a flat foot or a foot with excessively high arches.

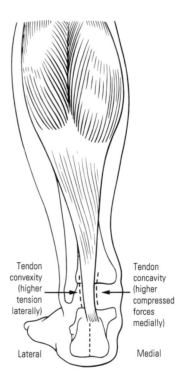

The Achilles tendon whips back and forth during normal walking. This "whipping effect" becomes magnified if the foot is too flat or too highly arched. It wrings the blood out of the critical zone in the tendon, making it more susceptible to tendonitis.
Saidoff DC, McDonough AL: *Critical Pathways in Therapeutic Intervention: Extremities and Spine*. St. Louis: Mosby, 2002.

CONTINUUM OF PATHOLOGY

Problems of the Achilles tendon initially affect only the inner and outer layers of the sheaths enveloping the tendon, but as the sheaths thickens, the tendon itself eventually becomes affected. This results in impaired gliding of the sheaths, causing friction and pain. This usually occurs in the critical zone, and the resulting inflammation may lead to structural disruption and degradation of the collagen fibers that make up the tendon. There may be micro-tears of the tendon, priming it for a partial or complete *Achilles tendon rupture.*

CONTRIBUTING FACTORS

Achilles tendon disease may result from physical training in cold weather, running on very soft surfaces such as sand, changing the running surface (for example, from grass to concrete), changing from flat to spiked shoes, or changing from long-distance endurance running to sprinting. Running in general, especially up or downhill, focuses force at the insertion of the Achilles tendon on the heel bone and places it at increased risk for injury. Other contributing factors include tight gastrocnemius and hamstring muscles, insufficient warm-up before exercise, sudden increases in mileage, changes in footwear, and running after a prolonged layoff.

SIGNS AND SYMPTOMS

During the first two weeks (the acute stage), you might feel a dull aching pain after exercise, which is a signal to take it easy and not provoke further injury. However, if activity continues, during the subsequent 3 to 6 weeks (the sub-acute stage), the tendon will feel painful during and after activity. This condition will worsen with each day that exercise continues. Climbing stairs may be painful. The tendon may be tender or bumpy to touch. After six weeks of continued exercise, pain is present even when not exercising or walking. Running becomes impossible.

CONDITIONS TO RULE OUT

Rupture of an Achilles tendon is easily recognized, but tendonitis is more subtle and may be confused with some of the following conditions:

- **HAGLUND'S DISEASE:** This disease is known as *pump bumps* or *posterior calcaneal tendon bursitis.* It is an inflammation of the *bursa* lying between the skin and the Achilles tendon. While this often happens in persons with a high instep, it most commonly occurs when wearing new shoes that have low-cut high heels and a rigid leather heel

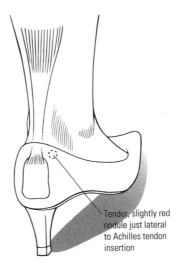

Tender, slightly red nodule just lateral to Achilles tendon insertion

A "pump bump" occurs when the bursa near the Achilles tendon swells up from irritation. This condition commonly occurs from wearing high-heeled shoes that have a rigid heel counter. Saidoff DC, McDonough AL: *Critical Pathways in Therapeutic Intervention: Extremities and Spine.* St. Louis: Mosby, 2002.

counter that rubs on the skin over the Achilles tendon. This condition is common to adolescent females and both male and female ice skaters. Inflammation at the site of the calcaneal tuberosity and subsequent excessive frictional stress on the bursa will result in swelling, redness (erythema), pain, and sometimes nodular thickening of the Achilles tendon. A blister develops that is followed by a reactive thickening of the bursa, leading to a bony enlargement (exostosis) of the heel bone.

- **ALBERT'S DISEASE:** This disease involves inflammation of the more deeply placed bursa between the Achilles tendon and heel bone. Because of the way the Achilles tendon attaches to the heel bone, part of the tendon's length stretches across the heel bone before attaching into its base. Albert's disease is common to young, female dancers who spend a lot of time on their toes. It results from friction to the bursa where the tendon attaches to the bone. Pain, swelling, and warmth are felt in the front of the Achilles tendon attachment rather than the tendon itself. Management of this condition includes avoiding standing on tip toes; not wearing shoes without a back, such as clogs, or shoes with a low shoe counter; wearing heel-lifts; applying ice; and taking non-steroidal, anti-inflammatory medications.

- **PLANTAR NERVE ENTRAPMENT:** This condition occurs when the lateral plantar nerve becomes compressed in persons lacking a sufficient arch. This nerve courses around and under the inner side of the heel. The flat foot may cause it to be repeatedly compressed with each step, causing tenderness and tingling. Treatment involves wearing an arch support within shoes and wearing shock-absorbing shoes.

- **BRUISED HEEL:** This condition involves an injury of the *fat pad* located beneath the heel bone, which acts as a cushion to absorb the impact of each heel strike during walking. This fat pad may be injured by repetitive jumps when landing on the heel, which typically occurs with hurdling and long and triple jumping. This type of severe impact imparts shear forces to the fat-

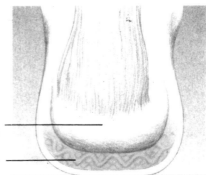

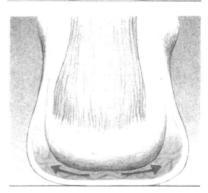

Heel bone (calcaneus)

Heel cushion

Left: normal heel cushion, in which the heel bone is protected by fatty tissue. Right: a painful heel cushion where the protective fatty tissue is pressed outwards toward the sides of the heel; this impairs protection of the heel bone. Peterson L, Renstrom P: *Sports Injuries: Their Prevention and Treatment,* Chicago: Yearbook Medical Publishers, 1983.

filled septa (the enclosed membranes within the soft tissue) and may rupture them. The cushioning effect is slowly lost even without trauma to the fat pad, because deterioration of the fat pad occurs naturally after age 40. Persons with a rigid foot and a high instep are more likely to develop a bruised heel. Wearing shoes with a firm, well-fitted heel counter helps maintain the compactness of the fat pad and buffer the force of impact.

- **SEVER'S DISEASE:** This disease is a painful condition of the heel that affects physically active boys (10–12 years old) twice as often as girls (8-10 years old). The immature heel bone is comprised of two portions glued together by the soft cartilaginous growth plate. Jumping activities such as basketball, gymnastics, track, and soccer may break the cartilage attachment. The pull of the tendons may be so strong while children are still growing that it pulls the bones apart. This is what happens in Sever's disease. Students may require an elevator pass to prevent climbing or descending the stairs in school. The foot may be immobilized in a cast for several months to minimize the strong pull of the Achilles tendon and allow the affected portions of the heel bone to fuse together again. An alternate treatment involves using heel pads in shoes to alleviate the pull of the Achilles tendon on the heel, as well as periodic stretching of the gastrocnemius muscle.

■ PREVENTION AND TREATMENT

The following measures will help prevent and heal problems of the Achilles tendon:

- **REST:** It is essential to rest an inflamed or sore Achilles tendon. Rest will prevent the disease from progressing. Avoiding or limiting the activity that led to the injury is recommended. Symptoms are the body's way of saying "Please rest!" Inflammation may spread from the tendon sheath to the tendon itself without sufficient rest. Once this happens, a vicious cycle of inflammation may occur in which the tendon excursion within an inflamed sheath contributes to more tendon inflammation. The best type of rest for Achilles tendon disease is to avoid activities that aggravate the pain. When the pain begins to subside, you can slowly increase those activities that were originally painful.

- **ICE APPLICATIONS:** The application of ice can mask pain, decrease inflammation, and provide

an analgesic effect that will alleviate many symptoms. Ice massage may be used 4 to 5 times per day for up to 25 minutes for the first two days. Ice is very helpful during the acute state when used with elevation.

- **HEAT:** Applying heat may provide relief after Achilles tendonitis passes beyond the acute stage (10 to 12 days). Ultrasound is a method of applying deep heat using electricity that passes though special crystals, which vibrate at high frequencies. This vibration penetrates deep into tissues as heat energy and may provide relief. Ultrasound therapy may help by organizing the orientation of scar tissue fibers that occur within the Achilles tendon so that they are more capable of resisting stress. Ultrasound applied in the pulsed mode may deliver pain-relieving medications to the inflamed Achilles tendon. Using a moist heating pad provides superficial heat to the tendon. Be sure to wrap the heating pad in multiple towels to avoid burning the skin. The application of heat allows for better stretching of the tendon.

- **STRETCHING:** It is important to stretch the triceps surae muscles prior to engaging in any activity. Passive, gentle stretching via wall *push-ups* is one of the most important strategies in the management of Achilles tendon disease. Stretching by way of a wall lean stretch with the knee in full extension is best performed gently, slowly, and without bouncing (see figure on next page).

- **INCLINE BOARDS:** These boards are indispensable for use in proper stretching of the triceps surae complex and the Achilles tendon. Begin by standing near the top of the board with the knees in full extension, making sure that the heels are flat and touching the board at all times. The feet should be gradually worked to the base of the incline board. If you do not have an incline

Below: Stand on your toes for 10 seconds and then come down flat on the floor. Repeat until you feel real fatigue in your calf muscles.

As the calf muscles begin to strengthen, you can put all your weight on the affected leg and keep the other leg off the floor. Then you can hold dumbbells or a barbell to increase your body weight. Use the affected leg for balance, but do not do all of the lifting with the affected calf.

Right: Place one foot as far away from the wall as you can and still keep your rear heel flat on the ground and the other leg a few inches from the wall. Bending your elbows, lean into the wall and support yourself with your hands, but don't let your rear heel come off the ground. Hold the stretch for 10 to 15 seconds and push back up. Reverse legs and repeat. Levy AM, Fuerst ML: *Sport Injury Handbook: Professional Advice for Amateur Athletes.* New York: John Wiley & Sons, Inc., 1993.

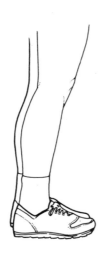
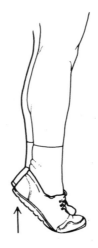
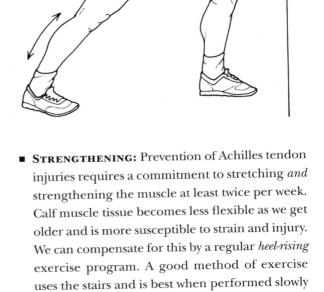

board, you may substitute a book. This exercise is known as a *heel drop*. This exercise should be performed for 3 to 5 minutes 6 to 8 times per day. Multiple, short periods of treatment daily are more effective than one prolonged period. Move farther down toward the base of the board while leaning your back against a wall as more and more stretching and flexibility are achieved. Alternately, stretching may also be performed using the "foot-on-chair" method or by employing stairs. Aggressive hamstring stretching is an indispensable part of the flexibility program because tight hamstrings may contribute to triceps surae and Achilles tendon tightness. (Please see figure 21-6 in Chapter 21 on page 179.)

- **STRENGTHENING:** Prevention of Achilles tendon injuries requires a commitment to stretching *and* strengthening the muscle at least twice per week. Calf muscle tissue becomes less flexible as we get older and is more susceptible to strain and injury. We can compensate for this by a regular *heel-rising* exercise program. A good method of exercise uses the stairs and is best when performed slowly at least 10 times each exercise period.

- **MEDICATION:** Oral non-steroidal, anti-inflammatory drugs are very helpful in controlling the pain and inflammation associated with Achilles tendonitis. Over-the-counter medications include those containing ibuprofen: Motrin®, Advil®, Nuprin®, and Medipren®, and prescription medica-

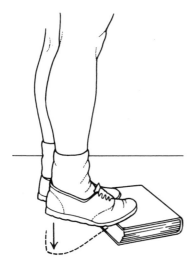

Stand with your forefeet on a raised surface, as if you were going to do a back dive off a diving board. Let your weight take your heels down below the level of the surface so that the back of your calf is stretched. Hold for 10 to15 seconds and come back up. Repeat until your calf is fully fatigued.

Levy AM, Fuerst ML: *Sport Injury Handbook: Professional Advice for Amateur Athletes.* New York: John Wiley & Sons, Inc., 1993

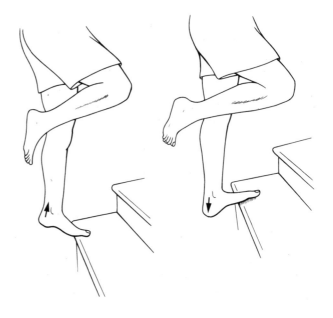

Strengthening and stretching of the calf muscle and the Achilles tendon are accomplished by careful exercising at least twice per week. Saidoff DC, McDonough AL: *Critical Pathways in Therapeutic Intervention: Extremities and Spine.* St. Louis: Mosby, 2002.

tions: Naprosyn®, Indocin®, Feldene®, and Relafen®. All medications should be used under the direction of a doctor because of potential side effects.

- **WARMING UP:** Adequate warm-ups should be performed for the entire body, particularly the dominant arm, for 10 minutes before engaging in physical activities such as volleyball. Warm-ups include stretching and gently moving the joints in the ankle and foot through the entire range of motion in a relaxed manner. Range of motion and stretching exercises should also be performed after athletic games.

- **ORTHOSES:** An orthosis is placed within a shoe to help mold the foot so that it is better capable of withstanding the stress of walking. An orthosis can maintain the arch of the foot in a position

known as *subtalar neutral*; this is the foot posture in which the least amount of Achilles tendon excursion occurs with each step. Additionally, using a heel lift will relieve the stress on an already aggravated Achilles tendon. Lifts should be used in both shoes to prevent one foot from becoming longer than the other.

- **THERAPEUTIC MASSAGE:** Massage of the Achilles tendon is often helpful and involves rubbing either back and forth or in a circular motion. This may actually increase pain at the time it is performed, but it is nevertheless helpful to the healing process because it increases local blood flow. The local fluid collection known as *edema* and the accumulated pain chemicals caused by inflammation are pressed out by massage. This deep form of massage also stretches the fibers and allows them to heal in a stretched manner. This is desirable because healthy Achilles tendons must stretch to their fullest capacity in order for normal walking to occur. Massage must be performed on the back and both sides of the tendon. It should be done for 15 minutes at a time every other day for 1 to 2 weeks. Therapeutic massage for an Achilles tendon problem is best done by a physical therapist.

- **EDUCATION:** Education is essential in preventing Achilles tendonitis and in preventing flare-ups. Wear good shoes and make changes in running surfaces or mileage gradually. Know what type of foot you have. Whether you have a flat foot, a high instep, or something in between, have your podiatrist perform an orthotic assessment if your feet hurt. Make sure to stretch and warm up before exercising, even if you do not exercise regularly.

- **INJECTIONS:** Steroid injections may be recommended when the above measures are not successful or if the pain is severe. Typically, a shot of cortisone is injected into the sheath and not into the tendon itself, followed by a week of rest. Occasionally, a second shot is necessary. No more than three shots should ever be administered because the steroid can weaken the tendon and cause it to rupture! Avoid cortisone shots until you've tried everything else. Consider it a last resort, never a first-approach solution.

TENDON RUPTURE

The final stage of Achilles tendon disease is *tendon rupture*, which may occur as the final insult to the degenerated Achilles tendon. It may also occur with no prior warning. There are two separate groups of people who strain their Achilles tendon to the point of tearing. Each is characterized by its own mechanism of injury:

- **MECHANICAL FAILURE:** Active, young males without any prior symptoms may tear their Achilles tendon due to excessive force that causes the tendon to undergo *mechanical failure*. This usually occurs from a sudden jump or lunge on the sports field, where immense and sudden recruitment of the muscle fibers comprising the triceps surae is necessary for sudden, explosive effort. For example, the take-off start of a 100-meter springing dash may impose force that exceeds the limit of the tendon and causes it to rupture.

- **CHRONIC DEGENERATION:** Middle-aged adult males with a history of Achilles tendon pain and weakness may rupture a tendon due to *chronic degeneration*. Changes in the fibers making up the

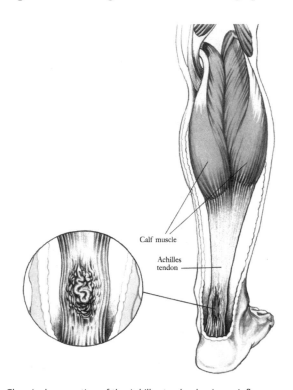

Calf muscle

Achilles tendon

Chronic degeneration of the Achilles tendon begins as inflammation and then gradually causes a slowly developing tear in the critical zone of the tendon. Peterson L, Renstrom P: *Sports Injuries: Their Prevention and Treatment.* Chicago: Yearbook Medical Publishers, 1986.

Achilles tendon may begin at the early age of 25 to 30 years old, making the tendon more prone to disease or tears with each passing year. A trivial event such as accidentally missing a step while descending a stairwell or walking off a curb unexpectedly may exceed the tendon's tolerance limit for tension and cause a tear. Tears often occur in parents, who may have been athletic in their younger years, when they take on too much, too fast with their adolescent children and participate in athletic activities that involve sudden acceleration or jumping.

Typical athletic activities that result in Achilles tendon rupture include volleyball, tennis, basketball, or other racquet sports. Sporting activities with explosive run-ups and take-offs increase the likelihood of tendon rupture. Ruptures are more common in males with a *mesomorphic* physique (a hard, heavy body type). Tears may also occur from a direct blow to the Achilles tendon or from too many steroid injections. For some unknown reason, persons with Type O blood seem to have a higher incidence of tears in the Achilles tendon.

PARTIAL VS. COMPLETE STRAIN

People with a torn Achilles tendon often report an audible pop or snapping sound accompanied by a sudden sharp and severe pain, as if they had received a blow from behind. The classic tale of Achilles rupture is one in which someone turns around and punches the person standing behind them in retribution for a perceived kick when, in fact, no one has kicked them. *Full thickness rupture* of the tendon results in an immediate inability to walk or stand on the toes. This is known as a positive *heel drop sign*. There will also be pain; the normal contour of the tendon will be obliterated by swelling; and a gap may be felt. The entire triceps surae may

appear more bunched up. Walking and standing on the toes may be possible if only a *partial rupture* has occurred, but there will be pain and swelling. Stiffness after rest or sleep is a common complaint when a tear is partial. Tear of the Achilles tendon is diagnosed based on history and examination. However,

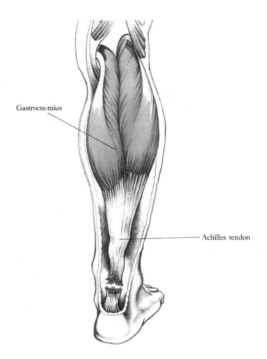

Gastrocnemius

Achilles tendon

Total rupture of the Achilles tendon.
Peterson L, Renstrom P: *Sports Injuries: Their Prevention and Treatment.* Chicago: Yearbook Medical Publishers, 1986.

if too much time passes after the original injury, it may be difficult to determine the problem. Magnetic resonance imaging is the standard for diagnosing and treating a torn Achilles tendon.

TREATMENT

Treatment of a completely torn Achilles tendon may be either conservatively or surgically managed. However, *immediate* non-surgical management is

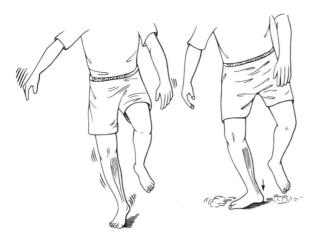

Positive heel drop sign is almost certain confirmation that the Achilles tendon has totally ruptured.
Saidoff DC, McDonough AL: *Critical Pathways in Therapeutic Intervention: Extremities and Spine.* St. Louis: Mosby, 2002.

best for the non-athletic injured person over age 50. Waiting longer than seven days often leaves surgery as the only option. Management of this condition involves the application a cast below the knee for four weeks with the foot postured so that the toes point downward. This position approximates the torn ends of the tendon. Intensive physical therapy is essential to stretch the Achilles tendon and strengthen the triceps surae after the cast is removed.

Surgery is best for those younger and more athletic. However, if a decision to operate is made, it is essential to do it as quickly as possible. The two ends of the torn tendon will have a shredded appearance similar to two untidy shaving brushes, and the surgeon will bring them together under local anesthesia for percutaneous (through the skin) repair. Open repair involves general anesthesia or a spinal epidural and is less likely to re-rupture than percutaneous repair. Intensive physical therapy after surgery will help restore the tendon as closely as possible to its pre-injury level of function.

Management of a partially torn Achilles tendon is usually conservative and involves wearing a cast for several weeks followed by physical therapy. However, if the tendon is inflamed, the accompanying cyst and scar formation may need to be surgically removed.

TENNIS LEG

Tennis leg refers to a sudden tear or strain in a portion of the gastrocnemius muscle. It commonly occurs in persons who participate in racquet sports, running, basketball, or skiing, especially when straightening the knee rapidly from a crouching position. Tears typically occur in the inner belly of the gastrocnemius muscle when a player lunges forward to meet a ball or anticipate the movement of an opponent player. This type of strain may also occur in a middle-aged person who misses a step while descending a stairwell. The result is sudden, intense, tearing calf pain that may be followed by swelling, cramping, and discoloration at the inner calf due to internal bleeding at the site of the torn muscle fibers. Rising up on the toes is possible, but

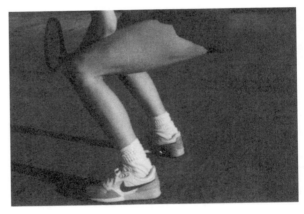

Tennis leg can occur when rapidly straightening the knee from a crouched position so that the gastrocnemius muscle is suddenly and painfully stretched.
Baxter D: *The Foot and Ankle in Sports,* St. Louis: Mosby, 1995.

painful. Strain of the gastrocnemius muscle is managed by applying a cold compress, elevating the leg, and avoiding contraction of the muscle. Crutches may be needed. Physical therapy will help restore the muscle back to its original, pre-injury level of functioning.

Tennis leg involves a tear of the inner gastrocnemius muscle. Peterson L, Renstrom P: *Sports Injuries: Their Prevention and Treatment.* Chicago: Yearbook Medical Publishers, 1986.

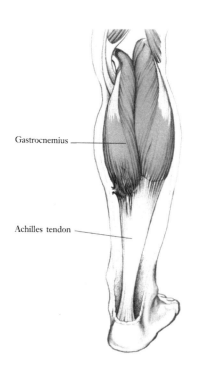

Gastrocnemius

Achilles tendon

9 Ankle Joint Sprain

After coaching a weekly game of soccer for his 5-year-old twins, a 44-year-old man came home on Sunday and played basketball with his teenage son and his son's friends. He attempted to block a shot by a member of the opposite team by leaping up toward the basket. His right ankle violently twisted inward when he landed and he collapsed to the floor, holding his exquisitely painful ankle in both hands with his eyes shut. Unfortunately, he has most likely suffered a sprain *of his right ankle joint.*

THE ANKLE JOINT

THE WORD "ANKLE" means *bent* or *crooked* in Greek. It is that part of the leg that deviates from the linked long bones comprising the thigh and shin bones, and creates a forward bend at the foot. The ankle joint actually refers to two separate joints known as the upper and lower ankle joints. The upper ankle joint is known as the *talor joint* (derived from the Latin *talo*). The more complex lower ankle joint is known as the *subtalor joint*.

The *talor joint* is made up of the two shafts of the shin bones known as the *tibia* and *fibula*, and an oddly-shaped bone called the *talus*. The anatomic relationship of the three bony components of the ankle joint is similar to that of a mortise and tenon joint, which is used in carpentry; it means putting a square peg in a square hole. The two-pronged, fork-shaped structure of the two shin bones tapers as it descends downwards; the head of the talus projects and inserts upward into the concavity above. The

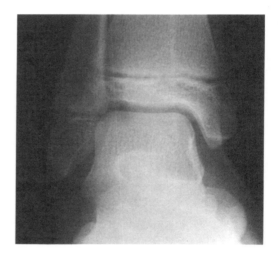

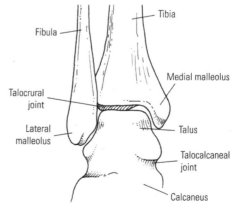

The two ankle joints: talar (talocrural) joint and the subtalar (talo-calcaneal) joint, and the surrounding bones.
Couglin MJ, Mann RA: *Surgery of The Foot and Ankle,* 7th Edition. St. Louis: Mosby, 1999.

anatomic arrangement of these three bones allows the upper ankle joint to work like a hinge joint and is often responsible for lateral ankle sprains. The two ends of the shin bones at the ankle are known as the *malleoli.* They do not taper off at the same level, making sprains of the ankle joint more likely than if they tapered off equally.

The bumps of bone on the inner side of each ankle are known as the medial or *tibial malleolus,* and those on the outer side are known as the lateral or *fibular malleolus.* The lateral bump extends a bit further downward, which means the ankle bends inward more easily than outward. Imagine getting the side of your foot stuck in a crack in the sidewalk in such a way that it suddenly and painfully twists inward. Too much inward bending is the motion that can sprain the outer ligaments and cause the most common type of ankle sprain: a *lateral ankle sprain. Medial ankle sprains* are far less common, but they are much more serious injuries.

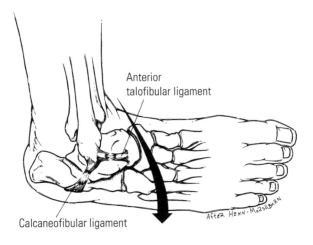

The lateral collateral ligaments become sprained when the foot rolls inwardly.
Malone TR, Hardaker WT: *Rehabilitation of Foot and Ankle Injuries in Ballet Dancers,* JOSPT 11:8, 1990.

◼ LATERAL LIGAMENT COMPLEX

A *ligament* connects one bone to another bone, and the many ligaments that span a joint together make up a *ligamentous capsule.* The ankle joint is enveloped by a ligamentous capsule that provides stability to the joint. Covering the capsule is a second group of protective ligaments along the inner and outer side of each ankle joint known as *collateral ligaments* because they provide "collateral" (side-to-side) stability to the ankle. These collateral ligaments are distinct thickenings of the joint capsule and are individually named according to their origin and insertion. These ligaments serve collectively as a guide in directing motion. They stabilize the joint and aid in proprioception, which is the awareness of where your limbs are in space. The collateral ligaments reinforcing the inner ankle are known as the *deltoid ligaments* and those protecting

the outer ankle are known as the *lateral collateral ligaments.*

The three lateral collateral ligaments, listed in order of increasing strength as well as the order of likely injury, are the *anterior talofibular ligament,* the *calcaneofibular ligament,* and the *posterior talofibular ligament.* They are easily remembered by their abbreviations: the ATFL, CFL, and PTFL, respectively.

When the ankle is in the vulnerable position known as *plantar flexion* (in a position in which the toes are pointed downward) and *inversion* (a position in which the ankle is pointed inward), the ankle bones are engaged so as to be virtually helpless in preventing an ankle sprain. Instead, the lateral ligament complex tightens to prevent excessive inversion and plantar flexion. However, when the inversion and plantar flexion happens too strongly or too fast, these ligaments will tear, resulting in an *ankle sprain.* When a ligament is stretched excessively or torn, it is called a *sprain.* The ATFL has the weakest yield force of the lateral collateral ligaments and is often the first to tear. Therefore, it is the most commonly injured ligament with an ankle sprain.

INCIDENCE OF SPRAINS

The ankle complex is the most frequently injured joint by athletes, both professional and recreational. Every day, approximately 23,000 people sustain an ankle sprain in the United States. The national annual incidence of this injury has been estimated at 4.5 million with restricted-activity days calculated at 20.7 million per year; bed bound disability days at five million per year; and 5.8 million days lost from work or school. Up to 85% of these injuries involve sprains of the lateral collateral ligaments. Studies indicate that playing basketball is the most common cause of injury. Ankle sprain has also been reported in football, soccer, skiing, cross-country running, volleyball, and falling from heights. Ankle sprain is the most common acute injury afflicting ballet dancers. Children's ankles often break rather than sprain because their ligaments are stronger than their growing, soft bones.

CAUSES OF ANKLE JOINT SPRAIN

Imagine the outer side of your foot lands on a crack in the sidewalk and instead of pushing off into the next step, your ankle twists to the inside, causing the lateral ligament complex on the outer complex to stretch and possibly tear. This is one example of a typical ankle injury. In this situation, however, you may have time to prevent a serious injury.

Another very common situation that may cause ankle joint sprain is when a basketball player jumps up high toward the basket and lands on the outer border of the foot. The ankle may violently tilt inwards from the force of impact, causing sudden and very painful stretching or tearing of the lateral

ligament complex. This type of injury can be excruciatingly painful.

Women who wear high-heeled shoes are significantly more susceptible to inwardly twisting of the ankle because the outer edge of the shoe may get caught in a crack in the sidewalk. The lateral ligament complex is placed at risk for excessive stress during the running, cutting, twisting, tackling, and collisions in football, when the foot is on the ground and the body twists above it.

BACK TO FRONT AND OUTER TO INNER

Some people are more likely to sprain their ankles than others because of the type of foot they have. Having a high instep makes you more likely to sustain lateral ankle sprains than someone with flat feet. This has to do with the way in which force is distributed along the sole of the foot during normal walking. The manner in which a child walks begins to mature between 13 to 14 months and is characterized by heel-to-toe walking. As discussed in Chapter 6, instead of walking entirely on the soles of the feet, the foot relates to the ground in three different phases. The foot initially strikes the ground with the heel; this is known as the *heel strike* phase. This is followed by the entire sole of the foot contacting the ground; this is known as the *foot flat* phase. The third phase is the *heel off* phase, because the entire weight of the body is momentarily balanced on the ball of the foot.

The weight of the body is focused at the back of the foot near the outer heel during the heel strike phase. It then moves toward the mid-foot during the foot flat phase. Finally, it moves toward the inner front portion of the foot where the big toe is located because the big toe thrusts the body forward. However, people with a high instep (arch) tend to walk on the outer sides of their feet, causing an imbalance in the distribution of body weight. This makes it more likely that a foot will twist inward and cause an inversion injury.

■ DIFFERENT GRADES OF ANKLE JOINT SPRAINS

- **GRADE I:** Mild sprains involve stretching and some fiber tearing of the ATFL without significantly disrupting the ligament. Quantitatively, this may be classified as having less than 25% of the fibers torn. Symptoms include mild swelling and point tenderness, little or no internal bleeding in the outer ankle, and mildly restricted range of motion. There is no instability when examining the ankle, although you may have difficulty walking.

- **GRADE II:** Moderate sprains involve moderate injury to the lateral ligament complex, frequently with complete rupture of the ATFL and partial tear of the CFL. Quantitatively, this may be classified as having 25 to 75% of the fibers torn. You may hear an audible "pop" when the injury occurs. Examination of the ankle shows limited range of motion with localized swelling, bruising, and tenderness at the front and outer ankle, although a defect of the ATFL is not palpable. Localized swelling and bruising become more diffuse and within a few days it may spread as far as the toes. Mild or no ankle instability may be present, but you may not be able to toe rise or hop on the injured foot. You may walk with a limp or may be unable to bear weight without the assistance of a cane or crutch. A grade II injury may be indistinguishable from a grade III injury in the acute phase due to the severe pain associated with both. Injury to the intermediate dorsal cutaneous nerve (a sensory skin nerve) may also occur because it crosses directly over the ATFL, resulting in numbness to the upper surface of the foot.

- **GRADE III:** Severe sprains involve a complete tear of the ATFL and capsule as well as rupture of the CFL. Quantitatively, this may be classified by having more than 75% of the fibers torn. This injury is referred to as *ankle subluxation*, whereas additional tear of the PTFL is classified as *ankle dislocation*, although this occurs infrequently. Swelling is rapid with a severe sprain; it may be egg shaped; and it is often located over the outer ankle at the lateral malleolus (bump at the end of the fibula). Examination of a grade III injury reveals severe pain, diffuse swelling, and bruising on the lateral side of the ankle and heel, tenderness, and an inability to bear weight. Black-and-blue discoloration may often spread to the opposite, inner side of the ankle within 24 hours. The *peroneal nerve* crosses the ATFL and may be stretched or torn during a severe sprain, resulting in weakness of the ankle muscles that move the ankle outward to the side.

■ DIAGNOSIS OF ANKLE JOINT SPRAIN

If an ankle sprain makes it difficult to walk or causes significant swelling or pain, it is advisable to see a doctor to evaluate the severity of the sprain and to make sure you have not fractured a bone. Your doctor will evaluate the severity of a potential sprain by doing a hands-on examination that involves tilting the ankle in different directions in order to identify excessive motion. He can determine which and how much of each ligament has been injured by selectively tilting or drawing apart the bones of the ankle. He may order stress x-rays if he is unsure of the extent of your injuries because of swelling or pain. Regular x-rays can only image bone, not ligaments. However, by stressing the ankle with weights, the amount of distance that the ankle bones move can accurately indicate which ligament is torn and to what degree.

■ PREVENTION AND TREATMENT

A supervised rehabilitation program will help make sure a sprained ankle heals properly. Ignoring this type of injury may contribute to possible future ankle sprains because the ankle may have residual instability. Athletes with a history of ankle sprains are at high risk for re-injury. The first 72 hours of the treatment program includes rest, ice, elevation, compression, and controlled motion using passive and active range of motion, gait training, and using an incline board to stretch the Achilles tendon.

- **PROTECTION:** Protect an injured ankle by using a splint and crutches or a cane. Use the cane or single crutch on the side opposite the injury.

- **REST:** Avoiding walking during the acute state when pain and swelling is at its worst.

- **ICE:** Application of ice using a slush bath or a cold pack should be used as soon as possible after injury to numb pain, limit swelling, and reduce the inflammatory process. The level of water should reach the base of the calf; the leg may be immersed for 15 to 20 minutes. Wearing a sock or neoprene cover over the toes may be helpful in retaining toe warmth.

- **MEDICATION:** Non-prescription medications may reduce inflammation and pain. Narcotics and other prescription strength drugs are rarely necessary.

- **COMPRESSION:** The injured ankle may be compressed in order to limit the amount of swelling and pain. Use an elastic wrap or bandage as soon as possible after the injury. It is especially important not to take the compressive wrap off and then put it back on. Doing this for even a short time provides a window for significant *rebound swelling* to develop. Placement of an elastic wrap should occur so that it is tightest (but not too tight!) at the toes and then get progressively looser as you move up the leg in a figure-eight wrap.

- **ELEVATION:** Keeping the injured ankle above the level of the heart will help prevent the swelling from getting worse because it helps drain the extra fluid (edema) back into the blood stream. The ankle should be elevated continuously, even during sleep. This may be accomplished by placing telephone books under the foot of the bed or by inserting a dresser drawer at the foot of the bed between the mattress and box spring. Using a whirlpool bath is not a good idea because it places the foot in a position below the heart. This will make the swelling worse.

- **RANGE OF MOTION:** Reducing stiffness and swelling can be accomplished by passive movement of the ankle joint. This is when someone moves your ankle for you. Range of motion exercises that involve bending and straightening the ankle can begin once symptoms subside. These exercises should only be done in those directions of movement that are not painful. As pain further recedes, side to side motion may also begin.

- **STRENGTH PROGRESSION:** The muscles around the ankle should be actively strengthened as the pain recedes. Begin with *isometric* exercises in which the joint does not move, but the surrounding muscles alternately tense and relax. *Concentric* exercises in which the muscles tense in order to move the ankle joint may begin as pain and swelling progressively diminish. More and more force using an elastic band or cuff weights may be progressively applied.

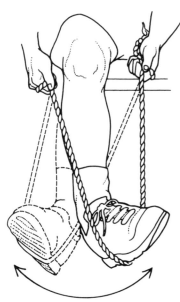

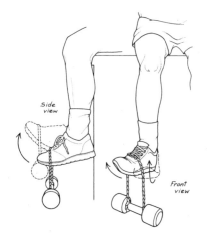

Dorsiflexion exercises of the pretibial muscles.

Resistive side to side (inversion-eversion) ankle exercises using rope as resistance.

- **WEIGHT-BEARING EXERCISES:** These exercises are helpful for ankle sprains, provided pain is kept to a minimum. *Closed kinetic chain* exercises can be performed after the injury has begun to heal. These are exercises done with the foot fixed on the ground. The benefit of this type of exercise is that the ankle joint is exercised in the same way that it normally functions in walking, running, and climbing. As a result, the scar tissue within the healing ligament is remodeled consistent with the applied stress, making them more resistant to future stress.

- **SUPPORT:** Although wearing a cast for simple ankle sprains has fallen out of favor, wearing a brace or case supports the ankle during healing and controls potential instability, preventing the ankle from sustaining further stress or being re-injured. Ankle sprains normally take about 6 weeks to heal.

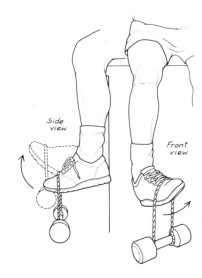

Open-kinetic chain inversion exercises of the ankle joint.

- **BALANCE EXERCISES:** These exercises are essential to preventing future ankle sprains. Normally, receptors in our ligaments called *proprioceptors* sense the position of the ankle and provide the brain with three-dimensional information about where the ankle is located in space. If these proprioceptors are damaged during a sprain, you are more likely to put your foot in an injury-provoking position. Ligaments in the process of healing are often weaker than before they were injured, resulting in an ankle that is very untrustworthy on rough terrain and likely to twist again. The more times you sprain your ankle, the less stable it will be in the future. It is possible to re-train damaged proprioceptors with specific balance exercises, once pain and swelling have subsided. One way to retrain proprioceptors is to balance on a wobble board—a circular disc with a ball attached beneath it. You can also dribble a ball while standing on the injured leg or toss and catch a ball with someone while standing on the injured leg.

- **PREVENTION:** Ankle sprains may be prevented by being aware of those situations or mechanisms that can cause ankle sprain and by wearing the appropriate footwear. Avoiding shoes with high heels or soles may prove helpful in preventing sprains or re-sprains. Wearing high top shoes or sneakers is also a good idea because they provide external support to the lateral ligament complex, thereby protecting against lateral ankle sprain. Stretching of the heel cord is also helpful in preventing ankle sprains. Taping the ankle prior to sports can be very helpful because it provides additional support external to the lateral ligament complex. The use of shoes with molded soles and multiple cleats, rather than shoes with fewer spikes, also helps decrease the likelihood of injury when playing sports.

SEVERE SPRAINS

Sprains that do not. respond to therapy—or are very severe from the outset—may require a surgery called *ligament reconstruction*. This procedure involves a small incision in the lateral side of the ankle. A portion of the *peroneal brevis tendon*, which runs parallel to the lateral ligament complex, is used as a surrogate ligament. Afterwards, the ankle is placed in a cast or brace for 6 weeks to allow for healing. Physical therapy can begin once the cast or brace is removed.

10 Shin Splints

A 42-year-old, hard-driving attorney made partner in her prestigious law firm and decided that she would run every day to get in shape. She began her day by jogging 3 miles each morning before work along the foothills of her suburban neighborhood wearing her old, worn out tennis shoes. Three months later and 11 lbs lighter, she complained of right medial leg pain and tenderness along the area corresponding to the right front area of her shinbone of three weeks duration. The painful area was warm and tender. She experienced pain when she bent her toes downward and simultaneously turned her foot outward manually with her hand. She also felt pain when she pointed her toes upward and bent her foot inward against resistance. Walking on her heels caused similar pain in the area of her right shin. This woman has anterior shin splints *of her right leg.*

THE SHIN BONES

THE *tibia,* also known as the shin, is the long bone in the front of the leg that connects the knee to the ankle. When we say we "got kicked in the shin," we are referring to the tibia. The tibia is a strong bone that bears the majority of body weight. Most of the muscles that move the foot are attached to the tibia. The *fibula* is a long slender bone that runs beside the tibia on the outer portion of the lower leg and bears little weight. Because the tibia is the principal bone of the lower leg in terms of bearing weight, those muscles which lie just in front of it are called the *pre-tibial muscles,* whereas those muscles that lie behind it are known as the *post-tibial muscles.*

◼ TIBIALIS ANTERIOR/POSTERIOR MUSCLES

Many of the musculoskeletal muscles are described by their attachment or function. The *tibialis anterior* is the muscle that attaches to the front or "anterior" portion of the tibia bone. It causes the toes to point upward (extension) and inward (inversion). The tibialis anterior is the muscle primarily affected by *anterior shin splints.* The *extensor hallucis longus* is an important muscle that points the big toe upward. "Extensor" refers to any muscle that extends a joint; "hallucis" refers to the big toe; "longus" means that it is a long muscle that begins in the upper portion of the leg, not in the foot. The *extensor digitorum longus muscle* also begins in the upper portion of the leg and allows the toes to point upward. These three muscles all attach to the upper front portion of the tibia bone in what is known as the *anterior compartment* of the leg and may be affected by anterior shin splints.

Posterior shin splints involve the muscles of the *deep posterior compartment,* which is located behind the shinbone. The main muscle is the *tibialis posterior,* which together with other muscles, points the toes inward. Other muscles in this compartment include the *flexor hallucis longus,* which allows the big toe to bend (flex) downward, and the *flexor digitorum longus*, which allows the four little toes to bend downward.

SHIN SPLINTS DEFINED

Viewed as a spectrum of related disorders, the term *shin splints* or *shin splint syndrome* encompasses the various stages of pain resulting from overuse that develop between the knee and ankle, especially in the lower two-thirds of the leg bone. This pathology first involves the tendon (*tendonitis*). If the condition is allowed to get worse, it will begin to involve the muscles (*myositis*). If there is further overuse, the stress will focus on the muscle attachment to the bone at the *periosteum* (the outer covering of the bone) resulting in a condition called *periostitis*. This may then lead to a *periosteal avulsion*, a condition in which the periosteum is peeled off the bone.

Shin splints are relatively benign and often get better, unless they are ignored or the body is pushed beyond its limits. In this case, the problem may worsen and evolve into worse conditions. Shin splints are the bane of many athletes, runners, tennis players, and dancers, especially as they approach middle age. Shin splints highlight the importance of not pushing oneself too hard. There are three different categories of shin splints, which are divided according to the muscles and tendon involved. Each category is from a different compartment in the lower leg: anterior, posterior, and lateral.

The lateral compartment of the lower leg contains the two peroneal muscles known as the *peroneal longus* and *peroneal brevis*. These muscles run down the outer (lateral) side of the leg close to the long fibula bone and enter the foot, attaching to its outer side. Contraction of the peroneal muscles move the foot outward in what is known as *eversion*. A broad band of tissue known as the *peroneal retinaculum* tethers the peroneal tendons against the upper ankle and thereby prevents bowstringing during peroneal contraction. Overuse of the ankles may rub the peroneal tendons against this retinaculum and the ensuing friction may cause irritation and inflammation of the tendons, which may develop into full-blown *lateral shin splints* if ignored.

THE DYNAMIC DUO

Despite originating from different parts of the leg, tibialis anterior and posterior share a common attachment on the inner side of the foot. Thus, contraction of these muscles helps the long arch of the foot reassume its arch-like shape during supination. Because of this dynamic arch support, the tibialis anterior and tibialis posterior do not work against each other, they help each other. When two muscles work together, they are said to be working together in *synergy*. Tibialis anterior and posterior work together as a dynamic sling to help reconstitute the long arch of the foot during certain portions of the gait cycle. This happens when both muscles simultaneously contract during late stance phase, when the heel comes up and the big toe thrusts back in anticipation of the next step.

ECCENTRIC ENERGY AND ABSORPTION

Simultaneous, concentric muscle contraction of the tibialis anterior and posterior helps rebuild the long arch of the foot during late stance because the muscles actually shorten. Shortening of the muscle is what happens in concentric contraction when the entire muscle pulls together and exerts a pulling force. For example, when you lift a gallon of milk, the biceps in your upper arm shortens to perform the lift. Something very different happens during the kind of contraction known as *eccentric* contraction.

Imagine lowering a gallon of milk to the table. It must be done slowly, carefully, and without too much speed, lest the force of impact break the container and spill the milk. This task is accomplished by a lengthening contraction of the biceps muscle known as an *eccentric contraction*. Eccentric activity is a force-dissipating strategy that is also utilized during locomotion to cushion against potentially injurious forces. During early stance, just after heel strike, tibialis anterior and posterior work in synergy by eccentrically contracting. This has the effect of dampening the jarring effect of heel strike by slowing down the rate at which the long arch of the foot collapses. This process is known as *pronation*. (See Chapter 6.) The forces of impact are dissipated by decelerating pronation of the foot, and the energy of the foot landing during heel strike is partly absorbed and diluted without the injurious ground-reaction forces disrupting the bone or soft tissue of the foot and leg.

FACTORS THAT CONTRIBUTE TO SHIN SPLINTS

Shin splints are a classic *overuse syndrome* resulting from tissue overload that may be caused by several factors. The most common cause of shin splints can be expressed in just four words: too much, too soon. Contributing factors include wearing worn or ill-fitting shoes, jogging or running on banked surfaces, over-striding on level surfaces, hill running, and suddenly increasing the distance covered.

People with feet that have flattened arches are especially vulnerable to developing both anterior and posterior shin splints. The flattened foot places excessive tension along the anterior and posterior tibial tendons during walking and running, which can cause the tendons to elongate. If activity continues, this tension is more likely to exceed the tensile capacity of the tendon, leading to further and perhaps more serious injury

The feet strike the ground between 600 and 750 times per mile when jogging, which is usually done on hard surfaces. It is often pursued by middle-aged people beyond physical prime who desire the shapely physique of youth and the carefree ease of movement of earlier years. However, these middle-aged adults often push their bodies beyond the limit of endurance and overuse injuries such as shin splints are often the result.

SIGNS AND SYMPTOMS

As discussed in Chapter 9, the tibialis posterior tendon curves around a bump of bone known as the *medial malleolus* as it travels down to the foot. The curvature of the tendon around this bony bump acts as a simple pulley. It also increases friction to the tendon, which might cause tendonitis, fraying of the tendon, or eventual tendon rupture. Therefore, posterior shin splints cause pain to be felt closer to the foot, along the inner and backside of the leg. Pain may be reproduced by resisting the foot from pointing inward into inversion, or while stretching

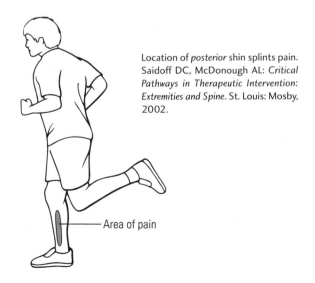

Location of *posterior* shin splints pain. Saidoff DC, McDonough AL: *Critical Pathways in Therapeutic Intervention: Extremities and Spine.* St. Louis: Mosby, 2002.

Area of pain

the foot into a position in which the toes point downward (plantar flexion), upward (dorsiflexion), or outward (inversion). Walking on the toes may also be painful.

In contrast, the tendon of the tibialis anterior muscle passes into the foot under the *extensor retinaculum*, which is a flat sheet of tough tissue that binds the tendons down along the contour of the foot and prevents them from bowstringing upward during contraction. Muscle-tendon overuse of tibialis posterior due to overpronation leads to stress

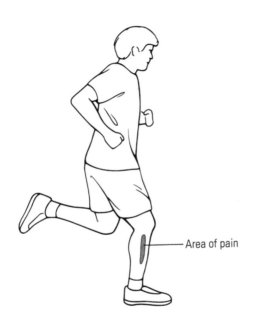

Location of *anterior* shin splints pain.
Saidoff DC, McDonough AL: *Critical Pathways in Therapeutic Intervention: Extremities and Spine.* St. Louis: Mosby, 2002.

and inflammation of the muscle. Eventually, inflammation may spread further, to the point where the muscle attaches to the bone, and the muscle fibers will tear away from the bone. Because of this, the symptoms of anterior shin splints are felt in the front and outer side of the mid-leg region where the muscle bulk of the tibialis anterior is located. Resist-

ing the foot from moving inward (inversion) and upward (dorsiflexion), as well as stretching the position in which the toes point downward (plantar flexion) and outward (eversion), may reproduce pain. Walking on the heels may also be painful, and the skin over the pretibial muscles may be warm and tender.

■ CONDITIONS TO RULE OUT

Shin pain does not always mean you have shin splints, but it might be a sign of one of two other problems that may be mistaken for shin splints. Often, one of these two conditions may develop when shin splint syndrome is ignored:

■ **COMPARTMENT SYNDROME** is a potentially devastating condition caused by exercise without proper rest. Following excessively strenuous activity, the muscles within the three compartments in the lower leg may swell to the point of becoming so constricted that they receive insufficient blood. This is a potentially dangerous situation because the oxygen-starved muscles may undergo irreversible damage if this continues for too long. The lower leg will appear swollen, red, and glossy. Initially there is cramping that may be accompanied by weakness or numbness. Symptoms will ordinarily resolve within a few minutes if the activity is immediately stopped, but may persist much longer if the activity is continued. The individual should stop exercising, rest, have his limb packed in ice, and be observed very closely. This condition often occurs in the right leg (reason unknown) of males in the second decade of life. Exercise-induced compartment syndrome is an emergency that must be managed by a doctor. Surgery may be required to release the pressure. Laser Doppler flowometry (LDF) is a new diagnostic technique that enables doctors to differentiate compartment syndrome from ordinary shin splints.

- **TIBIAL STRESS FRACTURES** are tiny cracks in the tibia that occur when overuse of the leg exceeds the ability of the tibia to withstand stress. Stress fracture may occur when a poorly conditioned athlete suddenly increases mileage or speed too rapidly, or does not rest and allow the soft tissue to recuperate after an injury. Stress fractures can end a season for an athlete and are often precipitated by participation in new forms of activity, overtraining, or a change in the way the sport is performed. This change may be as trivial as wearing a new pair of jogging shoes or changing the direction of a regular jogging route. Bone represents the body's last defense when soft tissue has been stressed beyond its capacity to cope, resulting in bone failure in the form of a *stress fracture.* These fractures are hard to detect early and only become visible on an x-ray after 3 to 4 weeks. Diagnosis is based on clinical findings, including point tenderness and pain that occurs with activity but subsides during rest. The pain of a stress fracture is confined to a smaller area than that of shin splints. Swelling may also be present. Technetium 99m bone scans show increased radioisotope uptake into the region of new bone formation as early as 3 days following injury. This testing method is considered the gold standard in early detection of a stress fracture. Management of a stress fracture involves resting the leg and using crutches or a cast if pain is severe. Healing may take 10 to12 weeks.

PREVENTION AND TREATMENT

- **REST:** It is best to eliminate sports such as jogging and playing tennis after an injury because shin splints are often brought on by overuse. Periods of inactivity may range from one to two days, or many weeks in severe cases. Players returning from a rest period should be allowed to practice when they are free of pain. Rest is imperative, because without it shin splints will only get worse.

- **ICE:** The application of ice can decrease inflammation and provide an analgesic effect. It is most helpful when used during the acute state and can be applied 4 to 5 times per day for up to 25 minutes for the first 2 days. Ice should be used in conjunction with elevation.

- **MEDICATIONS:** Oral non-steroidal anti-inflammatory drugs are very helpful in controlling both the pain and inflammation associated with shin splints. Non-prescription medications include ibuprofen (Motrin®, Advil®, Nuprin®, and Medipren®) and prescription medications (Naprosyn®, Indocin®, and Relafen)®. All medications should be used under the direction of a doctor because of potential side effects. Local steroid injections are not advisable.

- **ULTRASOUND:** Ultrasound is a method of applying deep heat using electricity that passes though special crystals, which vibrate at high frequencies. This vibration penetrates deep into tissues as heat energy and may provide relief. Once shin splint syndrome passes beyond the acute stage, applying deep heat may provide relief. Ultrasound applied in the pulsed mode may deliver pain-relieving medications to the inflamed extensor tendon. This is known as *phonophoresis.*

- **ORTHOSES:** An orthoses is placed within a shoe to help mold the foot so that it is better capable of withstanding the stress of walking. An orthoses can maintain the arch of the foot in a position known as *subtalar neutral,* which is the foot posture that exerts the least amount of stress on the muscles and tendons originating on the shin bone. Alternately, the podiatrist may recommend a heel lift or heel wedge. It is often helpful to have two pairs of shoes and alternate wearing them so as to vary the stresses on your feet and legs.

■ **MASSAGE:** Inflammation of muscles may occur with shin splints, accompanied by adhesions that bind the muscle fibers together and prevent the muscle from contracting fully. Deep transverse friction massage rids the muscle of these adhesions, allowing it to broaden during contraction.

■ **STRENGTHENING:** It is important to strengthen the pre-tibial and post-tibial muscles. This may be accomplished using cuff weights or elastic bands. Walking on the heels of the feet helps strengthen the pre-tibial muscles. Eccentric exercises are especially important because they absorb the injurious forces that may occur during jogging or running.

■ **STRETCHING:** It is important to stretch both before and after exercise. Gentle stretching of the inflamed muscles (the pre-tibials in anterior shin splints) also helps gain soft tissue extensibility. Stretching of the anterior compartment musculature may be accomplished by sitting on the heels. This is best done on a carpeted surface, legs and feet together, toes pointed directly backward. Slowly sit back onto your calves and heels until you feel tension in the shin muscles. Hold for 20 seconds, relax, and then repeat several times.

Many people with anterior or posterior shin splints have tight calf muscles and a tight Achilles tendon. Stretches are best performed gently and slowly, keeping the heel on the floor, and without bouncing. The use of an *incline board* is helpful in proper stretching of the triceps surae complex and the Achilles tendon. The feet should be gradually worked to the base of the incline board. Begin by standing near the top of the board with the knees in full extension, making sure that the heels are flat and touching the board at all times. This regimen may be performed 10 to 12 times per day, 5 minutes per session, for a total of 1 hour. Multiple limited treatments are more effective than lengthy sessions. As stretching and flexibility are achieved, you may move down toward the base of the board while leaning your back against a wall. Alternately, stretching may also be performed with the "foot-on-chair" method or by employing stairs. (See illustration in Chapter 8, page 79.)

■ **EDUCATION:** Jogging or running should be done on a level, soft surface, wearing good running shoes such as air sneakers with cushioned inserts. Initially, speed and mileage should be limited, and then increased incrementally. It is essential that athletes participate in sports that do not stress the injured musculature while they are waiting for shin splints to heal. Bicycling (using the heel to push off), swimming in a pool without kicking or using a kickboard, simple exercise in a pool, stair-climbing, rowing, cross-country skiing, or circuit weight training are excellent for maintenance of muscle tone, cardiovascular fitness, and aerobic capacity. Try to avoid jogging on uneven, hilly, or hard surfaces until shin splints are completely healed. Introduce jogging or running very slowly after an injury, opting for running on grass or a soft surface. Always cool down after exercise by gently stretching.

Knee

THE KNEE JOINT is one of the largest joints in the body, and it is extremely complex. The knee joint is very important because it must bend and straighten during walking, at the same time that the entire weight of the body is balanced above it. The many ligaments and muscles that attach to the knee serve the purpose of stabilizing the knee and ensuring balance. These ligaments and muscles must remain healthy in order to maintain the length and tension necessary for the knee function properly.

11 Meniscus Injury

A 45-year-old man felt a sharp pain in his right knee when he was up to bat during a Sunday morning baseball game. As he swung hard at the oncoming ball, his body came around with the bat. It is a good thing he hit the ball into the woods because he hobbled slowly around the bases. "I twisted my knee and now it clicks and locks," he complained after the game. While he can still walk, his knee clicks, occasionally locks, and feels like it is going to give way. He has sustained an injury to the meniscus *in his knee.*

■ DONUTS ON THE KNEE

THE TWO MENISCI are "c-shaped" washers between the thigh (femur) and shin (tibia) bones. The front portion of the meniscus (the upper portion of the "c") is known as the *anterior horn,* and the back curve is known as the *posterior horn.* The meniscus on the inner side of the knee is known as the *medial meniscus,* and the one on the outer side of the knee is known as the *lateral meniscus.* There are only two menisci because the end of the thighbone at the knee has two bony bulbs (known as *condyles*) that are protectively cushioned from injury by the meniscus under each bulb. The medial meniscus is attached by knee ligaments more securely than the outer, lateral one and is not as free to move around. This lack of maneuverability makes the medial meniscus more vulnerable to becoming pinched between the femur and shinbones, especially the thicker posterior horn. A pinched meniscus may become frayed or torn and, if ignored, may eventually cause arthritis at the knee.

■ SHOCK ABSORBERS

Menisci are made up of soft cartilage and are easily compressed, much like rubber. They resemble a donut sandwiched between the shin and thighbone and play an important role in dampening the bone-crunching collision of these two bones that occurs with each step. At one time, the menisci were routinely removed, as were the tonsils and appendix. However, doctors have learned the hard way that a meniscus is an irreplaceable cog in knee machinery of vital importance.

■ GASKETS INSIDE THE KNEE

Which exerts more pressure: a human wearing high heels or an elephant's leg? Believe it or not, although an elephant's leg pushes down with more force to the ground, high-heeled shoes exert more pressure. This is because pressure measures the amount of force over an area, while force does not. So, if both were standing on plain earth, the high heels would indent a small hole into the earth, whereas the elephant's wide feet may not even leave marks. What does this have to do with the knee? Everything!

The knee joint is designed so that the round end of the thighbone connects to the flat surface of the shinbone. From an engineering standpoint, this is not a good design strategy because the thigh bone would simply slide right off the tibia, and that would not work well at all. Also, the body weight pushing down on the flat top of the shinbone would mar the joint surface of the knee joint because the concentration of pressure would be too great for the joint to tolerate. The menisci lie on top of the flat shinbone and solve this problem by creating a concave socket that accepts the round end of the femur from above, thereby making the knee joint more stable. In this way, the menisci create a shallow socket at the knee that improves stability and prevents too much pressure from damaging the joint.

The menisci act like a gasket inside the knee because they are flexible. They actually stretch in different directions during walking to accommodate the peculiar round-on-flat relationship between the two long bones at the knee. In this manner, the menisci spread out the forces transferred between the two bones and actually reduce the pressure to the joint surfaces.

YOUNG VS. OLD MENISCI

The menisci in younger people are very flexible. As we grow older, the ongoing compression of the menisci causes them to become like old rubber that has been exposed to air. This process begins after age 40, when the menisci begin to become hard, less flexible, and more brittle, to the point of developing cracks, which are known as *degenerative meniscal tears*. These cracks may occur without injury from something as minor as the up and down motion of squatting to the level of a young grandchild. Because more and more people beyond age 40 are involved in sports, degenerative tears of the menisci occur more commonly than they did in the past.

TWIST 'N' TURN

Injury to the meniscus can occur in any age group from non-contact or contact stress. However, the *non-contact mechanism* of meniscal injury in younger people usually occurs because of forcefully rotating the knee while bearing weight. The meniscus can be injured because it gets stuck between the two bones. The meniscus may also tear because the twisting motion at the knee causes a *shear force* to the meniscus. Body tissues are very vulnerable to injury from shear forces, which impart two forces moving in the opposite direction from the affected body part. When you rotate your knee with your foot planted on the ground, your thighbone rotates one way and your shinbone rotates another. Shear forces occur at the contact point of these two bones, which is right where the meniscus is located!

Meniscus injuries are common to ballet dancers, who assume and hold certain positions. A partial or complete tear can occur during basketball or tennis when quickly twisting or turning while the foot stays planted on the ground. It can also happen during sideways cutting motions to avoid collision with an opposing player while playing football. This can happen during rapidly speeding up (acceleration) or slowing down (deceleration). The meniscus will stay connected to its untorn portion if the tear is tiny. If the tear is large, the meniscus may be left hanging by no more than a thread of cartilage.

Another common way that the menisci may be injured in any age group is from violent blunt trauma to the knee. This is known as a *contact mechanism of* injury. Even though the menisci are deeply located within the knee, they are physically connected to the many ligaments surrounding and protecting the knee and are therefore vulnerable to injury.

■ IMAGINE YOUR FINGER IS STUCK IN A DOOR!

Meniscal injuries in younger people are quite common because they are so active. The meniscus can be injured by twisting the knee while the knee is bent (flexed). These injuries often happen during skiing activities, but they may also occur from sudden sideways cutting maneuvers during running. These activities can cause a part of the meniscus to become caught between the shin and thighbone in the same way as getting your finger caught between door hinges.

■ PIRATES PARROT-BEAK AND BUCKET HANDLE

The different varieties of meniscus tears give rise to colorful sounding names such as parrot-beak and bucket-handle that help describe what the tear looks like. A small tear may develop into a degenerative tear where a portion of the meniscus becomes frayed and torn in many directions. A tear of the meniscus can become serious over time because the loss of a normally functioning meniscus allows excessive rubbing (degeneration) of the

bones in the knee joint resulting in early arthritis.

Unfortunately, the menisci do not heal easily. Injured tissue needs a blood supply to be able to heal, and the inner two-thirds of the meniscus has no blood supply. Because of this, a deep meniscal tear will usually fail to heal and get worse with time, although an injury to the outer rim may heal.

■ SIGNS AND SYMPTOMS

A torn meniscus will hurt at the side of the knee joint, especially during complete bending or straightening of the knee. The pain may be vague or felt even when the knee is at rest. Locking of the knee may occur at times because a torn fragment of the meniscus may become pinched between the two long bones of the knee. Locking often occurs while trying to straighten the knee out of the bent position. The knee will feel "rubbery." The knee often unlocks on its own with gentle movement. This unlocking will be accompanied by a click or snap. However, if the knee does not unlock easily, do not try to force it into the straight position or walk while it is locked. Doing so will cause the meniscal frag-

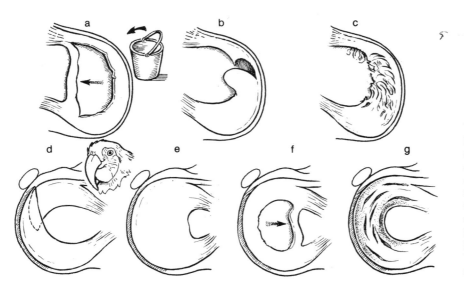

Type of meniscus lesions: (a) bucket-handle tear; (b) flap tear; (c) degenerate tear of the medial meniscus; (d) oblique "parrot-beak" tear of the lateral meniscus; (e) discoid lateral meniscus; (f) locked bucket handle tear of the lateral meniscus; and (g) cystic or myxoid degeneration of the lateral meniscus.
Dandy DJ: Essential *Orthopaedics and Trauma*. Edinburgh: Churchill Livingstone, 1989.

ment to mar the delicate surface of the knee joint, creating craters that may lead to premature arthritis. A knee that will not unlock requires immediate medical attention.

If knee locking is not a serious problem, a person may continue simple activities such as walking. When attempting to perform strenuous activities such as sports or climbing stairs, the knee may catch as the fragment moves around inside the knee. The knee may feel weak and react by unlocking itself, causing it to buckle. Swelling may also occur in the joint, especially if the tear nips a small blood vessel at the peripheral edge of the meniscus. If a meniscus injury is ignored for a long time, the knee may become weak to the point that the muscles around the knee shrink. This is called *muscle atrophy*. It most often affects the muscle on the inner portion of the thigh adjacent to the kneecap (known as the *vastus medialis muscle*). The knee will not be able to fully straighten, due to weakness of this muscle.

DIAGNOSIS OF MENISCUS INJURY

Your doctor will begin her diagnosis of a meniscus injury by listening to the story of the injury and symptoms, followed by a physical examination, during which she will perform certain movements of your knee. These tests include bending the leg and rotating the leg outward and inward while trying to straighten it, which may manipulate the fragment back into its rightful place. These hands-on tests are rarely performed on children with meniscal injury because they are so flexible. Swelling may occur on and off with both children and adults, and there may be mild limping.

X-rays will not show whether a meniscus is torn or not, but they are useful to help rule out other conditions that may cause similar symptoms. Magnetic resonance imaging (MRI) uses magnetic waves rather than x-rays to show damage to body tissues. This test is about 90% accurate in diagnosing meniscal tears. However, some doctors may elect to do an arthroscopy because an MRI is so expensive; this is a procedure in which a slim, fiber-optic cable goes directly into the knee to view what is going on using a super-miniaturized video camera on its tip. The advantage of arthroscopy is that the doctor can diagnosis *and* fix or remove the torn piece of meniscus with a miniaturized scalpel, also located at the tip of the cable.

CONDITIONS TO RULE OUT

Several different conditions may mimic meniscus injury and should be ruled out by a health professional. Conditions to be ruled out might include:

- **DISCOID MENISCUS:** Most people have a meniscus that is shaped like a half-moon. However, about 5% of people have a differently shaped meniscus that is shaped like a circular disc. This type of meniscus is thicker than an ordinary meniscus, which causes the bulkier outer rim to be more easily pinched by the shin and thigh bones. These round menisci are more common in children under 10 years old, and they are often discovered during arthroscopic examination after injury. Treatment involves surgically contouring the round meniscus into a more crescent-like shape.

- **CYSTIC MENISCUS:** This condition involves the outer (lateral) meniscus and may occur in young adults. The cyst is a bubble on the surface of the meniscus that occurs from a horizontal tear to the meniscus, allowing fluid from the joint to leak outward. This may feel like a dull ache on the side of the knee that may worsen at night. Treatment involves the use of an arthroscope.

- **POPLITEUS TENDONITIS:** This condition involves inflammation of the small tendon behind the knee that is responsible for unlocking the knee during walking. It is more common in people who have flat feet. Excessive exercise may cause stress and friction to this tendon. This condition is medically diagnosed by manually pinpointing the inflamed tendon. Treatment consists of icing and rest, followed by heat in the form of ultrasound. It is also important to avoid running on hills or banked surfaces. Strengthening the pes anserine—the insertion on the inner knee—will also help to prevent re-injury. Regular stretching of the quadriceps and hamstring muscles, as well as the use of an arch support, is also helpful.

- **PLICAE:** These are folds in the knee left over from the embryonic stage of development that usually disintegrate after birth. In some people, however, they remain after childhood as bands of tissue that rub painfully against the bones within the knee during walking and become inflamed. Unlike meniscus problems, in which pain is felt at the joint line, plica-related pain is slightly above the knee joint line. Arthroscopy is the best way to identify whether a torn plica is causing knee problems.

- **JOINT MICE:** Some people have small pieces of bone fragments loose within the knee joint. They move about, hence, the analogy to mice. These bone fragments may occasionally cause the knee to lock or catch. They are most common to males in their 20s who are right leg dominant. Symptoms include knee pain, knee collapse, joint swelling, locking, and a catching sensation; these are all symptoms similar to meniscus injury. Joint mice can often be seen on x-ray.

- **LIGAMENT SPRAINS:** Sprains of the *meniscotibial ligament* may occur from a blow to the outer knee while the foot is planted to the ground. Symptoms are identical to a medial meniscus injury, and differentiating one from the other requires an arthroscopic examination.

- **AVULSION FRACTURES:** These occur when a fragment of bone from the top of the shin bone, known as the *tibial spine,* presses down on the medial meniscus. These fractures can be easily missed on x-ray, although a careful review may reveal them.

- **FAT PAD SYNDROME:** There is a pad of fat in the knee that increases the leverage to the powerful quadriceps muscle of the front thigh. This fat pad may be rubbed too hard during excessive knee activity, or it may be injured by a blow to the knee. The fat pad may become inflamed and undergo a roughening of its surface, which causes it to become trapped and pinched between the kneecap and thigh bone during straightening of the knee. The knee may buckle and feel painful, but locking will not occur. Treatment with physical therapy is usually successful.

PREVENTION AND TREATMENT

About one-third of all meniscus injuries can be treated *without surgery* if the tear is small (less than 5 millimeters in length) and not too thick. These injuries are best treated with time, medications, bracing, and exercise. A muscle-strengthening program designed to build up the quadriceps and hamstring muscles may help the meniscus after the initial symptoms have been relieved. Strengthening these muscles helps the menisci because the anterior horns of both menisci are connected to the quadriceps muscles, and the posterior horns are connected to the hamstring muscles. Working these muscles with an elastic band or weights (resistive exercises) helps enhance the way the menisci move within the knee, making a torn fragment less likely to get jammed between the bony surfaces. Before resistive exercises begin, however, other gentler exercises should be performed in accordance with an individually designed physical therapy program.

These same principles can be applied in the prevention of meniscus injuries. Avoid sudden cutting-motions when running, especially if you are over 40 years of age. Be careful when you step down. Take the time to strengthen and stretch the muscles around the knee.

Strengthening exercises designed to increase quadriceps and hamstring strength may include:

- Warming up the knee joint by riding a stationary bicycle in a relaxed easy manner

- Raising the leg up and down while lying on your back (avoid a totally straight knee)

- Extending the leg while sitting, first without and then with an ankle cuff weight

- Raising your leg while lying on your stomach

- One-third knee bends

Knee joint forces can be reduced during impact loading and during walking and running by building up muscle bulk. The more force the muscles absorb, the more they are able to protect the joint from abnormal rotations. Traditional strengthening exercises are important in building muscle bulk, and working a muscle as it elongates is particularly helpful in absorbing injury-causing forces. This type of exercise involves *eccentric contractions*. Any exercise plan for strengthening the knees should be designed by a physical therapist, who will make sure the exercises are done properly and without risk of new or repeated injury. Pool exercises such as gen-

tle, small flutter kicks while holding the side of the pool are especially helpful early on.

Proper flexibility through stretching of these muscle groups is an essential part of keeping knees healthy. This same strategy of muscle building and conditioning is important in the *prevention* of soft-tissue injuries such as a meniscal tear. The passage of time is also important in dealing with a meniscal tear. About 1 to 3 months of physical therapy is a reasonable time expectation for significant improvement following injury. The best results occur in people who do not have an arthritic knee and who have intact cruciate ligaments.

WHEN IS SURGERY NECESSARY?

Your doctor may recommend surgery if you have had a serious knee injury caused by direct trauma. However, if only the meniscus is injured, surgery depends on several factors: your age, where the tear occurred, and how active you are. Generally, if the tears are small and close to the periphery of the meniscus, it is okay to rely on exercise and physical therapy, especially if the knee does not lock up. If the knee does not respond to therapy after 2 to 3 months, and is still bothersome, then surgery may be considered. If the tear is deeply located and generally not bothersome, it may be reasonable for a person under age 40 to have arthroscopic surgery, especially if the tear cuts through the entire thickness of the meniscus. Older people who are not active may decide to skip the surgery if they are directed to do so by a doctor, because older, degenerative-type tears are usually not repairable.

As discussed above, arthroscopic surgery involves a small incision in which a thin tube enters the knee. There is a scalpel on the end of this tube that removes or trims the part of the meniscus causing the problem. Total removal is avoided because it causes long-term problems to the knee joint.

Sometimes, the surgeon may be able to stitch up the torn meniscus with biodegradable sutures that dissolve in about 6 to 8 weeks. Removing part of a meniscus takes 10 to 20 minutes, while repairing it takes about an hour and a half. The success rate (50 to 90%) of meniscus repair depends on the age and location of the tear, the age of the injured person, and the expertise of the surgeon. If the tear is beyond repair, partial menisectomy is performed and the torn flap is removed. Although short-term satisfaction is pretty high after partial meniscal removal, removing as little one-third of the meniscus causes the contact between the shin and thigh bone to increase by as much as 300 to 400%! The long-term consequence may be premature arthritis if the knee is worked too hard and not properly cared for by appropriate exercises in the years following surgery.

After surgery, crutches or a walker for up to 1 week may be used, although the patient may need to use it for up to 1 month if the meniscus has been repaired. Crutches are best used until the injured person can walk without a limp. It is very important to perform knee and leg exercises during this time according to the doctor's orders or therapy instructions.

If the meniscus is repaired, the knee will often be covered by a hinged brace that allows only certain motions for about 8 weeks (with or without weight bearing) according to the particular doctor. After this time, a full eccentric training program utilizing elastic cords and other exercises may be started in a physical therapy setting.

12 Knee Sprain

A 38-year-old teacher dared herself to ski down an intermediate slope while on vacation in Aspen, Colorado. Unfortunately, she lost partial control and veered off the trail, impaling the tip of her right ski in a snow bank. Her legs went in opposite directions; she lost her balance; and she fell backwards. Her right leg became stuck in the snow and turned clockwise. She was able to extricate herself from this contorted posture, release her bindings, and gingerly hobble down the slope. She complained of a tearing sensation and sharp pain in her knee when she got back to the ski lodge infirmary, but heard no audible "pop." She was not able to ski again for the remainder of her trip and continues to complain of soreness with activity. She is unable to straighten or bend her knee fully due to pain. This woman has sprained the collateral ligament *of her right knee.*

A 20-year-old college sophomore football player got tackled from behind in such a way that the full weight of the other player hit his right shinbone while he was standing still. His shinbone moved forward relative to his body and he heard a loud "pop." Then he experienced excruciating pain and collapsed immediately. It required two men to assist him off the playing field and he needed crutches the next day to get around. Within 12 hours, his knee was hot to the touch, very swollen, black and blue, and slightly bent from muscle spasm. He is not able to walk downhill or on a cobblestone street even with crutches. This man has sprained his cruciate ligament *at the knee.*

▍THREE JOINTS IN ONE

THE KNEE JOINT is one of the largest joints in the body and the most complex. It is actually three joints in one. The meeting of the long shin (tibia) and thigh (femur) bones are correctly referred to as the *knee joint* or *tibiofemoral joint*. The kneecap covering the distant part of the thighbone is a separate joint known as the *patellofemoral joint*. The tibiofemoral joint works like a hinge to bend and straighten the leg.

The distal portion of femur meets the top of the shinbone in a unique way. Instead of simply connecting, the distal femur has two flared, bony bulbous ends that connect to the shinbone in such a way that the knee joint is actually comprised of two half-joints. These two bulbous ends are not identical, as you might expect; one is larger and extends farther out than the other, causing subtle but important differences between the inner and outer side of the knee. This is normal in the healthy adult knee and has a slight appearance of "knock-knee" when standing. This asymmetry between the inner and outer side of the knee is an example of an anatomic

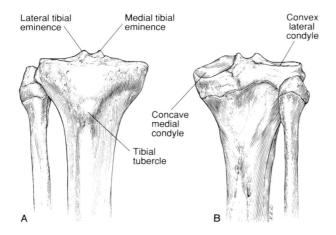

Lateral tibial eminence

Medial tibial eminence

Convex lateral condyle

Concave medial condyle

Tibial tubercle

A   B

Front and back views of the distal end of the right thighbone show-ing how the inner (medial) bulbular head projects farther out than the outer head. This normal in the healthy adult knee and imparts a slight amount of knock-knee when standing.
Tria AJ, Klein KS: *An Illustrated Guide to the Knee*. New York: Churchill Livingstone, 1992.

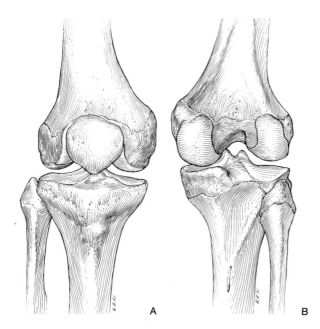

A   B

Front (A) and back (B) view of the human knee.
Tria AJ, Klein KS: *An Illustrated Guide to the Knee*. New York: Churchill Livingstone, 1992.

predisposition, since this discrepancy causes slightly uneven weight bearing and may be one contribut-ing factor in arthritis of the knee.

DESIGN STRATEGY

The best way to describe a stable joint is the "ball-and-socket" model in which one end of the joint is rounded and protrudes like a "ball," and the cor-responding "socket" is concave. This type of joint occurs at the hip and shoulder, and to some degree, at the elbow. It allows for a stable, reliable fit. As previously discussed in Chapter 11, this is not the case at the knee, where the round end of the thighbone connects to the flat surface of the shin-bone at the knee, with the meniscus between them for cushioning.

COLLATERAL LIGAMENTS

The knee is stabilized by four very strong ligaments. These ligaments bind the knee together by anchor-ing the two ends of the thigh and shinbones together. The *collateral ligaments* on the sides of the knee support and reinforce the knee joint by pre-venting too much side-to-side movement. The term "collateral" is another way of saying "security," as referred to in banking when collateral is used to guarantee repayment of a loan. The two collateral ligaments are located along the inner and outer side of the knee and provide security by preventing *lateral instability*; this is a situation where the shin and thigh bone may move excessively sideward.

The *medial collateral ligament* (MCL) is a broad band of ligament that straddles the inner (medial) side of the knee and provides stability to the inner side of the knee. The outer restraining ligament is known as the *lateral collateral ligament* (LCL). This very strong, cord-like ligament spans the outer (lat-

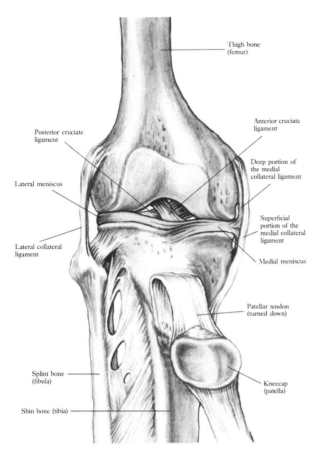

Posterior cruciate ligament

Lateral meniscus

Lateral collateral ligament

Thigh bone (femur)

Anterior cruciate ligament

Deep portion of the medial collateral ligament

Superficial portion of the medial collateral ligament

Medial meniscus

Patellar tendon (turned down)

Splint bone (fibula)

Shin bone (tibia)

Kneecap (patella)

The thigh and shinbones are held together at the knee by a series of outer (collateral) and inner (cruciate) ligaments.
Peterson L, Renstrom P: *Sports Injuries: Their Prevention and Treatment.* Chicago: Year Book Medical Publishers Inc., 1986.

eral) side of the knee and provides stability to the outer side of the knee. The MCL is more prone to injury than the LCL.

Cruciate Ligaments

To prevent the shin and thighbones from sliding over each other from front to back, two remarkable ligaments located in the middle of the knee joint anchor the ends of the two bones together. They are called *cruciate ligaments* because they cross each other and provide extra stability. This cruciform design prevents the knee from bending or straightening beyond a certain point. In this way, the knee ligaments set a limit on exactly how much movement can safely occur at the knee joint. This is essential when you consider the enormous forces passing through the knee during walking. The cruciate ligaments are especially important when athletes suddenly cut and run at an angle to their original direction in order to avoid an opponent. Both ligaments are named for their position in relation to each other. The anterior (front) cruciate ligament (ACL) limits rotation of the knee and the amount the knee can straighten. The posterior (behind) cruciate ligament (PCL) also limits rotation of the knee and the amount of bending at the knee.

Sprain

This arrangement of ligaments at the knee works pretty well during normal movements such as standing, walking, and running. Ligaments are pretty strong and have almost as much tensile strength as steel. Problems occur when you forcefully run into objects or people; when others crash against you; or when your foot gets positioned in such a way that your knee undergoes an unusual twisting motion. The ligaments protecting the knee are strong, but they can certainly reach a breaking point. Even steel cables have a breaking point. When a ligament stretches, becomes frayed, or is torn following injury, it is called a *sprain*. More than 4.1 million people seek medical care each year for knee problems, according to the American Academy of Orthopedic Surgeons. Many of these problems are knee sprains, which are more likely to occur in young to middle-aged adults. Ligament sprains at the knee joint are unlikely to occur in children and adolescents, who are more susceptible to bone injury.

The ACL is about 50% weaker than the PCL and this accounts for why sprain of the ACL is more common. Women sprain the ACL more often than men, although exactly why is unknown.

SKIING

There are both *contact* and *non-contact mechanisms* for injury to the ligaments of the knee. Skiing is a common type of non-contact mechanism for knee sprain. Downhill (alpine) skiing is a popular sport, but it can be dangerous. Accidents can happen from crashing into other skiers or otherwise getting your limbs positioned in such a way that you may cause serious injury to your ligaments, especially at the knee joint. Approximately 5% of all skiers have to be rescued each winter because of injury. The number of accidents involving novice skiers is three times higher than injuries to expert skiers. The collateral and cruciate ligaments as well as other structures such as the meniscus can be injured during ski-related injuries. When this happens, it is called a *combined sprain.*

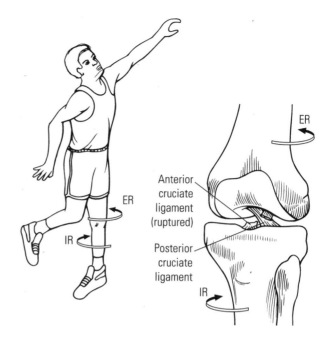

A basketball player descending from a jump-shot can land in such a way that the thigh bone externally rotates (ER) or the shinbone internally rotates (IR), causing a tear to the anterior cruciate ligament. Saidoff DC, McDonough AL: *Critical Pathways in Therapeutic Intervention: Extremities and Spine.* St. Louis: Mosby, 2001.

CAUSES OF INJURY

Injury to the anterior cruciate ligament from a twisting motion during which the feet are planted one way and the knees get turned another way represents a major injury to the knee. The non-contact mechanism often involves a twisting injury from landing on one leg and suddenly changing direction at the same time. This can occur following a basketball jump-shot. The player descending from a basketball rebound may land a little off balance, with one knee nearly straight, and tear the ACL when the thighbone rotates one way and the shinbone rotates the other way. A *contact mechanism of injury* to the ACL may occur if you're tackled from behind and the shin bone of your stationary foot receives a blow that pushes it forward. In American football, an all-out effort by a running back to avoid a tackle by pretending to run one way while planting and cutting in the opposite direction (known as a "plant-and-cut strategy") can result in a torn ACL.

The most common mechanism of injury to the posterior cruciate ligament is a blow to the anterior tibia with the knee flexed to 90 degrees. A non-contact mechanism of injury to the PCL may occur from stepping into a crack in the sidewalk or a hole in the ground while walking or running. Extreme straightening of the knee may cause hyperextension when the knee moves in a direction beyond straight. This is normally prevented by the PCL, but if stepping into a crack or pothole occurs quickly and forcefully, the PCL may sprain. The collateral liga-

...prain because of a lateral ...al ligament injuries most ... to the side of the knee, ... in sports such as football

... at the knee have typi- ...njury such as a tackle or ... ...ay feel something give way or hear a "pop," although the latter occurs more readily with cruciate sprain. The knee may buckle sideways during a collateral ligament sprain. The pain is often excruciating and causes immediate knee collapse. This type of knee injury is often so painful that it is remembered for many years. If the injury occurs while you are skiing or playing basketball, you may not be able to continue playing and your knee may feel very unstable when you try to stand up. Swelling occurs immediately in the front

of the knee with an ACL injury, in the back of the knee with a sprain of the PCL, and on either side of the knee if the collateral ligaments have been injured. The knee feels very hot and the muscles surrounding it will prevent normal movement. Once the acute phase has subsided, the knee may collapse whenever you try to put weight on it, twist it, or walk on uneven ground or on cobblestones.

■ CLASSIFICATION OF SPRAINS

One way to classify sprains is based on where along the length of the ligament the injury occurred. For example, a sprain can occur along the midsubstance of the ligament; this is known as a *midsubstance tear*. It can also tear near the shin or thighbone attachment. Another way to classify a sprain is by the *amount of fibers* that were stretched or torn. This is a very good way to classify sprains and it correlates well with the amount of knee instability the doctor discovers during a stress test.

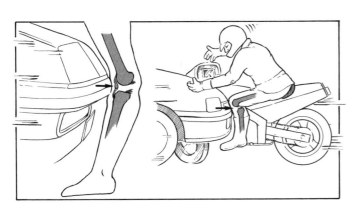
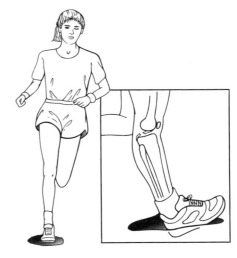

Above left: An injury to the upper portion of the shin bone violently shoves the shin bone backward and tears the posterior cruciate ligament. Dandy DJ: Essential *Orthopaedics and Trauma*. Edinburgh: Churchill Livingstone, 1989.

Above right: Stepping in a pothole while running causes the straightened knee to abnormally bend forward, causing a tear of the posterior cruciate ligament. Saidoff DC, McDonough AL: *Critical Pathways in Therapeutic Intervention: Extremities and Spine*. St. Louis: Mosby, 2001.

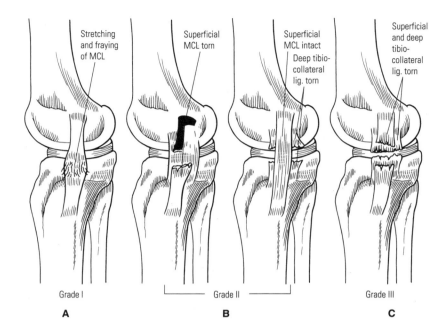

Classification of sprain of the medial collateral ligament. A. Grade I sprains involve ligament stretching and micro-tearing; B. Grade II sprains involve partial or incomplete tearing; C. Grade III sprains involve a complete tear of the ligament.
Saidoff DC, McDonough AL: *Critical Pathways in Therapeutic Intervention: Extremities and Spine.* St. Louis: Mosby, 2002.

There are three grades of sprains:

- **GRADE I SPRAINS** involve stretching of the ligament without any obvious tear of fibers, although *micro-tears* may have occurred. There will be tenderness locally at the knee, a bit of swelling, and no obvious instability of the knee during a stress test. You will be able to return to a normal level of functioning within a few days, provided you take it easy for awhile, apply ice, elevate the affected leg, and apply compression to the injury.

- **GRADE II SPRAINS** involve a ligament that is partially torn with local tenderness, more than a little swelling, and mild instability of the knee during a stress test. The activities of daily living may be difficult with a grade II sprain, and a cast or brace might be required for a couple of weeks in order to limit the amount of movement at the knee so that the ligament is not stressed further. Walking with a cane after the injury begins to heal may provide relief and hide the limp associated with this level of sprain. You will be able to return to your normal activity level after an appropriate period of rehabilitation.

- **GRADE III SPRAINS** represent complete rupture of the ligament, serious swelling, and tenderness. The ligament may be stretched so much that it is useless in maintaining stability at the knee. This level of sprain is quite painful and may cause a person to fall to the ground when it occurs. A stress test will show serious instability, especially if it is done before the surrounding knee muscles have a chance to go into a protective spasm. The use of crutches and rehabilitation will be necessary. Surgery may also be necessary, depending on the age and activity level of the injured person.

■ DIAGNOSIS OF KNEE SPRAINS

Your doctor will take a medical history, including the details leading up to the injury, how the injury occurred, and the symptoms you experienced right after the injury. This is very important in diagnosing a knee problem. As discussed in Chapter 11, simple x-rays may show nothing more than soft tissue swelling, whereas stress x-rays filmed under anesthesia are quite revealing in showing the degree of joint instability. The joint is stressed during a stress x-ray by applying pressure in such a way that the doctor can see whether a ligament has been torn.

These *stress tests* can determine whether the different parts of the knee joint stay properly aligned when pressure is applied in different directions. A positive test indicates an injury occurred and what ligament was torn or stretched. Pressure is applied to the tibia by moving it forward and backward when testing cruciate ligaments. The doctor will exert pressure on the side of the knee when collateral ligament injury has occurred.

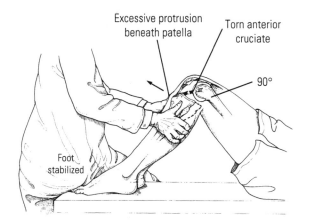

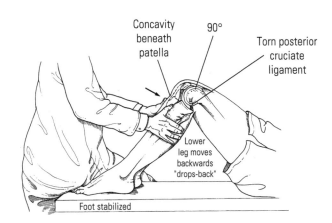

The *anterior drawer test* (above left) pulls (draws) the shinbone forward (anteriorly), and the *posterior drawer test* (above right) pushes the shinbone backward (posteriorly). Scuderi GR, McCann PD, Bruno PJ: *Sports Medicine: Principles of Primary Care*. St. Louis: Mosby, 1997.

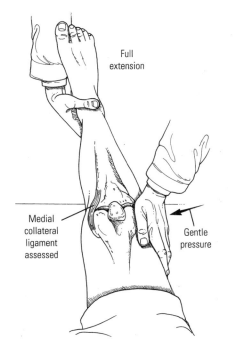

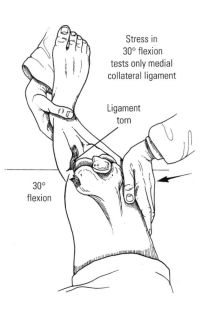

Left: Applying direct pressure to the outer portion of the straightened knee tests whether the medial collateral ligament is torn on the inner side of the knee. Scuderi GR, McCann PD, Bruno PJ: *Sports Medicine: Principles of Primary Care*. St. Louis: Mosby, 1997.

The hands-on evaluation of the doctor can be easily confirmed by the use of x-rays, magnetic resonance imaging (MRI), and computerized axial tomography (CAT scan).

CONDITIONS TO RULE OUT

Unfortunately, many people with cruciate ligament rupture are often told they only have a sprained knee after x-rays taken in the local emergency room appear negative. Making the correct diagnosis may not be easy if time passes following an acute ACL tear because stress testing will be difficult due to pain and muscle spasm. Therefore, it is essential to examine the injured person immediately after injury, before pain, swelling, and muscle spasm get worse. If delay is unavoidable, then specialized diagnostic aids such as arthrography, arthroscopy, or examination of the knee under anesthesia are appropriate. The opportunity to repair a severe anterior cruciate ligament sprain may be lost unless detected within the first few days following acute injury. (There is more leeway with collateral ligament injury.) Doctors should be highly suspicious of an ACL injury if the history and clinical examination suggest a sprain. Typically, arthroscopy and examination under anesthesia are not carried out unless the diagnosis is not clear from the history and clinical examination.

Even without x-rays or other forms of imaging, a clinical diagnosis can be as high as 85% simply by the history and clinical presentation, including these four essential components:

- A "pop" at the time of injury

- Inability to continue activity

- Gross swelling of the knee

- Maximal swelling within 12 hours after injury

CONDITIONS TO RULE OUT

- **MENISCUS INJURY:** (See Chapter 11.) The events leading up to a meniscus injury are quite different from the injury of a knee ligament. Meniscus injuries typically occur during low-speed activities when the knee is bent, while knee sprains occur from high-speed collisions or twisting of the knee while the knee is in a straight position. You rarely collapse from a meniscus injury, nor is there usually a single episode that stands out in your mind as having caused it. A memorable event usually occurs that causes a sprain of the knee ligaments. It is often hard to stand upright once this type of injury has occurred.

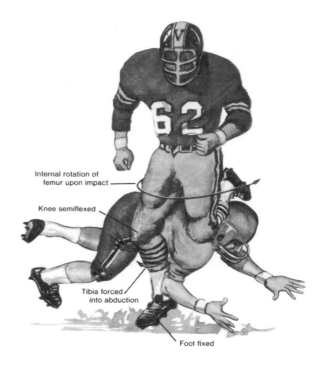

Internal rotation of femur upon impact

Knee semiflexed

Tibia forced into abduction

Foot fixed

A clipping-type tackle is an infraction of the rules of football. It can cause devastating injury to both the collateral and cruciate ligaments as well as the meniscus. Healey JE, Jr: A *Synopsis of Clinical Anatomy*. Philadelphia: WB Saunders Co, 1969; See also: Moore KL: *Clinically Oriented Anatomy*, 2nd Edition. Baltimore: Williams & Wilkins, 1985.

- **UNHAPPY TRIAD OF O'DONOHUE:** O'Donohue was an orthopedic surgeon who described an injury that most commonly occurs in American football. This type of injury has to do with an infraction of football rules in which "clipping" is performed. Typically, a football player carrying a football is clipped (blocked) from the rear by a running lineman. The lineman's hip will hit the runner's knee from the side during a flying tackle, and because the runner's leg is firmly planted in the turf, severe disruption of the knee occurs. This is considered a serious injury because it can cause tearing of the MCL, the ACL, and the meniscus. Currently, it is believed that these injuries often involve the lateral meniscus. People with these types of injuries are encouraged to undergo magnetic resonance imaging and arthroscopic examination of the knee to determine the extent of injury, with particular attention paid to these triad structures.

- **HOUSEMAID'S KNEE:** This is another name for *bursitis* at the front of the knee. It is also known as "water on the knee." Several bursae are located around the knee that allow for efficient movement without too much friction building up. The bursa located at the front of the knee is known as the *pre-patellar bursa* because of its location. Sometimes, the fluid inside the bursae may become infected and inflamed, which will appear as a round swelling on the front of the knee. In the past, this problem was the occupational hazard of housemaids who got down on their knees to scrub the floor and wore away the skin over their knees, thus introducing germs into the bursa just underneath the skin more easily. Plumbers, carpenters, and carpet layers are also at risk for this problem, which can be prevented by wearing kneepads.

- **COMMON PERONEAL NERVE INJURY:** The *peroneal nerve* branches off the sciatic nerve trunk and passes just underneath the skin at the outer aspect of the knee joint. It may become stretched when a collision occurs along the inner knee, or it may become compressed and bruised if a blow is delivered to the outer knee. A sudden violent kick of the foot straight out with the toes pointed inward can stretch the nerve to the point of injury. This nerve allows you to point your toes upward (dorsiflexion) and bend your ankle sideways (eversion). It also provides sensation to the outer and upper portion of the foot. These motions will become difficult to perform if this nerve is injured, and you might lose sensation in your feet.

- **PATELLAR INSTABILITY:** (See Chapter 14.) Instability of the kneecap may occur from a blow to the inner knee that deflects off the kneecap. The force of this blow may cause the kneecap to dislocate or move out of its groove. Although the kneecap usually goes back into place on its own, it may be tender to touch and the soft tissue surrounding the kneecap on the inner (medial side) may be tender and painful.

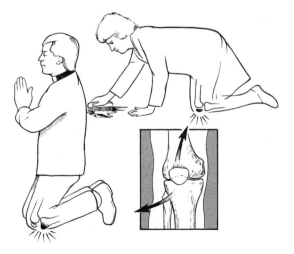

Housemaid's knee affects the prepatellar bursa located in front of the kneecap; the kneeling position that causes clergyman's knee irritates the bursa located behind the kneecap. Dandy DJ: *Essential Orthopaedics and Trauma*. Edinburgh: Churchill Livingstone, 1989.

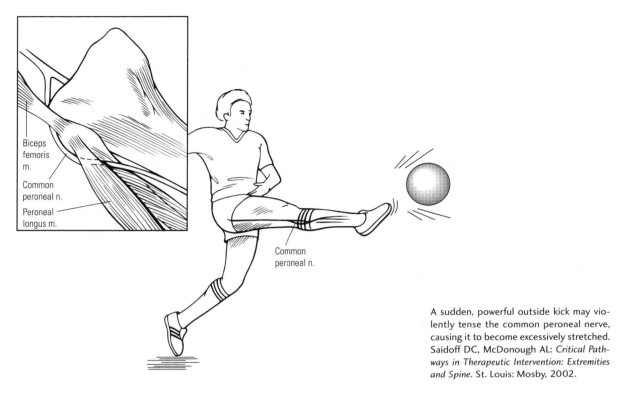

Biceps
femoris
m.

Common
peroneal n.

Peroneal
longus m.

Common
peroneal n.

A sudden, powerful outside kick may violently tense the common peroneal nerve, causing it to become excessively stretched. Saidoff DC, McDonough AL: *Critical Pathways in Therapeutic Intervention: Extremities and Spine.* St. Louis: Mosby, 2002.

■ IMMEDIATE CARE

Swelling at the knee from a grade II or III sprain may reach a maximum at 12 hours following injury because the ligament bleeds from its torn ends. Not a whole lot of damage can occur, however, because the collateral ligaments lie outside the knee joint proper. On the other hand, bleeding can erode the inside of the joint very quickly because they lie inside the joint. Blood contains enzymes that can literally digest the delicate articular cartilage, requiring weeks to heal. In addition, blood within the joint will clot, thereby acting like glue that causes the structures within the joint to stick to each other; this limits joint motion. In addition to resting, elevating, compressing, and cooling the sprained knee, it is essential that a doctor remove the blood from within the knee by aspirating it with a needle. This procedure will save the cartilage. It will also detect whether or not the underlying bone is broken, based on whether the withdrawn blood contains any fat, because bones contain fat.

■ PREVENTION AND TREATMENT

Ignoring a knee sprain may soon lead to debilitating instability and arthritis of the knee joint. Because the knee contains so many structures, most of which are necessary for normal activities, injury to one major structure often means that other structures, such as the meniscus or knee cap, will be substantially affected. Over time, this might result in recurrence of an old problem or new problems at the knee. Early protection, followed by rehabilitation and activity modification, is extremely important when it comes to recovery from injuries to the knee.

Most grade I and II collateral ligament sprains heal well following about 4 to 6 weeks of physical therapy. Grade III sprains require more bracing and therapy before you can get back to full, unrestricted activity. The mainstay of treatment for collateral ligament injuries is early motion and controlled stress of the torn ligament, which will help the ligament heal stronger and faster. The knee should be protected by wearing a sleeve-type brace for protection and stabilization. Range of motion exercises and muscle strengthening exercises may be performed in a variety of settings, such as in a whirlpool bath. Exercises may be done with the foot attached (closed chain) and unattached (open chain) to the ground, or with muscles operating at the same speed throughout the range of motion (isokinetic), such as when exercising in a pool. Stretching of the tight muscles around the knee and calf and balance training to retrain the balance receptors and improve agility are also very important. Treatment is best performed under the supervision of a physical therapist.

Cruciate ligament injuries are more serious and require more attention. While all of the treatments described above are appropriate for cruciate ligament injuries, strengthening several muscles is essential as they can actually compensate for torn cruciate ligaments. Studies have shown that working the quadriceps muscles (the front of the thigh) helps compensate for a weakened PCL, while exercising the hamstring muscles (the back of the thigh) protects the ACL from stress.

■ When Is Surgery Necessary?

Surgical repair of medial collateral ligament injuries are recommended when other structures in the knee have also been injured. Otherwise, collateral ligament injuries are best managed with aggressive physical therapy. Lateral collateral ligament injuries take longer to heal than medial injuries and usually require surgery if they are fully torn.

Many factors determine whether the right treatment for cruciate sprain is surgery, including: age, associated knee injury, past history of knee injury, work demands, athletic activity level, injury of related structures, and motivation to participate in physical therapy, both before and after surgery.

People who are less than 25 years old at the time they sustain a cruciate ligament injury generally have a poor prognosis if treated non-operatively, compared with a good prognosis for those older than age 35. People younger than 25 years of age are best managed by a more aggressive, surgical approach, because this group tends to be more active and more likely to sustain re-injury.

On the other end of the spectrum, older people with isolated ACL injury who are willing to modify their activities and avoid running, jumping, and cutting movements might do well without surgery. However, if the injured person finds modification of activity too restrictive or troublesome, he might be better suited for surgery. Each case of knee sprain must be considered individually, based on lifestyle and need. The decision to operate or to conservatively manage an ACL sprain is best reached by agreement between the doctor and the injured person.

Surgery involves reattaching the frayed ends of the ligament or reconstructing the torn ligament by grafting a portion of healthy ligament from somewhere else in the body. Successful recovery after surgery requires that a rehabilitation exercise program recommended by the doctor or physical therapist be followed for several months.

13 Arthritis of the Kneecap

A 31-year-old recently divorced woman has been spending her Saturday mornings serving as the catcher in her eight-year-old son's little league baseball team. Squatting for long periods in the catcher's position has begun to cause a dull ache in the front of her knees that seems to be getting progressively. Climbing and descending stairs has become difficult. She is also having trouble getting up from a low couch after sitting for long periods. Her effort is accompanied by a grating sound and grinding feeling in both of her kneecaps. Walking down hills is also not easy. Sometimes her knees feel as if they are going to give way, although she cannot understand why, because she can freely and painlessly kick her legs and feet in the air and it does not bother her at all. Since childhood she has had mild knock-knees and the arches of both of her feet are flat. The source of this woman's problem is arthritis of the kneecap, also known as chondromalacia.

■ CHONDRO — WHAT?

CHONDROMALACIA is a condition that affects the *patella* (kneecap). The patella ("shallow dish" in Latin) is a small triangular shaped bone located within a tendon of the quadriceps muscle. It glides back and forth over the front of the knee whenever the knee is bent or straightened. The outer portion of the patella is easily felt by touching the kneecap and tracing its upside-down triangular outline. The inner portion of the patella is covered with cartilage, which glides against the cartilage at the end of the thighbone during knee motion. This cartilage against cartilage gliding enables motion to occur freely and with little friction. Problems start occurring when the cartilage on the undersurface of the patella undergoes too much uneven pressure, causing one portion of its undersurface to break down. This wearing away of cartilage and the symptoms it causes is known as

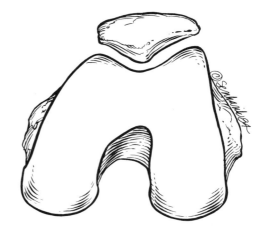

The kneecap or patella sits atop the groove at the far end of the thighbone (femur) as the *patellofemoral joint*. Nicholas JA, Hershman EB: *The Lower Extremity and Spine in Sports Medicine*, 2nd Edition. St. Louis: Mosby, 1995.

chondromalacia. *Chondro* means "cartilage" in Greek and *malacia* means "abnormal softening."

Chondromalacia is also known as *Runner's Knee* because it often occurs in runners.

WHY ARE KNEECAPS NECESSARY?

Aside from protectively capping the front of the knee with a bit of bony armor, the patella plays an important role in the biomechanics of the knee joint. The large muscle group of the front of the thigh is called the *quadriceps muscle*. This massive muscle is made up of four different sections ending in the *quadriceps tendon*, which envelops the patella and travels beyond it to attach to the tibia bone. The knee straightens when the quadriceps muscle contracts.

People who have had their patella surgically removed must work much harder to bend or straighten their knee because they have lost the mechanical advantage of the patella. They also have a rather flat-looking knee rather than the pleasantly rounded front portion attributed to the kneecap. The patella acts as a *pulley* for the quadriceps tendon and amplifies the leverage of the quadriceps muscle by as much as 30% so that knee extension happens more efficiently than it might otherwise without the benefit of a kneecap.

PATELLOFEMORAL FORCE

The cost paid for having a patella and the leverage it confers to the knee is that the huge forces generated by the quadriceps muscle are transmitted through the kneecap and compress its underside against the tips of the thighbone. For example, when you start from the squatting position and try to stand up, it is your quadriceps muscles that withstand the weight of your body in order to move you into the upright position. These enormous forces must pass through the patella and, therefore, the underside of the kneecap endures large forces known as *patellofemoral joint compression forces*.

Regular activities that involve bending and straightening the knee, such as walking or stair climbing, will increase patellofemoral compressive joint forces 0.5 to 3.3 times body weight. When bending the knee beyond 90 degrees, such as when performing a deep knee bend, stress is narrowly focused at only one aspect along the inner side of the kneecap, resulting in patellofemoral compressive joint forces 7 to 8 times normal body weight. Thus, for a person weighing 170 pounds, about 1,190 pounds of compressive force is imposed on the patellofemoral joint during prolonged squatting activities! Those enormous forces must be borne by a little fleck of bone known as a *facet* that is located along the inner border of the kneecap. Just imagine the patellofemoral forces in obese people! It is no wonder that obesity is a risk factor for chondromalacia.

CARTILAGE BREAKDOWN

The patellar surface must be prepared to regularly sustain forces close to 500 pounds per square inch. This magnitude of force helps explain why the *hyaline cartilage* lining the patellar surface is the thickest in the human body and may range anywhere from ⅔ inch thick. These forces are multiplied in the overweight individual. The cumulative effect of years of micro-trauma leads to a wearing down of the cartilage and degeneration of the underside of the patella, especially its inner (medial) border. The early stages of degeneration manifest as cartilage softening known as *chondromalacia*. The problem may get worse and eventually progress to *patellofemoral osteoarthritis* if steps are not taken to relieve the pressure.

It does not always take years or decades to develop damaging changes to the underside of the patella. Very active children, for example, as well as young adults between 10 and 25 years of age may damage the articular surface of their patella due to excessive involvement in sports.

■ CLASSIFICATION

Malacia (softening) of hyaline cartilage may occur anywhere in the body, but due to years of unabated patellofemoral pressure, it develops almost exclusively in the patella, with the exception of Asian people who, for unknown reasons, rarely develop chondromalacia. When these changes on the underside of the patella occur, they may be classified according to how the changes appear.

- **STAGE I:** Softening of the cartilage on the undersurface of the patella and inflammation of the patellofemoral joint.

- **STAGE II:** Loss of water and resilience of the cartilage, causing blistering of its normally smooth surface.

- **STAGE III:** Blisters develop into fissures, giving the cartilage the appearance of crabmeat; hence the term "crabmeat changes."

- **STAGE IV:** The cartilage on the undersurface of the patella is either dead or worn away, leading to *patellofemoral arthritis.*

■ WHO IS MOST LIKELY TO GET ARTHRITIS OF THE KNEE?

In addition to developing slowly from excessive force over many years, chondromalacia may occur soon after acute trauma from a direct blow to the patella—for example, during a motor vehicle accident in which the patella is forcefully and suddenly

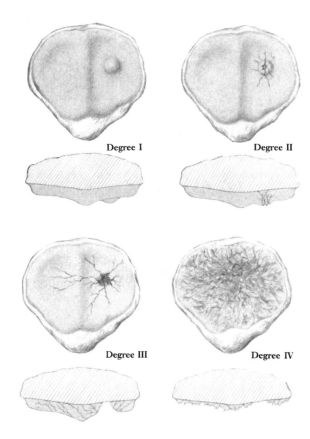

Stages of Chrondromalacia. Peterson L, Renstrom P: *Sports Injuries: Their Prevention and Treatment,* Chicago: Year Book Medical Publishers Inc., 1986.

pressed against an automobile dashboard. People who spend a lot of time in the squatting position are predisposed to chondromalacia because this knee posture places the maximum pressure at the patellofemoral joint. Chondromalacia is considered an occupational hazard for baseball catchers because they spend so much time in the squatting position.

Some people seem to be more susceptible to cartilage breakdown than others—for example, someone who is born with a patella that develops with less than ideal alignment in relation to the tip of the thighbone. This causes abnormal alignment and tracking of the patella during bending and straightening of the knee, focusing pressure along the inner side (known as a facet) of the patella, which wears it thin, resulting in chondromalacia. Chondromalacia may temporarily occur in female adolescents during the pubescent growth spurt because the hips widen during puberty.

Some people have an imbalance in the strength of the four quadriceps muscles. Typically, an important part of the inner quadriceps muscle known as the *vastus medialis oblique* becomes atrophied and weak in what is known as *quadriceps dysplasia,* which is a common condition in adolescents. This causes the stronger portions of the quadriceps muscle to pull outward on the patella, thereby altering its balanced tracking across the femoral head. The result is excessive wear on the inner facet, which eventually leads to chondromalacia.

Excessively *tight hamstring muscles* may also contribute to chondromalacia because the quadriceps muscles must work especially hard to overcome this tightness when straightening the knee. In addition people with *pronated* (flat) feet will be particularly at risk for developing chondromalacia because the foot, shin, and knee are all linked together. The bones and joints of the foot and leg work in a complex synchrony of various motions, including rotation. The excessive pronation of the foot that often accompanies flat-arched feet causes rotation of the shinbone in one direction at a time, when it should optimally be rotating in the opposite direction. This causes *maltracking of the patella,* and its outer facet may wear thin and soften.

WHAT DOES IT FEEL LIKE?

Chondromalacia of the kneecap feels like a dull ache or soreness on the front of or under the kneecap, especially after moving around a lot. The inner side of the kneecap may feel especially tender. Pain and stiffness may be felt when sitting for long periods of time—for example, during a long car ride, in a theatre, or when getting up suddenly from a sitting or squatting position. On the other hand, activities such as walking downhill, climbing or descending stairs, jogging on hills, or pushing the clutch while driving a stick shift may all provoke pain. It may hurt the most when squatting. Symptoms may be reproduced by firmly pressing the kneecap against the underlying thighbone. There may be some swelling and the knee may feel as if it is going to give way, especially when walking down an incline or descending stairs. Many people experience a

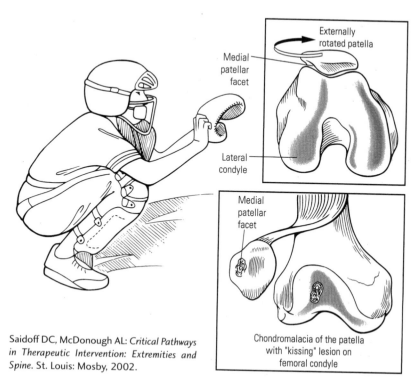

Externally rotated patella

Medial patellar facet

Lateral condyle

Medial patellar facet

Chondromalacia of the patella with "kissing" lesion on femoral condyle

Saidoff DC, McDonough AL: *Critical Pathways in Therapeutic Intervention: Extremities and Spine.* St. Louis: Mosby, 2002.

grating sound when the knee is straightened or bent. Often, the quadriceps muscle above that kneecap is weak, especially the inner portion known as the *vastus medialis oblique*. The inner knee will show a dimple if this muscle is weak.

The diagnosis of chondromalacia is based on the description of symptoms and an x-ray to view the undersurface of the patella.

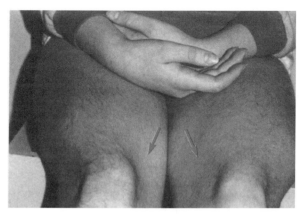

When the vastus medialis oblique is weak or poorly developed, a pronounced dimple (arrows) is seen on the inner side of the knee. Staheli LT: *Fundamental of Pediatric Orthopedics*. New York: Raven Press, 1992.

■ CONDITIONS TO RULE OUT

■ **PATELLAR OVERLOAD SYNDROME:** Skeletal growth increases during late childhood at a steady rate until the onset of puberty, allowing children to grow in height. This happens so quickly in some children that the rate of growth between the long bones in the thigh and shin outstrips the rate of growth of the adjacent soft tissues such as the quadriceps muscles and patellar tendon. This causes tightness of the extensor mechanism, resulting in increased contact pressure between the kneecap and thighbone, resulting in pain and irritation when bending the knee. The affected child classically walks around with "high water pants," indicating that the hemline

of his pants needs to be lowered because of a recent growth spurt. The child may complain of a pain similar to a toothache over the front of their knee, especially near the outer border of the kneecap. This problem can be dealt with by initiating an active program of stretching the hamstrings and calf muscles.

■ **PES ANSERINE BURSITIS:** The term *pes anserine* literally means "goose's foot" in Latin. It refers to several tendons that have the appearance of a webbed foot that wrap around the inner side of the knee. Among their many roles, the *pes anserinus* help the kneecap track normally in its groove. Because of the potential for high friction and increased risk for developing tendonitis where these many tendons attach at the inner side of the knee, a *bursa* is located where the tendons attach. It reduces the friction in that area. However, sometimes the bursa can get inflamed from overwork. This may cause pain just below the inner knee, whereas pain from chondromalacia is typically felt at the front of the knee or along the inner side of the kneecap.

■ **FAT PAD INFLAMMATION:** The fat pad at the knee acts to fill dead space within the knee joint, lubricates the joint, and supports and cushions the many structures in and around the knee. Getting hit in the knee or undergoing knee surgery may traumatize the fat pad and cause it to bleed internally. Over time, this results in an enlarged and roughened fat pad that can no longer act as a shelf to hold up the patella, causing the kneecap to sag downward. Since the fat pad has many nerve endings, it can be painful, especially when straightening the knee because this position squeezes the fat pad.

■ **PLICA SYNDROME:** As previously discussed in Chapter 11, plica are delicate folds of tissue that are embryologic remnants of the fetal knee. The knee joint is divided by three separate compartments during gestation within the womb that merge into one by the time the baby is born. These three compartments sometimes persist as folds of tissue called *plicae* and may undergo rubbing as the knee bends and straightens. The cumulative effect of this rubbing is that the plicae become dry bands of tissue that may actually interfere with motion. Although uncommon, this condition causes pain at the knee after getting up from a prolonged sitting position, whereas chondromalacia usually causes pain during activity.

PREVENTION AND TREATMENT

Almost 95% of all people with chondromalacia experience some relief following physical therapy. A multifaceted approach is important in making sure relief of symptoms occurs. While it is important to reduce pain, it is just as important to get to the root of the problem, which is determining exactly why the knee cap is not aligned well enough to track without causing excessive friction. The focus of treatment is to realign the patella so that it tracks better and keeps patellofemoral forces to a minimum.

- **REST:** Take it easy. Try to avoid or minimize any activities that bring on symptoms.

- **MEDICATION:** Studies have shown that using salicitates such as aspirin helps prevent degeneration of cartilage. The prescription drug phenylbutazone has been found to be helpful in reducing the inflammatory response around the soft tissues of the knee. Steroid use is not recommended.

- **COLD AND HEAT:** During the period immediately follow the onset of pain, cold applied over the affected kneecap may help relieve symptoms. Later on, as symptoms subside, taking a nice hot bath before bed or when getting up after sleep may help.

- **STRENGTHENING:** It is essential to strengthen the entire quadriceps muscle group, particularly the inner portion known as the *vastus medialis oblique* portion, in order to manage chondromalacia. This can be accomplished by lifting the leg up straight in repetition. This is known as a *straight leg raise.* Cuffed weights may be added to the leg. These exercises can be done while lying on one's back, on either side, and on one's stomach. Some physical therapists may help strengthen these muscles by using electrical stimulation or biofeedback techniques.

- **STRETCHING:** It is very important in both prevention and treatment of chondromalacia to perform stretching exercises because tightness of the hamstring and calf muscles can act to compress the kneecap even more tightly against the femoral condyles. Thus, it is essential to stretch these muscles, the Achilles tendon, iliotibial band, and adductor muscles of the thigh.

- **ORTHOSES:** As discussed in previous chapters, an orthotic can be used to realign the arch of the foot, and the rear and forefoot in an ideal position so that it corrects the anatomical relationships between the different parts of the foot. In this manner, the foot and shin work together in the proper alignment. This, in turn, causes the kneecap to become realigned and able to track more normally without wearing out prematurely.

- **BRACING:** Various types of braces are commercially available to externally centralize the kneecap and realign it so that it tracks better between the femoral condyles. Many of these braces consist of elastic sleeves with a cutout in the front for the kneecap and a thickened buildup of material on the outer side known as a *lateral buttress*. In this manner, the elastic sleeve encircles the entire kneecap while avoiding direct pressure.

- **WEIGHT REDUCTION:** Because the patellofemoral forces are multiplied by excessive body weight, slowing down the progression of chondromalacia and perhaps even preventing it can be accomplished by participating in a safe weight reduction program designed for obese and overweight people.

- **TAPING:** This is a method of providing external support to the kneecap to ensure that it is properly aligned and can track better as the knee bends and straightens. This approach was introduced by Ms. Jenny McConnell, an Australian physiotherapist who correctly believed that the misaligned patella has several components that include glide, tilt, and rotation of the kneecap. All of these different problems can be addressed by her taping technique, which should be implemented under the guidance of a physical therapist.

- **ACTIVITY MODIFICATION:** Various activities and positions of the knee increase patellofemoral contact stress and pain. Running, jumping, and high-impact aerobics cause the large powerful quadriceps muscles to compress the kneecap against the underlying bone excessively, and these activities should be avoided. Riding a stationary or mobile bike with the seat in the low position causes the knee to be excessively bent so that too much pressure is focused beneath the kneecap. Instead, adjust the bike seat to the higher position. Activities that involve squatting positions should be avoided.

WHEN IS SURGERY NECESSARY?

Sometimes chondromalacia may not improve with physical therapy, in which case it can be surgically treated. *Arthroscopy* is a minimally invasive technique used to remove bony spurs from the inner surface of the kneecap. While this procedure has short-term benefits, chondromalacia usually comes back. This underscores the importance of identifying the cause of patellofemoral pain and abnormal function and initiating treatment with an eclectic program of physical therapy. Surgery can also be helpful in repositioning the kneecap, bringing it into better alignment..

14 Unstable Kneecap

Your 19-year-old daughter cleared her schedule of early morning classes and went jogging. As she approached a corner, she was bumped by a teenager on a bicycle whose front wheel glanced off her right inner kneecap before he applied the brakes. In addition to the pain from the collision, she felt something "give" in her right knee as if something were momentarily out-of-place. She sat down to examine her bent knee and noticed that it was not quite right. When she tried to straighten her knee, her kneecap moved back into its normal position. Later that day, her knee was tender and painful to touch at the inner side of the kneecap. It was also somewhat swollen. Your daughter has experienced a dislocation *of her right kneecap.*

■ THE PATELLOFEMORAL JOINT

THE *patellofemoral joint* is the joint between the *patella* (kneecap) and the far end of the thigh-bone or *femur* (not to be confused with the knee joint proper between the femur and tibia bones). As discussed in Chapter 13, the *patella* is a small triangular bone about the size of your nose that glides or tracks up and down a groove on the far end of the thighbone. The groove occurs because the far end of the femur terminates at the knee as two bulbous flares known as *femoral condyles*, creating a natural valley for the patella to slide up and down. As the knee joint straightens, the patella rides up, and as the knee bends, the patella slides down this groove.

■ PATELLAR INSTABILITY

We can compare this to riding down a slide into a pond. You will have good contact with the slide and enjoy the ride if your bottom is nice and round; this

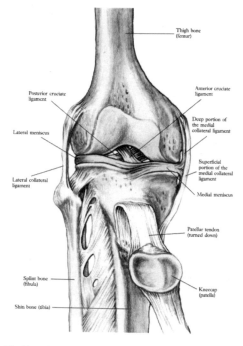

The Knee Joint: The underside of the patella is exposed to show the part that glides up and down cartilage at the end of the thighbone. This point of contact is known as the *patellofemoral joint*. Peterson L, Renstrom P: *Sports Injuries: Their Prevention and Treatment.* New York: Year Book Medical Publishers Inc., 1986.

is what occurs with most patellae. The undersurface of most patellae is convex (bumpy) and makes a good fit with the concavely-shaped femoral groove. This convex-in-concave fit works like a hand in a glove, providing stability that keeps the patella within the femoral groove during normal movement. In some people, however, the undersurface of the patella is poorly shaped or even concave, resulting in poor contact between the patella and the femoral groove. Because of this, the patella is likely to move (displace) sideways out of the groove. Like the waterslide example above, if the sides of the slide lack an upright flange on one side, you are more likely to fall off the slide as you ride down. Similarly, some people have a shallow groove or a groove where the outer side is shallower and the patella may "jump the track" and move outwardly. These variations are called *dysplasia* of the patella or the femoral condyles.

Patellar and *femoral dysplasia* are common causes of patellar instability. When this happens momentarily, it is known as a *patellar subluxation*, and the patella will return to the right place on its own. When this happens so often that the ligaments surrounding the patella tear, it may be considered a *dislocated patella*, which may cause the patella to lie outside its normal position within the groove.

■ QUADRICEPS EXTENSOR MECHANISM

Imagine a spider sitting in the center of a magnificent circular web. The web is very strong and capable when it is complete, whereas damage to one strand of the web will affect the stability of the entire web. This analogy can be applied to the patella and

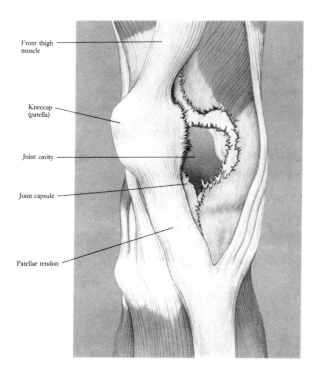

Above: Dislocated patella.
Peterson L, Renstrom P: *Sports Injuries: Their Prevention and Treatment*. Chicago: Year Book Medical Publishers Inc., 1986.

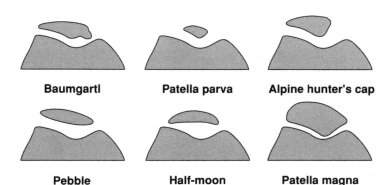

Baumgartl   **Patella parva**   **Alpine hunter's cap**

Pebble   **Half-moon**   **Patella magna**

Left: Differently shaped patella result in greater or lesser stability. Tria AJ, Klein KS: *An Illustrated Guide to The Knee*. New York: Churchill Livingstone, 1992.

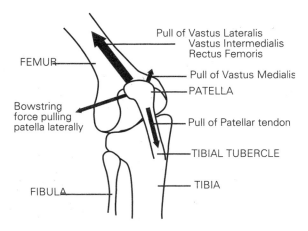

FEMUR

Pull of Vastus Lateralis
Vastus Intermedialis
Rectus Femoris

Pull of Vastus Medialis

PATELLA

Bowstring
force pulling
patella laterally

Pull of Patellar tendon

TIBIAL TUBERCLE

FIBULA

TIBIA

The *extensor mechanism* at the knee provides a balance of the forces around the knee. Weakness in any one component readily disturbs this precarious balance and may cause abnormal tracking of the patella. Staheli LT: *Fundamentals of Pediatric Orthopedics*. New York: Raven Press, 1992.

its function. The patella is held in place at the front of the knee by a variety of supports: the *quadriceps tendon* and *ligament,* and the bony shape of the patella and the bony valley in which it rests. One can imagine the patella centrally anchored by several cables all pulling on it at the same time so as to precisely balance it where it functions best, to track up and down the knee as the knee bends and straightens. This vital support system is known as the *quadriceps extensor mechanism* at the knee joint. If any one of these supports is pulled too hard (because they are overtight) or did not pull enough (because of weakness or laxity), then normal patellar tracking would be profoundly affected.

FACTORS AFFECTING THE QUADRICEPS MECHANISM

Many factors influence the quadriceps extensor mechanism at the knee joint. Some of these include the shape of the patella, the shape of the bony valley in which it rests, the strength of the ligaments

supporting the patella, and also the biomechanical status of the foot and hip joints; this means that a person who has an excessively flat or arched foot, similar to someone who has a hip joint that is excessively rotated one way or the other (known as *version*), is at greater risk for developing problems at the knee joint. This is because the knee, which is situated in the middle of the leg between the ankle below and the hip joint above, is in a precarious position. For the knee to work optimally, the joints above and below must be precisely oriented so as to create balance. Otherwise, excessive rotation of the long bones on either side of the knee, such as the thigh and shin bones, may cause the patella to slide outwardly, causing instability of the kneecap. Problems at the knee joint itself can also predispose a person to kneecap instability.

VMO SAVES THE DAY

Patellar instability typically occurs outwardly because of the shape of the bones at the knee and because the ligaments buffering the outer knee are usually weaker in the normal knee. Because of the angle of upward pull, the quadriceps muscles pulling outwardly are stronger. Because of this built-in anatomic over-pull, the human knee is considered anatomically predisposed toward outward instability of the kneecap. You can think of the patella as the object that two teams are pulling on in a tug of war, with the outer forces winning somewhat. One muscle in particular, known as the *vastus medialis oblique* (VMO), really pulls hard inwardly to counter those outward forces on the kneecap. The VMO can do this because of its unique location at the inner side of the thigh, just above the knee, and also because of the orientation of its muscle fibers. Unfortunately, weakness of this little slip of muscle is common.

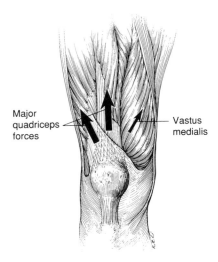

Although the outward pulling muscles are the major quadriceps muscles, the *vastus medialis* and its oblique portion pull inwardly to counteract the outward pull. Unfortunately, the anatomy of the human knee seems to have a design flaw in that the quadriceps mechanism favors outward pull. Tria AJ, Klein KS: *An Illustrated Guide to the Knee.* New York: Churchill Livingstone, 1992.

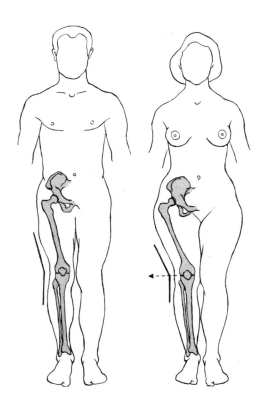

Redrawn from O'Donoughue DH: *Treatment of injuries to athletes*, ed 4, Philadelphia, 1984, WB Saunders. The comparatively wider pelvis in females predisposes women to swaying of the kneecap outwardly. Magee DG (ed.): *Orthopedic Physical Assessment*, Philadelphia: WB Saunders, 1997.

WHO IS MOST LIKELY TO HAVE KNEE PROBLEMS?

Instability of the patella more commonly occurs in adolescent girls and young women because the pelvis grows wider with maturation. The wider female pelvis makes the kneecap less stable where it rests between the two femoral condyles because it exerts more outward pressure that can more easily dislocate it out of its groove. In addition to the risk factors mentioned above, such as thighbone version, torsion of the shinbone, knock knees, and pronated feet, obesity is also a risk factor. Some people have knees that predispose them to instability of the patella, particularly with regard to the shape of the patella and the femoral groove.

Certain athletic maneuvers can traumatize the extensor mechanism so that the kneecap may dislocate outwardly—for example, when you suddenly twist sideways or quickly slow down (decelerate). A sharp sideways twist can also result in dislocation. A contact mechanism of injury would include a blow to the inner side of the kneecap or falling onto the inner side of the kneecap with the knee somewhat bent. Anyone who has had knee surgery is more likely to have an imbalanced extensor mechanism, which increases the chances of kneecap dislocation.

SIGNS AND SYMPTOMS

There may be complaints of sudden pain at the knee, as if it had suddenly gone out-of-place or momentarily slid over. A clicking sound or giving

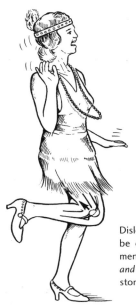

Dislocation of the patella: The patella can be dislocated by sharp twisting movements. Dandy DJ: Essential *Orthopaedics and Trauma*. Edinburgh: Churchill Livingstone, 1989.

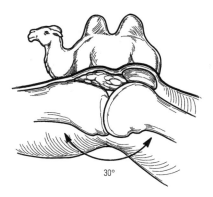

Camelback sign. Scott WN: The Knee. St. Louis: Mosby, 1994.

way sensation may accompany this feeling. The knee may appear quite normal, although feeling it with your fingertips elicits tenderness, especially on the inner border. The knee will most likely look normal because it usually and immediately returns to its normal position within the femoral groove. (In some cases, the kneecap may stay in an abnormal position, in which case the knee cannot straighten out of the bent position until a doctor puts it back into place.) Later in the day, the kneecap area may begin to swell a bit. A kneecap that has undergone this experience of instability will begin to take on a characteristic look when it is straightened. This is because the fat pad on which the knee rests becomes enlarged from being bruised every time the kneecap dislocates. This gives the knee the appearance of a double-hump camel known as the "camelback sign."

Many people have weak, flabby quadriceps muscles, particularly the inner portion of the VMO. This is known as *dysplastic VMO,* which can appear as a *dimple* about 2 inches above the kneecap on the inner side of the knee. Finally, many people with

patella that have subluxated or dislocated will have kneecaps that point inwards and face each other (known as *squinting patellae*), or they may point outwards away from one another (known as *owl eye patella*). When going up or down the stairs, people with this condition might complain that their knee occasionally gives way.

The classic way in which the doctor or physical therapist determines whether the kneecap is unstable is to try to reproduce instability using a procedure known as the *apprehension test* wherein the kneecap is forced outward while the knee is held straight out, and the person is watched to see if they become apprehensive (as noted by facial anxiety). If the kneecap moves outward very easily compared to the opposite, uninjured knee, there is damage to the restraints that normally prevent the patella from drifting outward. This result confirms subluxation or dislocation.

■ CONDITIONS TO RULE OUT

Several other possible problems should be ruled out, including:

- **PLICA SYNDROME:** Although uncommon, this condition causes pain at the knee similar to patellar instability after getting up from a prolonged sitting position, but it does not elicit tenderness around the patella. Also a dislocated patella, unlike plica syndrome, can happen from a blow to the knee. (See Chapters 12 and 13 for further discussion of plica syndrome.)

- **KNEE SPRAIN:** Sprains of the *medial collateral ligament* may be confused with dislocation of the patella because the inner knee structures are tender and injured in both conditions. However, whereas a blow to the inner knee might dislocate the patella, it would most likely sprain the restraining ligament on the outer side of the knee. Additionally, with a knee sprain, moving the kneecap around does not cause any tenderness as it might with a kneecap problem. (See Chapter 12.)

- **MENISCUS INJURY:** Injury of the meniscus is characterized by locking of the knee joint when the knee is either in the bent or straightened position. Meniscus injuries most often occur in people in their 30s and 40s, whereas kneecap dislocation occurs in younger people. Also, meniscus injuries will not score positive on an apprehension test.

■ PREVENTION AND TREATMENT

The conservative approach to management of patellar instability is recommended for those who fit certain criteria that categorize them as having an uncomplicated dislocated patella. These criteria include an absence of a underlying anatomic predisposition to dislocation, absence of any breakage of bone (known as *osteochondral fracture* or a *displaced fragment)*, an intact (untorn) VMO, and special x-rays (known as "Merchant-view" radiographs) that reveal central (normal) tracking of the patella within the femoral groove. People who do not meet these criteria are considered candidates for surgical intervention. Otherwise, the uncomplicated dislocated patella is managed by gently easing it back into its normal position within the femoral groove if it is still dislocated (which it will not be in most cases). Relocating the displaced patella is accomplished by manual pressure in full knee extension. The knee is then immobilized for several weeks, followed by physical therapy. The dislocation recurrence rate is approximately 30% in individuals younger than 20 years of age. This rate decreases to 5% in those over 40 years old.

The knee responds to patella dislocation by growing rough edges that look like bony spurs protruding out of the patella. These edges aid in stability and make repeated subluxation or dislocation unlikely with increasing age. This is one of those rare circumstances when advanced age is on your side. Because of this, age is also a determining factor in deciding whether or not to operate.

Subluxation of the kneecap will only worsen if ignored. It is therefore very important to start physical therapy right away. Rehabilitation of patellar instability has a success rate of about 80%.

The cornerstone of treatment of patellar instability remains *centralization* of the kneecap within the femoral condyles. This is accomplished by a variety of treatment options, the most important of which is strengthening the weakened inner muscles and stretching the taut outer muscles.

- **REST:** Take it easy. If you have identified what activity brings on symptoms, try to avoid or at least minimize that activity. Activities such as duck-walking, running up and down stadium stairs, squatting, and sideways cutting during running should be avoided because these activities can precipitate the symptoms that caused instability in the first place.

- **COLD AND HEAT:** Initially, when symptoms are painful after the provoking activity, cold compresses applied to both kneecaps may help relieve symptoms. Later on, as symptoms subside, taking a hot bath before bed or when getting up after sleep may bring relief.

- **STRENGTHENING:** It is essential to strengthen the entire quadriceps muscle group, particularly the inner portion known as the *vastus medialis* oblique, in order to manage patellar instability. This can be accomplished by repeatedly lifting up and straightening the leg. This is known as a *straight leg raise*, and cuffed ankle weights may be added to the leg to increase the effort. These exercises can be done while lying on the back, either side, or on the stomach. Some physical therapists may help these muscles strengthen by using electrical stimulation or biofeedback techniques. *Quadriceps setting* exercises are another approach to strengthening these powerful muscles. An exercise that is particularly helpful in strengthening the VMO is the *terminal knee extension* in which the bent knee is slowly raised until it is perfectly straight and held in that position before letting it down slowly. This should be repeated for up to five sets of 8–12 repetitions, as tolerated, or in accordance with physical therapy instructions. A cuff may be attached to the ankle to increase the effort.

- **STRETCHING:** It is very important for both the prevention and treatment of patellar instability to perform stretching exercises because tightness of the hamstring and calf muscles can act also tighten the soft tissue structures of the outer knee. To avoid an imbalance of pull at the quadriceps extensor mechanism, it is essential to stretch these muscles as well as the Achilles tendon, iliotibial band, and adductor muscles of the thigh.

- **ORTHOSES:** As discussed in previous chapters, wearing an orthotic device known as a "shoe cookie" can realign the arch of the foot and the rear- and forefoot into an ideal position so that it corrects the anatomic relationships between the different parts of the foot. In this manner, the foot and shin work in proper alignment. This, in turn, causes the kneecap to become realigned and thereby track more normally. Normal patellofemoral tracking means that the knee will be less likely to subluxate or dislocate.

- **BRACING:** Many types of braces are commercially available at local drugstores to externally centralize the kneecap and realign it so that it tracks better between the femoral condyles. Many of these braces consist of elastic sleeves with a cutout in the front for the kneecap and a thickened buildup of material on the outer side known as a *lateral buttress*. The elastic sleeve encircles the entire kneecap and keeps it in its tracks where it belongs.

- **WEIGHT REDUCTION:** Patellofemoral forces are multiplied by excessive body weight, and this increases the outward forces on the kneecap. Preventing or limiting instability may be accomplished by participating in a safe weight reduction program.

- **ACTIVITY MODIFICATION:** A common high school coaching technique frequently employed to build leg strength is running up stadium stairs. In a similar fashion, "frog-walking" involves squatting down to the ground with the hips and knees fully bent and walking 40 to 50 yards. Both of these activities can increase the tendency for patellar instability and should definitely be avoided.

WHEN IS SURGERY NECESSARY?

If a dislocation has occurred, the doctor or therapist should feel the inner side of the kneecap to determine whether or not the VMO has torn. People who have sustained a tear should be promptly referred to an orthopedic surgeon for surgical repair. Surgery is also appropriate when a fragment of the kneecap breaks off during dislocation and remains free to do more damage. In this case, the surgeon will excise the loose fragment. Surgery is also offered to those who experience recurrent subluxation or dislocation when 4 to 6 months of physical therapy has not helped much. The operation involves trying to correct any problems in the knee that predispose it to patellar instability, with an emphasis on releasing the tight over-pull of the ligament on the outer side (known as *lateral release*), and tightening of the flabby inner side using the tendon attachments so that the kneecap is better centralized for optimal tracking. Often, the line of pull of the patellar tendon is also redirected so that the patellar tracks in a more stable manner. After surgery, physical therapy is very important for the prevention of scarring, tightening of the released outer structures, and strengthening of the VMO.

15 Jumper's Knee

A 29-year-old new mother decided to get back into shape about a month after the delivery of her first child by taking up basketball with the all-female team sponsored by her church. She had not played basketball with a team since her college days, and she looked forward to the opportunity to slim down and become fit. After 2 weeks of playing 2 to 3 times per week, she began to feel pain at the front of her right knee, especially when landing after a jump shot. The higher or more forcefully she jumped, the more uncomfortable the pain was. The games were played during the late afternoon, and later in the evening she began to experience pain when walking upstairs, stooping, and kneeling. She has no swelling of her knee, although the area just below the kneecap is painful to touch. There is no locking or catching sensation, nor is there any buckling of the knee joint. She does not remember ever injuring her knee. This woman has developed jumper's knee, which is characterized by pain in the tendon just below the kneecap.

■ JUMPER'S KNEE DEFINED

JUMPER'S KNEE is an *overuse injury* in which the *quadriceps tendon* or *patellar ligament* becomes inflamed. It is the most frequent knee problem sustained by volleyball players because of the high frequency of jumping in volleyball. The quadriceps tendon undergoes severe forces throughout its length when landing from a jump, which if unabated, may tense the tendon beyond its capacity to withstand injury. Jumper's knee is not a self-limiting, benign type of injury, but rather a problem that can result in irreversible changes to the patellar tendon or ligament and eventually lead to tearing of these important structures if it is not treated when it first occurs. Therefore, prevention, early detection, and treatment are very important in the management of jumper's knee.

■ OPEN "SESAME"

To understand the function of the narrow, strong, and broad band of tissue known as the *quadriceps tendon* and the *patellar tendon*, we have to understand the function of the *sesamoid bone*, which is located

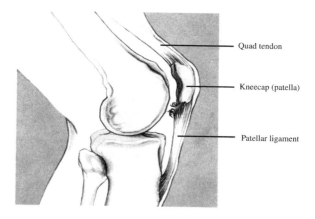

Jumper's Knee. Peterson L, Renstrom PP *Sports Injuries: Their Prevention and Treatment*. Chicago: Year Book Medical Publishers Inc., 1986.

between them. The sesamoid bone is named for its similarity to the sesame seed. It is unique in the sense that it floats in the few places where it occurs throughout the human body. Unlike other bones, which attach to the skeleton by ligaments, a sesamoid bone does not attach. The *patella* (knee-cap) is the largest sesamoid bone in the body, and its primary function is to allow the leg to straighten more easily, especially when the foot is in contact with the ground.

FOUR BELLIES

Getting up from the squatting position is accomplished by the massive muscle in the front of the thigh known as the *quadriceps*. "Quad" means "four," and the quadriceps has four separate muscle bellies. This four-in-one muscle tapers down at the knee into a common tendon that crosses the knee to attach on the shin bone. When the quadriceps contracts, it pulls the shin bone toward it, thereby straightening the knee joint.

Located in the middle of the quadriceps tendon is the kneecap, which basically ensures that the tendon has a ½ inch or so of leverage away from the knee joint. This leverage gain makes the work of the quadriceps much easier when opposing gravity, allowing a person to stand upright from the squatting position. This leverage gain also endows the quadriceps with about a 30% greater mechanical advantage. The kneecap is a very important bone that not only protects the front of the knee by "capping it," but it also helps us move around much better.

STRESSING THE TENDON

Locomotion refers to how we move around, which is mostly accomplished by walking. The patella rides up and down over our knee joint as we walk, and

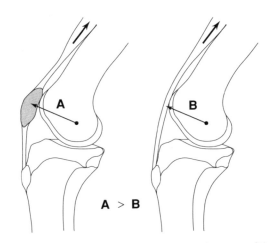

The kneecap in Figure A is farther away from the center of the knee, giving the quadriceps muscle more mechanical advantage to work the knee than that shown in Figure B. Tria AJ, Klein KS: *An Illustrated Guide to The Knee*. New York: Churchill Livingstone, 1992.

the tendon in which it is embedded must alternately elongate and relax. That part of the tendon above the patella is known as the *quadriceps tendon* or *suprapatellar tendon*, and the part below the patella, which attaches to the tibia, is known as the *patellar ligament* or *infrapatellar ligament* (even though it's not *really* a ligament).

Imagine jumping up and down repetitively over a short period of time. This typically occurs in games like volleyball and basketball, or during artistic endeavors such as leaping and landing during ballet dancing. The quadriceps tendon and patellar ligament undergo tremendous stress as they elongate (relax) and transmit tension generated by the quadriceps distraction. The muscle will start to fatigue after a while and may become inflamed or frayed if not rested. This inflammation is called *patellar tendonitis*.

TORSION AND VERSION

Normally, between the top of the quadriceps tendon and where it attaches below the knee is in fairly straight alignment. In this matter, the flat ribbon of tendon crossing the knee joint is well aligned to do its job. Some things, however, can change this alignment so that the tendon may become more easily irritated. Anything that causes the tendon to deviate from a relatively straight path across the knee joint, such as knock-knees or bowlegs, will increase the likelihood of sustaining jumper's knee.

Imagine holding a length of flat ribbon taut with two hands. Now, rotate one of your hands in one direction. What happens? The ribbon in the turning hand begins to twist on itself. This is what happens to the patellar tendon and ligament when the bone above (thighbone) or below (shinbone) rotates excessively. Normally, synchronistic rotations of these long bones occur as a normal part of move-ment. However, certain problems located in the hip or ankle joint can have far-reaching consequences on the patellar tendon and ligament. This occurs because the bones and joints of the leg work together. They are linked to each other like links in a chain.

Those with too much or too little *pronation* of the foot and ankle will have too much rotation of the shinbone (tibia), which will impart stress to that portion of the quadriceps tendon below the patella known as the *patellar ligament*. On the other hand, some people have excessive rotation of the thigh-bone (femur), which will excessively stress that portion of the quadriceps tendon above the patella known as the patellar tendon.

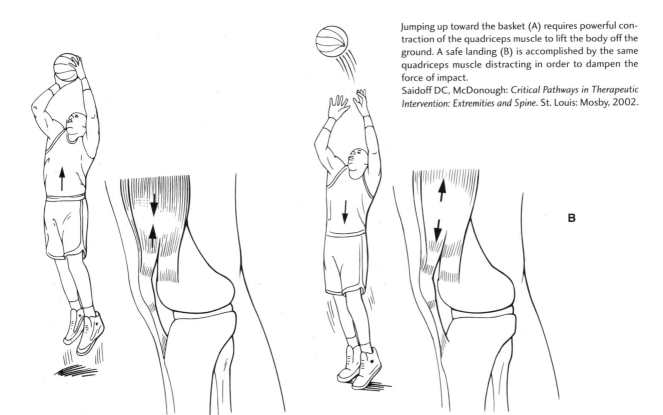

Jumping up toward the basket (A) requires powerful contraction of the quadriceps muscle to lift the body off the ground. A safe landing (B) is accomplished by the same quadriceps muscle distracting in order to dampen the force of impact.
Saidoff DC, McDonough: *Critical Pathways in Therapeutic Intervention: Extremities and Spine.* St. Louis: Mosby, 2002.

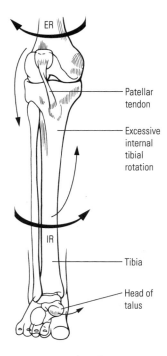

Overpronation of the foot causes the shinbone to rotate excessively during walking, which in turn causes torsion of the patellar ligament at the knee. In this manner, the patellar ligament undergoes stress, making it less capable of absorbing the enormous force passing through it and into the lower portion of the patellar tendon, making it more vulnerable to jumper's knee.
Saidoff DC, McDonough AL: *Critical Pathways in Therapeutic Intervention: Extremities and Spine*. St. Louis: Mosby, 2002.

WHO'S AT RISK FOR DEVELOPING JUMPER'S KNEE?

Runners, fast walkers, or joggers can also experience patellar tendonitis, but it is most likely to occur in jumpers. Having large, strong, quadriceps muscles is not necessarily protection against developing jumper's knee. One study has shown that athletes who generate the highest rate of force output, which enables them to jump higher and faster, also experienced the highest impact forces upon landing, making them more susceptible to jumper's knee. The higher and faster you jump, the more likely you are to develop patellar tendonitis. Players who bend their knees more than 90 degrees at take off will position their quadriceps for a stronger jump, as will those athletes who turn their lower legs and feet outward when they jump. Jumping on hard surfaces such as concrete or linoleum surfaces that do not absorb the impact of landing body weight, and springier surfaces such as wood or sand, will also increase the likelihood of injury.

STAGES

- **STAGE I:** A dull ache is felt after exercise or sports, although it doe not interfere with day-to-day activities. Medical attention is not usually sought at this early stage. This minor pain will usually resolve with rest in a few days to a week. On the other hand, if activity continues without rest, stage II will result.

- **STAGE II:** Pain is felt at the beginning of activity but disappears after warm-up. Athletic performance is still good, although pain reappears once the activity is over. Stage II pain is sharper and has a stabbing quality. Athletes as well as non-athletes will often seek medical attention at this stage because of persistent symptoms.

- **STAGE III:** Pain is experienced both during and after activity, and it actually gets in the way of both athletic involvement and day-to-day activities. Microscopic changes in the tendon occur at this stage, and the tendon may be irreversibly damaged to some degree. Stage III pain has gone untreated and has become constant. Climbing stairs, jumping, landing, sitting for prolonged periods of time with the knee bent, or in more involved cases, simply walking may exacerbate symptoms.

- **STAGE IV:** If the athlete continues to push herself despite symptoms, complete tendon rupture may occur if the knee is left untreated. Tearing of the tendon may be experienced as a sudden painful traumatic event associated with an immediate inability to extend the knee or perform day-to-day activities. This stage represents the catastrophic end stage of jumper's knee. It can be viewed with a lateral (taken from the side) x-ray, which will reveal that the kneecap is placed too high in relation to the femur bone. This condition is called a *patella alta* (from the Latin *altus*, which means "high").

SIGNS AND SYMPTOMS

Pain can occur anywhere along the patellar tendon or ligament, just around the patella, or where the patellar ligament attaches to the tibia. These areas are tender to the touch and are most easily provoked when the knee is straightened. The onset of symptoms may be insidious, and there may be no recollection of a specific traumatic event. A dull ache in the region just below the kneecap that is felt at the beginning of exercise or playing sports, such as jumping, running, climbing, kicking, deceleration cutting maneuvers, or kneeling, is a typical complaint. This ache usually lessens after warming up. Pain may then reappear after the activity or sport is stopped. Many people with patellar tendonitis have tightness of the hamstring and the Achilles tendon. Some may have overpronation of the feet. X-rays of the knee are usually normal. The physician or physical therapist will diagnose this problem based on the clinical examination. The person with persistent symptoms, particularly with tenderness along the inferior patellar pole, should be evaluated with a bone scan to rule out potential stress fracture and, therefore, be able to avoid potentially worse problems in the future.

WHEN CHILDREN EXPERIENCE JUMPER'S KNEE

Sinding-Larson-Johanssen disease is the adolescent version of jumper's knee. It was independently described in the early 1900s by Sinding, Larson, and Johansson as pain at the inferior or superior patellar poles, accompanied by x-ray findings of bone fragmentation of the pole. The upper border of the patella is known as its *superior pole,* and its lower border is known as the *inferior pole.* As discussed above, the patella is enveloped by a structure composed of tendons known as the *quadriceps tendon* above the tendon, and the *quadriceps ligament* below the tendon. The traction forces transmitted through the patellar tendon or ligament may be so strong during early puberty that the bony kneecap at the soft tissue attachments at either pole may be injured. Pain and swelling at either of the patellar poles and a relatively weak quadriceps mechanism are universally present. Tenderness is localized at the inferior patellar pole. Often, the quadriceps muscles show weakness. This condition is most common in normal males at puberty. It can be confirmed by an x-ray showing bone fragmentation at the inferior pole of the patella. Rest, stretching the hamstring muscles, and eccentric strengthening of the quadriceps muscles are recommended. Healing occurs over about 4 weeks. These children are not any more likely to develop jumper's knee as adults.

PREVENTION AND TREATMENT

Because jumper's knee is a progressive disease, early recognition is very important for successful treatment. The strategy of management is to interrupt and reverse tendon degeneration before irreversible damage has occurred. During the early stages of the disease, physical therapy plays a very important role in getting things back to normal, although this may take months of rehabilitation. A reliable indicator of whether healing has occurred is whether or not the tendon is still inflamed. This sign should be periodically re-evaluated and, if tenderness and swelling persist, further rest and activity reduction are recommended. The outcome of stage III jumper's knee is unpredictable, even with physical therapy. This potentially irreversible stage is managed similarly to the more benign forms of tendonitis and should include a prolonged rest period and avoidance of any activities that aggravate symptoms. Some of the treatment options for rehabilitation include:

- **REST:** Take it easy! Stop overworking your patellar tendon and ligament. If a particular activity provides relief from tension or stress, try switching to another activity. At the very least, reduce your involvement in the activity that provoked the injury to a bare minimum. Otherwise, you can do harm to the tendon in the long run and prevent physical therapy from making a difference in the healing process. Although this approach may not be practical for the highly competitive athletes who attend college on athletic scholarships or play professional sports, judicious selective rest should be balanced with other treatment modalities.

- **COLD AND HEAT:** Initially, when the symptoms are heat, pain, and tenderness, applying ice may help during the acute stage. After the first 72 hours, when the knee begins to feel better, applying a warm or hot compress may provide relief.

- **ULTRASOUND:** Ultrasound is a method of applying deep heat using electricity that passes through special crystals, which vibrate at high frequencies. This vibration penetrates deep into tissues as heat energy and may provide relief. Ultrasound applied in the pulsed mode may

deliver pain-relieving medications to the inflamed patellar tendon or ligament. This method of medication delivery is known as *phonophoresis*. Delivery of hydrocortisone using phonophoresis is performed by a physical therapist and may decrease the pain and inflammation of jumper's knee considerably.

- **MEDICATION:** Oral non-steroidal anti-inflammatory drugs are very helpful in controlling both the pain and inflammation associated with jumper's knee. Non-prescription medications include ibuprofen (Motrin®, Advil®, Nuprin®, and Medipren®) and prescription medications (Naprosyn®, Indocin®, Feldene®, and Relafen®). All medications should be used under the direction of a physician because of potential side effects. Steroid injections into the patellar tendon or ligament are not a good idea because the amount of steroid injected can harm and weaken the tendon and ligament, predisposing it to future rupture.

- **STRETCHING:** It is essential to stretch the tightened hamstring muscles in order to manage patellar tendonitis. This is because tightened hamstring muscles multiply the amount of stress delivered to the patellar tendon and ligament while running, walking, or when trying to fully straighten the knee. Stretching out tightened calf muscles and the Achilles tendon is also necessary. Rapid stretching or bouncing is not recommended. Stretching exercises should be performed slowly and sustained during the stretch for a count to ten before easing up slowly and letting go.

- **STRENGTHENING:** Exercise to build muscle bulk begins with quad sets and straight leg raising in the early phases of rehabilitation. It is important to perform exercises slowly and avoid those motions that cause pain. These exercises should be not be performed by bending the knee more than 45 degrees in order to avoid excessively tensing the quadriceps tendon and ligament. In the beginning, you can perform pain-free isometric exercises with quad sets and then progress to straight leg raising and terminal knee extension activities as the pain lessens. It may be helpful to rest between each cycle of exercise. As symptoms improve, one-half squatting exercises can be introduced. Eccentric exercises may be introduced later. Eccentric exercises of the quadriceps muscles may help prevent future recurrence as they elongate the muscle during contraction.

- **BRACING:** There are several commercially available braces that can prevent or help treat jumper's knee. A neoprene sleeve for the knee is helpful to some, while others use a strap to gently compress the patellar ligament beneath the kneecap. Such a strap attempts to redirect the pull of the patellar ligament by changing the direction of pull, thereby relieving some of the stress passing through the tendon and ligament.

- **ORTHOSES:** As discussed in previous chapters, an orthosis tailored to the specific needs of your foot can help prevent, and in some cases, may even cure jumper's knee. A custom orthosis alters the biomechanics of the foot, ankle, and leg so that forces are distributed more evenly, and the rotations of the shinbone that can cause torsion of the patellar tendon and ligament are reduced. If one leg is longer than the other, a heel lift can be applied to the shorter leg.

- **PATENT EDUCATION:** It is very important to modify your activities in order to avoid stressing the patellar tendon and ligament. Studies have shown that injury is less likely to occur on softer surfaces. Play volleyball and other games on grass, sand, or wood rather than on concrete or linoleum. Because high jumpers are more likely to injure their tendons, try to limit height-jumping, if possible. Try not to bend your knees more than 90 degrees when taking off or landing because this will generate more leverage and force through your quadriceps mechanism and stresses the tendon further. Athletic warm-ups and cool-downs are an essential part of prevention. Warm-ups have the effect of increasing circulation within the muscle and tendon, thereby increasing cellular metabolism. They are believed to decrease the incidence of any associated muscle soreness. A good way to warm up prior to athletic participation is by light jogging to the point of light perspiration. Cooling down can be done by rubbing ice over the knee following practice. Work-outs should be of limited duration and jumping and sudden deceleration should be eliminated completely.

WHEN IS SURGERY NECESSARY?

Surgical treatment for stage II and I jumper's knee offers gratifying long-term results, but should only be considered in the event of failed conservative treatment. A conservative management program of 4 to 6 months should be undertaken prior to surgical intervention for stage III. In the event of surgery, it is important to advance into the rehabilitation process slowly because the area of involvement is located at a point of relatively poor blood supply. Immobilization usually last about six months, followed by 4 to 6 months of limited activity before proceeding to more vigorous athletic activity. In the event of patellar ligament rupture, excellent function may be obtained, provided repair is performed early and normal tendon length is restored. Quadriceps tendon ruptures have a less favorable prognosis.

A brace is worn after surgical repair of the frayed tendons in order to immobilize the knee for about 2 weeks. After that, bending is allowed, although in a limited way in order to avoid stressing the tendon further. As the knee heals, the hinges on the brace can be adjusted to allow for more bending. Bending is very important because not letting the quadriceps muscles operate as they normally do can rob them of strength and cause atrophy. Most people with this type of injury eventually regain their normal activity level after healing, although they do have a higher risk of future rupture.

16 Runner's Knee

Your 26-year-old daughter came home for the holidays and decided to begin jogging around the neighborhood. She began to experience pain in her outer thigh at the end of a run and heard an audible "snap" that persisted, especially when going down a flight of stairs. Her twin brother, an avid cyclist who has been preparing for an upcoming race, complains of pain at the outer knee with each pedaling stroke as he rides around in your hilly neighborhood. He usually rides 15 miles a day and likes to raise his seat to the high position. What is going on here?

■ RUNNER'S KNEE DEFINED

THE THIGHBONE is long and slender along its length and bumpy and round at either end. Imagine a taut rubber band with one end stretched in front of the thighbone at the hip and the other end stretched just behind it down at the knee. Imagine the thighbone moving back and forth repetitively in a front to back direction, so that its bumpy round ends at either side bump against and rub along the taut band both at the knee and at the hip.

This is exactly what happens in the body in some persons, especially if they are middle-aged and athletic. When this happens near the hip it is called *snapping hip syndrome*, and when it occurs at the knee it is called *runner's knee*. Both conditions are a type of *repetitive strain injury* from friction at either end of an important structure known as the *iliotibial band*. Because the common denominator in what causes injury is friction, both conditions are collectively referred to as *iliotibial band friction syndrome*. Runner's knee is the more common form of this syndrome.

■ ILIOTIBIAL BAND

The thighbone is the longest and strongest bone in the body, running from your hip to your knee. The rubber band described in the analogy above is the iliotibial band (ITB). It begins at the *ileum* (a bone at the pelvis) and travels down the outer thigh to the *tibia* (shinbone). It is not a tendon, muscle, or ligament, but rather a special sort of soft tissue known as *fascia*. Fascia lies just underneath the skin and acts as an insulating cover to other types of soft tissue such as muscle. The iliotibial band plays a direct role in the musculoskeletal system. Several muscles attach to the iliotibial band as if it were a surrogate tendon, so that when these muscles contract, the ITB becomes tense and pulls on the hip and knee. This occurs every time we walk or run.

At the hip joint, the ITB rubs against a big protruding bump known as the *greater trochanter*, which is the site of attachment for many muscles. At the knee, the ITB passes across the outer side of the knee joint and attaches to the upper part of the shinbone. It passes across the flare or bump of the end of the thighbone, which is another site for potential friction before it attaches.

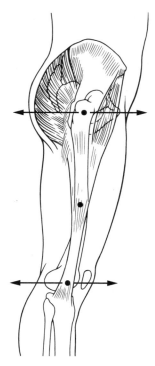

When the lengthy iliotibial band rubs across the bump at the thigh known as the greater trochanter, it is called *snapping hip syndrome*. When this happens at the outer knee it is called *runner's knee*. Saidoff DC, McDonough: *Critical Pathways in Therapeutic Intervention: Extremities and Spine.* St. Louis: Mosby, 2002.

■ WHO IS MOST LIKELY TO GET RUNNER'S KNEE?

Just about anyone who engages in athletic activities requiring repetitive bending and straightening of the knee is more susceptible to developing either snapping hip or runner's knee. Because of this, these conditions are common in downhill skiers, weight lifters, cyclists, and athletes who practice lots of jumping or circuit training. Saddle height and cleat position are the culprits for cyclists. Runners and joggers who run on very hard surfaces or crested surfaces, use new or inflexible running shoes, or who suddenly increase their mileage are prone to developing friction at either end of the iliotibial band.

Other reasons that make one more prone to these conditions include having a larger than average *greater trochanter*, which is a bulbous flare at the upper end of the femur. A similar bump also exists at the lower end of the thighbone near the knee and is known as the *lateral condyle* (outer bump). If either of these bony bumps are larger than usual, greater friction of the ITB can occur, making inflammation more likely. Persons with bowlegs have knees postured in such a way that they are more likely to develop problems. Also, persons with pronated feet are more likely to develop iliotibial band friction syndrome because they will have tightening of the iliotibial band. Similarly, people with a very high arch of the foot may also experience tightening of the ITB because a high instep causes excessive outward rotation of the shinbone, causing the ITB to be distracted at its attachment. This causes the ITB to become tensed along its length and more likely to undergo friction at either end. Some persons have a discrepancy in the length of their legs and, therefore, both legs are more likely to develop ITB friction syndrome.

Some people may have a relative rotation of their thighbone that originates at the hip. This condition is known as excessive *version*. These people typically have feet that point outward too much when standing or walking. Excessive outward version is known as *anteversion*. It stretches the ITB, making it more likely to sustain friction. Women have greater anteversion than men and are more likely to develop snapping hip syndrome because the wider female pelvis stretches the iliotibial band more than the narrower male pelvis. On the other hand, women are less likely to develop runner's knee than males because they are endowed with more subcutaneous fat, which acts to reduce friction between the ITB and the knee.

In the 1940s, a classification of body types was developed that categorized people according to body shape (not size), and particularly according to the amount of slenderness, angularity, and fragility. This identification of physique type is known as *somatotyping*. The people who develop iliotibial band friction syndrome are typically classified as *ectomorphs*. They have a light body build, are tall and thin, and have slight muscular development. This may be the result of having relatively less fat, because fatty tissue acts to reduce friction at points of high mechanical stress throughout the musculoskeletal system.

SIGNS AND SYMPTOMS

People with ITB friction syndrome usually complain of a diffuse pain over the outer aspect of the knee or upper thigh, which is provoked by running or cycling. This pain usually appears at the beginning of a sporting activity and gets better after playing for a few minutes. It may be worse when running along a crested surface or when ascending or descending stairs. The upper and lower sites of this friction syndrome may be tender to touch. People with tight or weak muscles of the hip joint are commonly associated with iliotibial band friction syndrome. There is usually no history of trauma or twisting injury, and pain is not usually felt during squatting, walking, sprinting, or playing racquet sports.

THE OBER TEST

One way to figure out if your ITB is tight enough to cause symptoms is to perform the *Ober test*. This is done by lying on your side on a bed with a hard mattress with the non-problematic side touching the bed and the leg that is causing the problem facing up toward the ceiling. First, the knee touching the bed should be bent to your chest. Then, have a friend gently take the straight upper leg, move it

behind you still extended, and let go so that it can sag down to the surface of the bed. The leg will not sag and snapping may occur if the ITB is tight, just as it does during sporting activities. This will be especially true if your friend tries to gently move your thigh down and it causes pain.

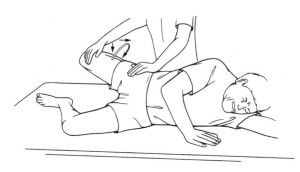

The Ober Test. If you feel uncomfortable during this test, your iliotibial band is tight.
Saidoff DC, McDonough: *Critical Pathways in Therapeutic Intervention: Extremities and Spine.* St. Louis: Mosby, 2002.

CONDITIONS TO RULE OUT

- **TROCHANTERIC BURSITIS:** A *bursa* is similar to a balloon filled with water that acts as a cushion in high stress areas of the body. It allows for movement and acts to cut down potential friction. The trochanteric bursa is located just underneath the skin at the widest part of the hips where a bump in the thighbone known as the greater trochanter protrudes sideways. Sometimes this bursa can become inflamed from too much legwork. Differentiating *greater trochanteric bursitis* from ITB tendonitis at the greater trochanter is often difficult because of the close association of the superficial trochanteric bursa with the TFL. Nevertheless, trochanteric bursitis is not accompanied by a snapping sensation, and the pain associated with bursitis is felt behind the greater trochanter and may even radiate into the buttock. Pressing directly on the greater trochanter may irritate the inflamed bursa and cause pain. (See Chapter 18.)

- **HIP POINTER INJURY:** This type injury is a direct contact injury to the pelvis that causes a severe bruise or an occasional bone fragment to chip off the pelvis. Because the injury can occur from a pointed blow to the hip or pelvis, this injury is called a "hip pointer." This is actually a misnomer because the site of injury is the pelvis and not the hip. This injury causes bruising and tenderness at the site of impact, and may also cause a limp. X-rays should be taken to rule out fractures. After icing, compression, rest, and oral medications, gentle stretching and strengthening of the abdominal muscles can begin about 48 hours after the injury, as pain recedes.

- **ILIAC CREST APOPHYSITIS:** This condition occurs in adolescents 13 to 17 years of age, who will complain of pain at the side bump of the pelvis known as the *iliac crest.* This overuse syndrome is most common in runners who do not have any history of injury or fall. Long distance or hill running generates shear at the pelvis bone, causing traction forces that shear away and detach the bones in the immature pelvis. Uphill running accentuates anterior pelvic tilt, and downhill running increases posterior pelvic tilt, hyperextends the spine, and curves it forward. Reciprocal arm swing across the trunk accentuates strain of pelvic rotation. This condition is suggested by a history of excessive running and tenderness at the iliac crest. Attempting to resist movement of the leg outward (abduction) causes pain. The condition usually resolves within 2 to 4 weeks. Rest, stretching, and strengthening of the muscles involved, with guidance from a physical therapist, is recommended once acute symptoms have begun to improve.

■ PREVENTION AND TREATMENT

Iliotibial band friction syndrome is a treatable condition, whether it presents near the hip or near the

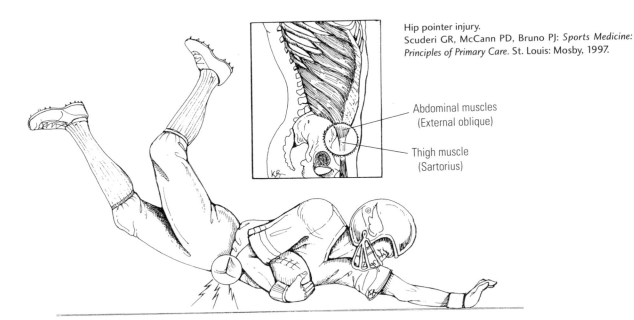

Hip pointer injury.
Scuderi GR, McCann PD, Bruno PJ: *Sports Medicine: Principles of Primary Care.* St. Louis: Mosby, 1997.

Abdominal muscles
(External oblique)

Thigh muscle
(Sartorius)

knee. However, it is often frustrating and difficult to stretch it adequately because the ITB is an extremely taut band. Physical therapy may be required for anywhere between 4 to 6 weeks; severe cases may require up to 8 weeks. Once local tenderness has gone away, athletic activity can begin again, slowly building up to the pre-injury level. Surgery is uncommon, if not rare, and is only reserved for recalcitrant cases that do not respond to conservative therapy.

- **STRETCHING:** Using stretching to gain extensibility of the ITB can be done in a number of ways. One way is to use the Ober test position described above, and to hold that position while the ITB undergoes a good stretch. Getting someone to help you makes this easier. The ITB may also be stretched while in the standing position without any assistance.

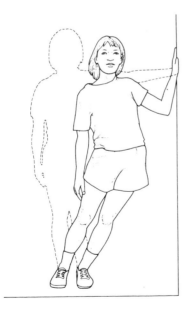

Stand sideways about 3 feet from a wall. Lean into the wall as if you were doing a one-handed push-up, and let your hip drop in toward the wall as far as it will go. This stretches the band on the leg closer to the wall. Hold the stretch for 15 to 20 seconds. Do three repetitions four to five times a day.

- **MASSAGE:** Deep tissue massage of the iliotibial band is helpful. Friction massage of the ITB is often helpful and pleasant when performed while taking a shower or bath. Friction massage involves rubbing where it hurts with the thumb or fingers either back and forth or in a circular motion. The level of pain may increase during deep tissue massage, but it will feel better afterwards.

- **ULTRASOUND:** Ultrasound is a method of applying deep heat using electricity that passes through special crystals that vibrate at high frequencies. This vibration penetrates deep into tissues as heat energy and may provide relief. Ultrasound applied in the pulsed mode may deliver pain-relieving medications to the inflamed patellar tendon or ligament. This method of medication delivery is known as *phonophoresis*. Delivery of aspirin hydrocortisone using phonophoresis is performed by a physical therapist and may decrease the pain and inflammation of runner's knee by considerably.

- **COLD AND HEAT:** When the pain is hot and tender during the acute phase, cold is very helpful in minimizing and controlling symptoms. Placing ice cubes in a plastic zipper lock bag and icing the area may reduce both the pain and inflammation. Later, when the acute stage has subsided, application of heat using a hot pack or hot bath can help relieve the chronic ache.

- **ACTIVITY MODIFICATION:** This may include avoidance of downhill running, decreasing mileage, and running on a level road instead of the drainage pitch or, alternatively, along opposite sides of the road. A steroid injection may be administered anterior, posterior, and deep to the iliotibial tract at the outer knee area known as the lateral femoral epicondyle by a doctor. Oral nonsteroidal anti-inflammatory medications may be taken for 14 days. A person with runner's knee should be encouraged to partially replace running with activities such as swimming with a minimal kick, or simply reduce their running stride length, overall running distance, and frequency of run.

- **ORTHOTIC CORRECTION:** As discussed in previous chapters, a custom orthosis alters the biomechanics of the foot, ankle, and leg so that forces are distributed more evenly. Wearing an orthosis can align the foot, ankle, shin, and knee in such a way that the tension on the ITB is diminished. If one leg is longer than the other, a heel lift can be inserted into the shoe of the shorter leg.

- **SHOES:** Switching from a hard shoe to softer running shoes can help ease the stress on the ITB.

Avoid running in sneakers with worn outer heels and switch to new running shoes. If one leg is longer than the other, the shoe on the short side can have a lift built into the heel.

- **BIKERS:** Cyclists should correct the cleat position of their bicycles so they are slightly bent outward in external rotation. For those cyclists who use fixed pedal systems, switching to floating pedals may afford relief. Adjusting the stance width using spacers placed between the pedal and the crank arm may reduce ITB stress by widening the cyclist's stance, thus improving the alignment of the entire leg.

17 Osgood-Schlatter Disease

Your 15-year-old son complains of pain in his right knee. Although he plays basketball and baseball with his friends every day, he has not fallen or collided with another player. He experiences pain primarily when he crouches in the "low defense" posture. He is usually the catcher and squatting down behind home plate makes the pain in his knee worse, as does bicycling home at the end of the day. It hurts him most right below the kneecap at the front of his shinbone where a bump has developed. The pain is aggravated by jumping, running, or going up or down the stairs. This young man has Osgood-Schlatter disease of his right knee, a sport-related condition common to active, growing adolescents.

OSGOOD-SCHLATTER DISEASE DEFINED

Osgood-Schlatter disease is a bone problem that causes pain in the front of the knee just below the kneecap where the patellar tendon inserts into the shinbone. Described in 1903 by Dr. Osgood in the United States and Dr. Schlatter in Germany, credit for its description is given to both doctors. This disease occurs primarily in boys 10 to 15 years of age during the pubescent and adolescent growth spurt. This very painful condition may affect one or both knees.

Understanding Osgood-Schlatter disease depends on understanding how the long bones grow. The ends of long bones like the shin bone (tibia) are still soft in growing children. They can be thought of as stretching and elongating. At the same time, the bone in the middle of the shaft becomes hard. Eventually, this hardening of bone (ossification) spreads from the center of the bone toward the ends, so that eventually the entire bone becomes hard. This system works rather well, but it leaves the soft growing ends (known as *endplates*) vulnerable to damage.

OSTEOCHONDROSIS

The soft ends of the growing long bones are called the *growth centers*. Children are quite active and the force exerted by their tendons and ligaments is sometimes so great that they may injure the soft growth center at the vulnerable end of these long bones, which may die and then grow back later. This process of disease and re-growth at the growth center is called *osteochondrosis*. Osgood-Schlatter disease is actually a type of osteochondrosis that occurs at the knee. (Osteochondrosis goes by other names when it occurs at other places in the body.) When osteochondrosis occurs because of a tendon pulling on bone, it is called an *apophysitis*.

BONY BUMP

As discussed in previous chapters, the *patellar tendon* originates from the heads of four muscles known as the *quadriceps muscle*. The forces imparted by the *quadriceps tendon* are extremely powerful because all

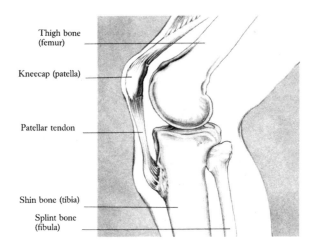

Osgood-Schlatter disease. The bone is inflames and broken up at the attachment of the patellar tendon to the shin bone. Peterson L, Renstrom P: *Sports Injuries: Their Prevention and Treatment*. Chicago: Year Book Medical Publishers Inc., 1986.

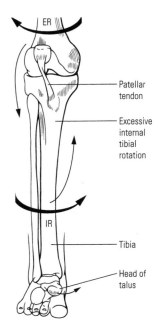

Overpronation of the foot causes the shinbone to rotate excessively during walking, which in turn causes torsion of the patellar ligament at the knee. In this manner, the patellar ligament undergoes stress so that it is less capable of absorbing the enormous force passing through it to the tibial tubercle, making it more vulnerable to Osgood-Schlatter disease. Saidoff DC, McDonough AL: *Critical Pathways in Therapeutic Intervention: Extremities and Spine.* St. Louis: Mosby, 2002.

four muscles share a single tendon. The quadriceps tendon envelops the front of the knee and continues down with a different name, the *quadriceps ligament*; it attaches to a bump of bone at the top of the shinbone. This bony bump is known as the *tibial tubercle*. It is relatively soft in growing children. Jumping activities cause enormous forces to be transmitted through the quadriceps muscles, tendon, and ligament. Those forces converge on one spot, the tibial tubercle. It is no wonder that this soft bump of bone reacts by lifting upward as a large, painful, and even more prominent bump.

RISK FACTORS

Osgood-Schlatter disease occurs often with jumping sports such as basketball or volleyball. The repetitive forces of jumping cause traction through the patellar ligament that pulls upward on the tibial tubercle. While Osgood-Schlatter disease occurs primarily in adolescent boys, it presents more and more often in adolescent girls (especially between

the ages of 8 to 13 years old) who are increasingly more active and athletic. Adolescents who have flat feet will undergo excessive *pronation* of the foot. *Overpronation* of the foot causes the shinbone to rotate excessively during walking, which in turn causes torsion of the patellar ligament at the knee. In this manner, the patellar ligament undergoes stress that makes it less capable of absorbing the enormous force passing through it to the tibial tubercle, making it more vulnerable to Osgood-Schlatter disease. Children with overpronated feet who develop Osgood-Schlatter during adolescence are more likely to develop an unstable knee cap as adults because the prominent tibial tubercle acts to increase the leverage of the patellar ligament. This, in turn, magnifies the rotational forces from the shin bone and causes more outer tracking of the kneecap. (See Chapter 14.) Both knees are involved in about one-half of all cases of Osgood-Schlatter's disease.

SIGNS AND SYMPTOMS

Osgood-Schlatter disease of the knee is indicated when a prominent, painful bump can be felt protruding from the top of the shinbone. There is no history of injury or popping sound. There may be some swelling, and the tibial tubercle will be quite tender, especially during or after an active game of basketball. Once traction of the soft tibial tubercle begins, pain can be provoked by squatting, because this posture causes the patellar tendon and ligament to be stretched tight, resulting in more pull on the tibial tubercle. For this reason, an affected adolescent may refuse to bend his knee to the maximum. Resisting straightening of the knee may also provoke symptoms. The quadriceps, hamstrings, and calf muscles may be tight. Pain may also be reported when running, climbing or descending stairs, or sitting for an extended period of time and then getting up. X-rays of the knee will show either a soft tissue swelling around the knee or bone fragmentation of the tibial tuberosity.

CONDITIONS TO RULE OUT

- **SINDING-LARSEN-JOHANSSON DISEASE** is another form of osteochondrosis, which is also known as *patella baja* or *high-riding patella*. This condition was independently described in the early 1900s by Sinding, Larsen and Johansson as pain at the upper or lower ends (poles) of the kneecap accompanied by x-ray findings of bone fragmentation of the pole. The patella (kneecap) is a small triangular-shaped bone whose upper border is

known as its superior pole. Its lower border is called the inferior pole. The patella is enveloped by group of tendons that are called the *quadriceps tendon* above the kneecap and the *quadriceps ligament* below the tendon. The traction forces transmitted through the patellar tendon or ligament may be so strong during early puberty that the bony kneecap at the soft tissue attachments at either pole may be injured. This condition occurs 1 to 2 years earlier than Osgood-Schlatter disease. It is similar to Osgood-Schlatter disease in that it is a problem of the growth plate of the inferior patellar pole or, less commonly, the superior patellar pole. Sinding-Larsen-Johansson disease may be considered the counterpart of Osgood-Schlatter disease at the patellar poles. Osgood-Schlatter disease is confined to the tibial tuberosity, and Sinding-Larsen-Johansson disease is a disorder involving both the bony and soft tissues at the bone-tendon junction. It is not unusual to see Osgood-Schlatter develop at the knee simultaneously with Sinding-Larsen-Johansson, although Sinding-Larsen-Johansson typically occurs 1 to 2

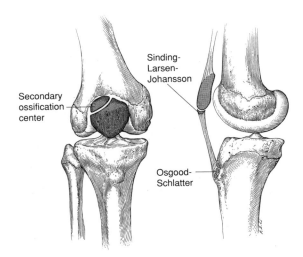

Sinding-Larsen-Johansson disease is considered the counterpart of Osgood-Schlatter disease. Tria AJ, Klein KS: *An Illustrated Guide to The Knee.* New York: Churchill Livingstone, 1992.

years prior to Osgood-Schlatter at approximately ages 8 to 13. This condition is most common in normal males at puberty.

- **JUMPER'S KNEE** is the adult version of Sinding-Larsen-Johansson disease. The difference between the two is that in jumper's knee the patellar tendon and ligament undergo stretching and fraying because the adult bones have hardened. Jumper's knee is a form of tendonitis (inflammation) of the tendon crossing over the top of the knee joint. It occurs commonly in adult athletes who jump, kick, run, and climb. It may progress to a patellar tendon or ligament rupture, if ignored. This condition is more likely to develop in people with a wide pelvis (females), knock or bow knees, or overpronation of the foot, because all of these conditions will angulate or twist the patellar tendon and ligament, making them more likely to develop tendonitis. Tremendous force is delivered through this tendon and ligament during activities such as badminton, weight-lifting, soccer, volleyball, and baseball. Certain vocations that involve a great deal of squatting, climbing, or kneeling are considered risk factors for jumper's knee.

TREATMENT AND PREVENTION

Osgood-Schlatter disease is a self-limiting, benign disorder that typically lasts 12 to 24 months and then usually resolves on its own. However, if a child continues playing despite pain, this condition may get worse and become more difficult to treat. Physical therapy is the best treatment for both Osgood-Schlatter disease and Sinding-Larsen-Johansson disease. Parents should not be alarmed by the serious sounding names of these two conditions because both of them are benign. Symptoms may be disregarded if they are only occasionally bothersome and do not limit activities. However, if symptoms are bothersome during sporting activities, the recommended treatment is rest, in order to give the body time to heal. Severe cases may require the use of crutches to help the child walk without pain. If the child complains of pain toward the end of the day but is without symptoms the following day, then only activity and exercise modification is recommended. An important approach to management of these conditions is to have the physical therapist identify patterns of muscle imbalance in the leg and thigh and address excessively tight or lax muscles. This is accomplished by appropriate stretching and strengthening exercises. The child may slowly return to his previous level of activity when the pain is completely gone.

OTHER TREATMENTS INCLUDE:

- **ICE MASSAGE:** Ice gently rubbed over the tibial tubercle for 10 to 20 minutes at a time may relieve acute symptoms. A compressive wrap may also bring relief. Combining cold therapy with compression using an elastic bandage and elevating the painful knee is helpful in relieving symptoms.

- **REST:** It is important to restrict activity so that the injured areas have a chance to rest and heal. Complete mandatory rest may be impractical for an active child, but it is important to encourage children with these conditions to take frequent rest periods during play. Some activity should be allowed, although strenuous or excessive exercise involving the knee should be avoided. Positions that require deep squatting or kneeling should also be avoided. It is helpful when parents take the time to discuss the child's problem with the coach or physical education instructor. It may be necessary for the child to sit out the remainder of the sporting season if he is limping.

- **STRETCHING:** Stretching of the hamstring muscles is very important because many children with these conditions have tight hamstrings and weak hip flexor muscles. The stretch should be gentle if the quadriceps is tight. Bouncing into a stretch is not a good idea. The amount of stretching should be slowly increased. Stretching may help minimize the excessive stress delivered to the tibial tuberosity during quadriceps femoris contraction. Stretching should be performed three times per day in accordance with instructions from a physical therapist.

- **STRENGTHENING:** Short-arc hamstring exercises can be done by forcefully bending the knee, but not throughout the entire range of knee motion. Instead, the knee should be bent in a short arc through a range of motion that is not painful. This can be done for approximately 6 weeks until symptoms subside in order avoid the risk of separation of the tibial tubercle. These exercises are best done three times per day for maximum benefit. Eccentric working of the quadriceps musculature makes muscles work in a way that involves lengthening of the muscle fibers. Eccentric quadriceps strengthening is very important because it helps unload the forces applied through the patellar tendon and ligament to the tibial tubercle. Other possible exercises include leg curls and straight leg raises. These exercises are best taught by a physical therapist.

- **MEDICATIONS:** Taking aspirin or other oral non-steroidal anti-inflammatory drugs such as ibuprofen or naproxen with a doctor's approval may help relieve pain. Corticosteroid medication is not advised as a form of treatment because of the potential for skin complications due to irritation to the relatively thin skin covering the tibial tubercle. Steroid injection is contraindicated because it provides little in the way of long-term relief and may cause patellar tendon deterioration.

- **IONTOPHORESIS:** This is a method of passing medicine through the skin into a specific area using electrical current. Typically, a small amount of analgesic is applied to the tibial tubercle in this manner in order to help reduce pain.

- **BRACES:** These can be worn if the pain is severe and the child limps when walking on level ground or when the sporting activity is over. Immobilization is rarely used and is reserved for children who cannot slow down or avoid the activities that aggravate these conditions. Protective kneepads may be purchased commercially and used to reduce traction on the tibial tubercle by applying direct pressure over the painful tubercle.

- **ACTIVITY MODIFICATION:** Avoid deep knee bending, excessive running, and especially jumping. Swimming and bicycling are good for strengthening the knee. Weight-bearing on the affected leg is permissible. Do not restrain a child from running. Gradual resumption of activity is allowed, once flexibility and strength are regained.

Hip

THE HIP JOINT is a ball-and-socket joint. It is the deepest joint in the body and is capable of an incredible range of movement. Two bones work together to form the hip joint. The "ball" is the end of the femur (thigh bone), which is the longest bone in the body. This bone is so strong that it can bear the weight of a compact car! It fits into the hip socket, which is part of the pelvis. The hip joints are vulnerable to overuse injuries and are often the first site of bone fracture in older women with osteoporosis. The hip joint is also often the site of arthritis due to age-related changes.

18 Bursitis of the Hip

A 51-year-old armchair executive complains of an ache at the side of her hip that is particularly bothersome when climbing the stairs, getting up from a deep chair and when running while playing tennis. In addition to playing tennis once a week, she also plays golf regularly. Unfortunately, she does not have much time to stretch routinely. The pain is never felt in the groin, but it sometimes wakes her up at night when turning over onto the painful side. Touching a particular spot on the outer side of her upper thigh is painful. She sometimes uses an icepack or non-prescription medications to relieve the discomfort. This woman has bursitis of the hip, also known as greater trochanteric bursitis.

▉ THE TROCHANTER

THE THIGHBONE (femur) is the longest, largest, bone in the body, and it is so strong that it can bear the weight of a compact car. It is structured on an engineering principle that says ounce for ounce, a tube is stronger than a rod. This principle endows the tubular thighbone with enormous strength to withstand the forces of walking.

Nevertheless, the thighbone has a weak spot related to how it was formed in the embryo. A large outward protruding bump of bone, which is known as the *trochanter*, is located in the upper one-third of the thighbone. It is known as the *greater trochanter* because it is the larger of the two bumps of bone on the otherwise slender, smooth thighbone. The trochanter breaks the continuous line of the tubular thighbone. It serves as the attachment site for the many powerful muscles that move the pelvis, thigh, and hip. The reason it protrudes outward is because this position affords the attaching muscles a longer lever arm and, hence, greater leverage to wield power.

▉ BURSAE

There is a good chance that friction can build up between the muscle attachments because so many muscles attach to the greater trochanter. Friction can cause inflammation and other problems. The body, in its wisdom, has developed a unique strategy: *bursa* (plural: *bursae*) to reduce friction.

As discussed in previous chapters, a bursa is a fluid-filled sac that is made up of synovial membrane, which is the same protective material that lines the inside of many joints. Compare a bursa to a balloon filled with water that is placed between two wooden boards moving in different directions. The balloon makes sure that the surfaces of the two boards are able to move close together without touching.

There are about 15 to 20 bursae in the area of the hip because it is an area of high friction. They may become injured if motion at the pelvis, hip, or thigh is excessive. The walls of the bursae may wear down, causing inflammation of the synovial walls. This is the body's way of telling us to slow down and

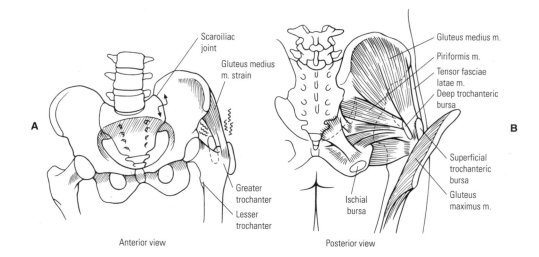

A. The bumps of bone on the outer thighbone near the pelvis known as the greater and lesser trochanters.
B. Bursae located where the muscles attach onto the trochanters.
Saidoff DC, McDonough AL: *Critical Pathways in Therapeutic Intervention: Extremities and Spine*. St. Louis: Mosby, 2002,

rest. Otherwise, the inflamed bursae will swell and hurt in what is known as *bursitis*. When this happens at the bursae of the greater trochanter, it is known as *greater trochanteric bursitis*.

ILIOTIBIAL BAND

The iliotibial band (ITB) is a long, flat strip of tissue between the pelvis and tibia (shinbone). (See Chapter 16.) It is located along the outer thigh and many muscles are attached to it, causing it to tense as the limb moves. The ITB also moves back and forth over the greater trochanter with each step forward. There is a bursa between the ITB and the greater trochanter known as the *greater trochanteric bursa* that lessens friction in that area. With excessive activity or overuse, the ITB will rub across the greater trochanter to the point of high-friction buildup, which can cause the underlying bursa to become inflamed.

WHO IS MOST LIKELY TO HAVE GREATER TROCHANTERIC BURSITIS?

Greater trochanteric bursitis is the most common source of hip pain after osteoarthritis of the hip joint. It is about twice as common in females. This may be attributable to the wider female pelvis, which tightens the ITB and compresses the underlying bursa. This condition typically occurs at middle age or older (4th through the 6th decades), although it can occur in all age groups. Young soccer players may injure the greater trochanteric bursa during a violent sideways fall, or it may be injured from repetitive soccer or karate kicks that cause the bursa to become flattened by the *iliotibial band* covering it.

Some people are predisposed to getting greater trochanteric bursitis for a variety of reasons, such as having one leg longer than the other. Bursitis can develop in either the shorter or longer leg. It can also happen to someone who has legs of equal length, but who creates an imbalance by running or jogging along a crested surface in such a way that one leg is higher than the other. A person whose foot is overpronated because of a flat arch, or who has a high arch, can tense the ITB band in such a way that it compresses the greater trochanteric bursa beneath it on either the longer or shorter leg.

Other problems that predispose a person to high friction at the greater trochanter include: running with the legs crossing at midline, having weak thigh muscles, or having thigh muscles that are too tight, especially the ITB. People who sit for long periods of time at work are more likely to develop these types of problems because the sitting position approximates the hip and knee ever so slightly and causes the ITB to accommodate to a shortened and, hence, tighter position.

■ SIGNS AND SYMPTOMS

The pain of greater trochanteric bursitis usually feels like an ache that comes and goes, unless it happens right after a fall onto the side, which will cause sharp pain when pressing the greater trochanter. You might walk with a slight limp if the pain is sharp. Turning your foot outward and moving your thigh away from the body is painful because it irritates the inflamed bursa. This motion causes the tendons to pull on the greater trochanter in such a way that it rubs against the inflamed bursa. Turning your foot inward and moving your thigh to midline will not cause pain, although crossing your thigh over midline will, because that posture also tightens the ITB against the inflamed, sensitive bursa. Certain activities of daily living, such as climbing stairs, getting up out of a deep chair or sofa, running, sitting cross-legged, or lying on the affected side, will irritate the inflamed bursa and cause pain. People often complain of pain that wakes them up when rolling onto the painful greater trochanter at night.

Positioning the thigh and leg into a posture resembling the number "four" will stress the greater trochanter bursa by causing the ITB to stretch tightly over it. This will provoke symptoms in at least half of all people with this condition.

If a fall onto the side of the body causes the greater trochanteric bursa to become directly injured, bleeding may occur in the bursa, resulting in clots that eventually calcify (turn into bone). There may also be a grating sensation at the greater trochanter. X-rays are usually advised.

■ SNAPPING HIP SYNDROME

Differentiating *greater trochanteric bursitis* from ITB tendonitis at the greater trochanter, which is also known as *snapping hip syndrome*, is difficult because of the close association of the trochanteric bursa with TFL. Nevertheless, trochanteric bursitis is not accompanied by a snapping sensation, and the pain associated with bursitis is felt behind the greater trochanter and may even radiate into the buttock. Pressing directly on the greater trochanter may, in turn, press the inflamed bursa and produce pain, which will aid in diagnosis.

■ PREVENTION AND TREATMENT

- **COLD TREATMENT:** Applying cold to an inflamed bursa can help provide instant relief from pain and inflammation during the acute stage.

- **STRETCHING:** A good way to get to the root of this problem is to stretch the ITB along its length. A moist hot pack may also be applied along the outer thigh for 20 minutes, using appropriate protective insulation to prevent a burn. Stretching of the ITB is accomplished by lying on your side on a bed with a hard mattress with the non-problematic side touching the bed and the leg that is causing the problem facing up toward the ceiling. First, the knee touching the bed should be bent to your chest. Then, have a friend gently take the straight upper leg, move it behind you still extended, and let go so that the leg can sag down to the surface of the bed. The leg can be gently pushed downward if it does not sag down easily, which will stretch the ITB. The ITB can also be stretched in the standing position.

■ **ORTHOSIS:** As discussed in previous chapters, someone who has one leg longer than the other can use an orthosis or heel lift to help even out the legs, thereby placing less stress on the ITB. An orthosis may also help the stress on the ITB caused by an overpronated foot, thereby lessening pressure over the greater trochanteric bursae.

■ **STRENGTHENING:** It is important to stretch the ITB, especially in cases where it is tight and the hip adductors are weak. The hip adductor muscles that make up the bulk of the inner thigh can be strengthened in either the sitting or standing position using elastic bands or pulleys. Strengthening exercises should be done in a manner that is not painful and does not irritate the greater trochanteric bursa.

■ **PHONOPHORESIS:** This method uses pulsed ultrasonic waves to move steroids or aspirin through the thin layer of skin covering the greater trochanter in order to penetrate the inflamed bursae and relieve symptoms. Iontophoresis is another method of passing medicine through the skin into a specific area using electrical current.

■ **INJECTIONS:** Steroid injections are sometimes helpful in relieving the pain of an inflamed greater trochanteric bursa, although too many shots may cause a bad reaction or damage the skin or nerves.

▪ WHEN IS SURGERY NECESSARY?

Recalcitrant cases of greater trochanteric bursitis may be helped by surgery that releases the tight fascia comprising the ITB that covers the greater trochanter, although this is rarely done.

19 Muscle Strain

A 40-year-old housewife ran down the stairs to answer the door and tripped on the last step in order to avoid stepping on her toddler's doll. She felt a sudden, sharp, pulling sensation in her calf muscles. Subsequently, she noticed swelling, cramping, and discoloration in her calf. Immediately after the injury she limped over to a nearby chair and sat down. She has experienced a muscle strain of the gastrocnemius muscle, which is located in her calf.

■ CONTRACTING - DISTRACTING

INJURIES TO MUSCLES are common, especially during sporting activities. Muscles and tendons are made up of minute muscle filaments that move together (contract) and move apart (distract). Individual muscle fibers may become stretched, frayed, or torn if they are forced to work beyond capacity. Muscles and tendons are strained if they are injured and there is no direct bruise or cut. A *muscle strain* occurs from sudden contraction or distraction of the attachments of a muscle, which may either result in a stretch or tear of muscle fibers. Common types of muscle strains include a pulled hamstring or groin pull injury, both of which occur in sprinters due to muscle overload. Muscle strains also occur more frequently with increasing age because the connective tissue comprising the muscle becomes less elastic and less capable of withstanding the excessive force that occurs in a short period of time.

The torn space is not filled in by new muscle tissue when a muscle tear occurs. Instead, a poorer quality tissue called *scar tissue* fills the gap. Muscle tissue works well because its fibers run parallel with each other, which distributes force evenly throughout the muscle. However, the fibers making up scar tissue do not contract and are randomly oriented. They represent a potentially weak site in muscle that is prone to further failure with excessive stretching or contraction. The injured muscle is considered weakened and more prone to re-injury because scar tissue is not as strong or capable as muscle.

The majority of muscle strains occur in the legs rather than the arms because of the enormous weight of the body on the legs and the ground reaction forces that pass upward from the ground into the legs. Thus, the lower limbs act as a transition point for potentially injurious forces during walking and running and are more likely to sustain muscle strain.

■ DISTRACTION TEARS

A distraction tear can occur when a muscle is suddenly and powerfully stretched beyond its limit—for example, when a football player performs a high kick. The hamstring muscles are located at the back of the thigh and may undergo a stretch so rapid that the fibers are torn apart. Another way that muscle fibers can be torn is if the muscular contraction is performed so quickly and with such force that the power generated by the activity exceeds the innate tolerance of the muscles, resulting in strain. For example, sudden acceleration of a sprinter during take off at the beginning of a race involves explosive concentric muscular effort in a short period of time. In contrast, sudden eccentric deceleration of a baseball player running to a base places high stress on muscle fibers. A combination of deceleration and acceleration may occur during sharp cutting movements in which a football player evades another player by suddenly slowing and then speeding up in another direction. These activities place great demands on muscle and often exceed the muscle's ability to cope, resulting in a strain injury.

TWO-JOINT MUSCLES

While most muscles span a single joint and attach to bone via only one tendon, certain skeletal muscles cross two joints simultaneously. Muscles that belong to this group are few, and yet these muscles disproportionately experience muscle tears because the demands of normal function often distract them more than those of single joint muscles. The majority of these two-joint muscles span the lower limbs and include the *rectus femoris* (one of the quadriceps muscles), the *gastrocnemius* muscle covering the back of the shinbone, and the *hamstring muscles* comprising the back of the thigh. The *biceps* is an example of a two-jointed arm muscle. These muscles are often saddled with the task of contracting while moving two joints simultaneously, especially in the legs. Two-joint muscles are more likely to experience injury because they juggle a more versatile task of contraction than single joint muscles.

ECCENTRIC CONTRACTIONS

Muscles work by either contracting or relaxing. If you were on a roof and wanted to pull up a heavy bucket of equipment, you would concentrically contract your biceps and the other muscles of your arms. The muscles work by shifting filaments closer together, with the overall effect of the entire muscle shortening and pulling the bucket upward against the downward pull of gravity. When muscle filaments *contract* to generate force, they are *contracting concentrically*.

Suppose you wanted to ease the heavy bucket back down to the ground. If you did this concentrically with your triceps extending your elbow, the bucket would fly down quickly and spill its contents when it crashed into the ground. However, you want the bucket to be lowered down in a graded fashion, bit by bit. This requires significant energy and effort. The muscle filaments *distract*, meaning they move away from each other in a steady, controlled manner. This is called an *eccentric contraction*. (The term *eccentric contraction* is a misnomer because the word "contraction" suggests that filaments are moving toward one another, when in fact they are distracting.) In this way, the heavy weight of the bucket pulled down by gravity is resisted little by little until the bucket reaches the ground safely.

Eccentric contractions are the muscular system's coping strategy in diluting the effects of forces, especially when heavy loads or high velocity is present. Eccentric contraction requires less energy expenditure than concentric contraction and is utilized (along with concentric contraction) during jogging and walking. Eccentric activity is very important when getting around because it helps absorb many of the potentially injurious forces that pass through the ankles, knees, hips, and spine.

COMMON TYPES OF MUSCLE STRAIN

While many different skeletal muscles may undergo strain, only the most common are mentioned here. Most strains occur in the leg muscles, especially those that cross two joints, as discussed.

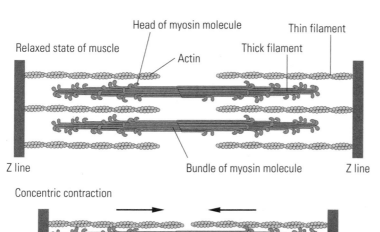

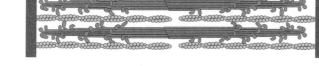

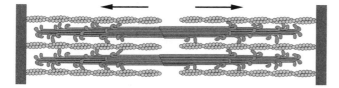

Myosin and actin filaments are actively engaged during concentric and eccentric contraction. In the former, the Z lines approximate; in the latter, they distract. During muscular activity the filaments chemicals interact when the heads of the myosin molecules (thick filaments) attach to the molecules (located along the length of the thin actin-filaments). This cross-bridging of the filaments results in swiveling of the head of the myosin molecules.
Saidoff D: *Critical Pathways in Therapeutic Intervention: Extremities and Spine.* St. Louis: Mosby, 2002.

■ **RECTUS FEMORIS STRAIN:** The rectus femoris muscle is one of the four quadriceps muscles. It is the most common muscle at the hip joint to get injured. Rectus femoris and the other quadriceps muscles act to flex (bend) the hip toward the face. This muscle may become strained during ice skating in the forward direction or running from a fast start. This strain may feel like a sudden stabbing pain or pulling sensation at the front of the thigh and groin area. The front of the thigh near the groin may be painful to touch. Resisting either hip flexion or straightening of the knee (knee extension) will be painful and indicates rectus femoris strain.

■ **GROIN PULL:** This injury is also known as an *adductor strain* because the adductor muscles may be injured. Located along the inner portion of the thigh between the hip and knee, the *adductor muscle* draws the thigh inward. It is the muscle responsible when you fold one leg over the other. Imagine two soccer players trying to kick the same ball at the same time with the inside of their feet. Although the forces cancel each other and the ball goes nowhere, they have both possibly strained their adductor muscles. Another example is trying to board a small boat with one leg, and having the boat move away from the dock with one leg still on the dock. The severe momentary contraction or overstretching of the adductor muscle may feel like a knife stab to the groin, preventing standing or walking. Resisting hip adduction or abduction (moving the thigh away from the other thigh) will repro-

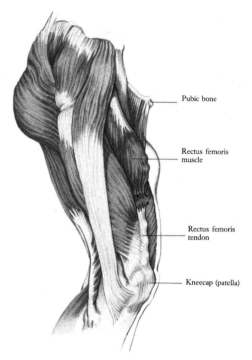

Strain of the quadriceps muscle.
Peterson L, Renstrom P: *Sports Injuries: Their Prevention and Treatment.* London: Martin Dunitz, Ltd, 1986.

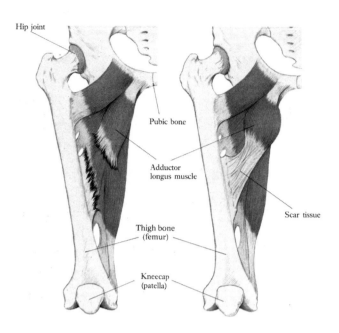

Total rupture of the adductor longus muscle from severe groin pull injury resulting in healing with a bump (from scar tissue) in the muscle.
Peterson L, Renstrom P: *Sports injuries: their prevention and treatment,* London, Martin Dunitz, Ltd., 1986 (Fig. 19-4).

duce pain. The groin will be painful to touch and swollen.

- **PULLED HAMSTRINGS:** The *hamstring muscles* are an important group of three muscles making up the back of the thigh. "Hamstring" is actually a veterinary term used to describe a large tendon above and behind the hock of a four-legged animal. A common and savage Roman method of subjugation of captured armies was to slice the hamstrings of captured soldiers so that they could not run away, and thus could be utilized as slaves. Thus, to be "hamstrung" is to become crippled. Strain of the hamstrings muscles may occur in sprinters or from jumping or playing tennis. A sudden and forceful kick of a ball may impart a high velocity stretch to the hamstrings, resulting in a tear. The person with a hamstrings sprain may feel or hear a popping sound and experience swelling about two hours after the injury. Black and blue marks indicating bleeding might be seen about 2 days after the injury. Resisting bending of the knee may cause pain, and it will be difficult to extend the knee because extension stretches the torn hamstrings.

- **BICEPS RUPTURE:** This is an uncommon injury that occurs most commonly in parachutists who incorrectly position the static line in front of the arm. Severe forces are applied to the biceps when the parachutist jumps, causing a tearing or popping sensation, followed by severe pain, swelling, and loss of strength. If the muscle is torn completely, a defect may be felt at the site of the strain.

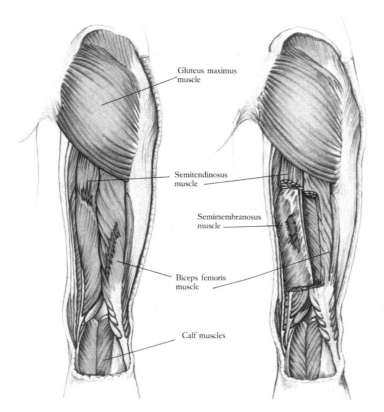

Gluteus maximus
muscle

Semitendinosus
muscle

Semimembranosus
muscle

Biceps femoris
muscle

Calf muscles

Tears of the various parts of the hamstring muscle.
Peterson L, Renstrom P: *Sports Injuries: Their Prevention and Treatment*. London: Martin Dunitz, Ltd., 1986.

■ CLASSIFICATION OF STRAINS

Strains are classified according to how much disruption occurs in the muscle and tendon fibers:

- **FIRST DEGREE STRAIN:** A *mild muscle strain* occurs from overstretching or minimal tearing of a muscle or tendon. It will often heal without treatment.

- **SECOND DEGREE STRAIN:** A *moderate strain* involves a more significant tearing of muscle fibers and must be treated with care so that it heals to its pre-injury level. The muscle can still contract with a partial muscle tear, although weakly and painfully.

- **THIRD DEGREE STRAIN:** If untreated, a moderate strain may lead to a third degree strain, which is total rupture of a muscle. A gap in the muscle may be felt by holding your fingers over the muscle with a third degree strain, and any attempt to contract the muscle is useless. Trying to contract the muscle does not generate any force, and it will look like there is a lump in the middle of the muscle.

■ MUSCLE SPASMS

One of the most common problems is muscle cramps that occur during or after intense or prolonged exercise. (See Chapter 2.) During activities that require brief, intense, bursts of energy, muscles attempt to generate more energy by drawing on stored sugars. They also utilize oxygen when they are working. Intense bursts of energy require more oxygen than readily available, and so muscles work *anaerobically,* meaning "without oxygen." This process is less efficient in the long run and allows for increased power at the expense of generating a waste product known as *lactic acid.* This by-product builds up in muscles and causes them to cramp. It is this buildup of waste material and its slow removal that causes discomfort to be felt for several days after intense or prolonged activities.

HEMATOMAS

Skeletal muscles in the leg or arm are organized in groups or compartments, with each compartment separated from the other by a sheath of tissue. Muscular *hematoma* refers to an isolated internal bruise from, for example, a blunt, hard blow to thigh muscle. The resulting bleeding within the muscle may slowly become reabsorbed or it may develop into one of two different types of hematomas. A significant bruise to muscle should be brought to the attention of a doctor. There are two types of muscular hematoma.

- **INTERMUSCULAR HEMATOMA:** When the injury occurs to the muscle *and* the sheath that separates

that muscle from other muscles, it is known as an *intermuscular hematoma.* This is the least problematic type of hematoma because the buildup of pressure from internal bleeding does not damage the muscle because the blood can spread over a large area. It eventually becomes reabsorbed.

- **INTRAMUSCULAR HEMATOMA:** This is a more serious condition that involves bleeding from a muscle or muscles within one compartment, in which the sheath enveloping that compartment is uninjured and intact. Blood from the injured muscle may cause pressure to build up within the compartment and literally strangulate the muscle so that no oxygen reaches it. This represents a medical emergency that requires immediate surgery to relieve pressure within the limb. Otherwise, use of the entire limb may be lost, because a muscle that is starved of oxygen cannot recover.

SIGNS AND SYMPTOMS

The signs and symptoms of a muscle injury include pain anywhere in the muscle that may go away somewhat during exercise, only to come back with a vengeance once exercise is over. Attempting to contract or stretch the muscle is painful and muscle weakness is prominent.

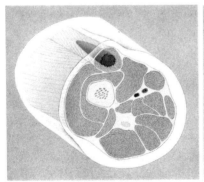 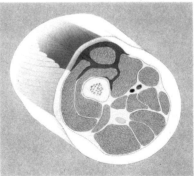

The left is an intermuscular hematoma. The right is an intramuscular hematoma.
Peterson L, Renstrom P: *Sports Injuries: Their Prevention and Treatment.* London: Martin Dunitz, Ltd., 1986.

■ PREVENTION AND TREATMENT

Different treatments are appropriate, depending upon whether the injury is acute (prior to 72 hours) or sub-acute (after 72 hours). Massage, stretching, strengthening, and range of motion should be avoided during the acute stage. During this time, the torn site within the muscle stops bleeding and begins to coagulate. Being overaggressive and doing any one of the aforementioned activities may cause bleeding to restart and should be avoided. A strained muscle can heal more quickly when rehabilitation is started early. Healing can take anywhere from 3 to 16 weeks. The return to athletic activity should be gradual.

■ **REST:** It is very important to rest in order to heal, although professional athletes do not easily accept the notion of rest. Sometimes, cross-training can act as a substitute to rest once healing is underway. However during the acute and sub-acute stage, rest is a necessity. Cycling and backstroke swimming are very good exercise substitutes for a person who has strained a leg muscle.

■ **ICE MASSAGE:** Ice gently rubbed over the affected muscle for up to 10 to 20 minutes at a time may reduce pain and inflammation, and also help reduce swelling.

■ **ELEVATION:** Elevating the affected limb helps reduce swelling and is best when done during the acute stage.

■ **COMPRESSION:** It is helpful to use compression in order to reduce swelling during the acute stage; this can often be applied using a compress or elastic bandage.

■ **PROTECTION:** The site of injury should be protected during the acute stage if there is a lot of pain. Use crutches or a cane on the side opposite to the injury if the injured muscle is in the leg. A sling may be worn if the injured muscle is in the arm. Walking carefully and using an elastic wrap may be helpful if the injured muscle is one of the muscles of the trunk.

■ **HEAT:** It is appropriate to apply heat during the sub-acute stage of injury (after 72 hours). The usual mode of heat delivery is a moist heating pad. Often, alternating cold and hot baths or compresses can help provide relief in the sub-acute stage.

■ **ULTRASOUND:** Ultrasound is a method of applying deep heat using electricity that passes through special crystals, which vibrate at high frequencies. This vibration penetrates deep into tissues as heat energy and may provide relief. Ultrasound applied in the pulsed mode may be used to deliver pain-relieving medications to the strained muscle. This method of medication delivery is known as *phonophoresis.*

■ **MEDICATION:** Oral anti-inflammatory medications can be used for short periods of time to help relieve pain and inflammation.

■ **RANGE OF MOTION:** These exercises include normal movements of the limb, as allowed by the joints. Passive range of motion is appropriate for the acute stage. This form of motion is done in such a way that another person moves the limb. The active range of motion exercises, where the individual actively moves his or her own limb, should only be performed after 72 hours have elapsed since the injury (sub-acute stage). All painful motions should be avoided. Performing these exercises in a pool can be very soothing.

- **STRENGTHENING EXERCISES:** Muscle strengthening exercises have the effect of organizing scar tissue so that it is aligned in such a way that it can better withstand stress. Begin with careful, isometric contraction exercises, followed by concentric and then eccentric exercises. Exercise progression should always be guided by pain. If it hurts, you are overdoing it. Backward walking and running is a good concentric exercise for the quadriceps muscles, whereas forward walking and running eccentrically works those muscles.

- **STRETCHING EXERCISES:** This type of gentle exercise involves strained muscles and may begin once the acute stage has passed. Stretching permits the muscle fibers to lie closer to each other and prevents the random alignment of new collagen fibers laid down at the site of injury. Instead, collagen is organized by the stretching activity, and it will become oriented in a way that best strengthens the injured muscle. A stretch of each muscle should last for at least 2 minutes at a time. The muscle on the other side of that joint, the antagonist muscle, should also be stretched.

- **MASSAGE:** Massage may benefit the healing muscle during the sub-acute state because it helps diminish swelling and stiffness. Massage should be done gently and should not be painful.

- **FRICTION MASSAGE:** Performing deep transverse friction massage is helpful in preventing sticky *adhesions*, which are congealed remnants of fluid resulting from the inflammatory process. These adhesions can develop between the individual muscle fibers and might restrict movement. This treatment is best performed by a physical therapist.

Back

ACK PAIN is the most common affliction known to humankind and causes quite a bit of misery. However, much of the pain and suffering resulting from back problems can be prevented by learning what movements cause injury and how to avoid them. Studies have shown that people who keep their backs in shape through proper exercise and stretching do not suffer from back pain.

20 Back Strain and Sprain

A 51-year-old, slightly overweight man set out to clear his driveway of 6 inches of snow from a recent storm. After about an hour and a half of continuous shoveling, he had finally cleared the driveway and was quite pleased with himself. The remainder of the day was uneventful, although he was very tired by bedtime. However, he felt severe pain in his entire back down to his buttocks the next morning when he woke up. He walked slowly and stiffly to the bathroom, taking small steps.
He could not bend over to wash his face or brush his teeth. Even standing up from sitting in a chair was very difficult. He has no recollection of having any pain while he was shoveling. However, afterwards his entire back was tender and his ability to move was limited and very uncomfortable. His leg strength was good and moving his legs was not painful. Lifting each leg up high, in turn, with the knee straight was not painful. This man has strained *his back muscles.*

A 39-year-old triage nurse at the local emergency room received a call alerting her that a person with severe bodily trauma was enroute via ambulance to the hospital. When the ambulance arrived, she went out to help lower the person to the ground. Instead of lowering the cot with two hands while facing it directly, she bent down with a twist to one side and gave it a tug to lift it up. She suddenly felt something snap in her low back, followed by severe pain that froze her in a bent over position. Hospital staff came to her aid and after several minutes she was able to gradually straighten up and the pain was considerably less. As she began to walk around again, the pain came back with an intensity that worsened as each hour of her shift dragged on. The pain was aggravated by any movement, and bending in any direction became impossible. Sitting down relieved her symptoms somewhat, although they returned when she tried to get up out of a chair. Lying flat on her back or on her side provided her with relief. She can point to the specific area in her low back that is most painful. She can raise herself off the ground when standing by rising up on her heels or standing on the ball of her feet. This is not painful, nor is standing or walking on the outer or inner borders of her feet. She can raise either leg, straight at the knee, very high without any pain. This woman has sprained *a ligament in her low back.*

BACK MUSCLES

THE MUSCLES that move the skeleton, including the bones of the back, are called *skeletal back muscles.* These muscles are quite small when you consider them individually, although they exert enormous force because they work together. The back muscles, together with the stomach muscles, move the back in various directions. They are known as *postural muscles* because they oppose gravity and work to hold the trunk up straight when sitting or standing.

BACK LIGAMENTS

Ligaments (from the Latin *ligare*, "to bind") are tough, fibrous bands that connect bones to each other at joints. Ligaments act as tie-pieces between bones, such as the ribs or the bones of the forearm, by fastening around or across bone ends in bands. In this way, ligaments serve to limit and guide the movement at joints, while preventing too much motion. They prevent injury if excessive motion occurs. The spine is a series of irregularly stacked bones that would fall apart into a confusing jumble, if not for the many ligaments that bind them together. Unfortunately, ligaments do not have a very good blood supply, which puts them at a disadvantage in terms of healing when a strain or tear occurs.

WORKING TOGETHER

The muscles and ligaments of the back are known as the *musculoligamentous complex*. They work hand-in-hand to brace the trunk and prevent injuries. The back is fairly stable when it is kept straight or arched backward. However, injury may occur when bending over in the forward direction because the bones connecting each segment at the spine disengage in the bent forward position, making the back especially vulnerable to injurious forces. Torsion forces that occur from backward twisting movements are even more injurious to the back.

When the back is bent over, it lacks stability. The disc located between the spinal segments is particularly vulnerable to becoming torn and damaged from twisting movements. The only protection to the back from injurious movements when the back

is in bent forward (in flexion) is the musculoligamentous complex, which protectively springs into action. However, even this complex may be bypassed by injurious forces if the bending or twisting movement is very sudden, or if the muscles are tired and fatigued. Injuries are likely to occur after excessive activity or if there is a lack of proper rest. Therefore, in order to avoid back injuries, beware of fatigue and quick bending or twisting movements of the spine.

MUSCLE STRAIN

Muscle and tendons are made up of minute muscle filaments that move together (contract and move apart (distract) in much the same way that a sliding door moves sideways into and out of a wall. Individual muscle fibers may become stretched, frayed, or torn if they are forced to work beyond capacity. Muscles and tendons are strained if they are injured and there is no direct bruise or cut. A *muscle strain* occurs from sudden contraction or distraction of the attachments of a muscle, which may either result in a *stretch* or *tear* of muscle fibers. Overworking the muscles of the spine may occur during labor-intensive activities such as snow shoveling. This activity is considered unusually stressful to the muscles of the back and may cause injury when performed to excess. Additionally, shoveling snow is implicated in severe injury of another important body muscle: the heart, as illustrated by the many middle-aged people who experience heart attacks while shoveling snow!

The torn space is not filled in by new muscle tissue when a tear of skeletal muscle occurs. Instead, a poorer quality tissue called *scar tissue* fills the gap. Muscle tissue works well because its fibers run parallel with each other, which distributes force evenly throughout the muscle. However, the fibers making up scar tissue do not contract and are randomly ori-

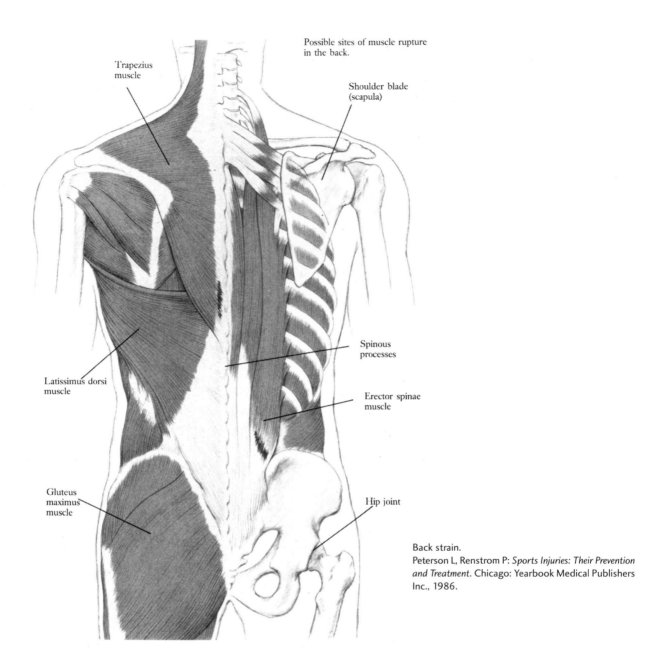

Possible sites of muscle rupture in the back.

Trapezius muscle

Shoulder blade (scapula)

Spinous processes

Latissimus dorsi muscle

Erector spinae muscle

Gluteus maximus muscle

Hip joint

Back strain.
Peterson L, Renstrom P: *Sports Injuries: Their Prevention and Treatment*. Chicago: Yearbook Medical Publishers Inc., 1986.

ented. They represent a weak site in muscle that is prone to failure with excessive stretching or contraction. The injured muscle is considered weakened and more prone to re-injury because scar tissue is not as strong or capable as muscle.

A *mild muscle strain* (1st degree strain) occurs from overstretching or minor tearing of a muscle or tendon and often heals without treatment. Back symptoms stemming from muscle strain are also caused by muscle spasms.

■ MUSCLE SPASMS

One of the most common back problems is muscle spasms (cramps) that occur during or after intense or prolonged exercise. (See Chapters 2 and 19.) During activities that require brief, intense, bursts of energy, muscles attempt to generate more energy by drawing on stored sugars. They also utilize oxygen when they are working. Intense bursts of energy require more oxygen than readily available, and so muscles work *anaerobically*, meaning "without oxygen." This process is less efficient in the long run and allows for increased power at the expense of generating a waste product known as *lactic acid*. This by-product builds up in muscles and causes them to cramp. It is this buildup of waste material and its slow removal that causes discomfort to be felt for several days after intense or prolonged activities.

■ LIGAMENT SPRAIN

In general, ligaments are not capable of stretching and are therefore able to bind the two ends of a joint securely, like taut adhesive tape. Ligaments are so strong that they are stronger even than bone, and they will occasionally pull away a fleck of bone where they attach rather than tear. When a force is applied to a joint, protective ligaments prevent the bones from separating. However, if the force is large or multiplied by speed, such as when quickly twisting or bending over, the force is just too much for the ligament to withstand, and it will tear.

A torn ligament is called a *sprain,* and it results in a less stable joint. Ligament injuries occur quite often, especially in the ankle and knee joints, and they are very painful. A mild sprain (grade I sprain) involves a tear of only a few ligament fibers, while a moderate sprain (grade II sprain) involves a tear of less than one-half of the fibers making up that liga-ment. A complete sprain (grade III sprain) involves a rupture of all of the fibers in the ligament. Aside from pain, a ligament sprain involves bleeding that will cause the neighboring joint to swell up after the injury. The affected joint will usually turn blue or purple the next day.

When a ligament tear occurs, the torn space is not filled in by new ligament tissue. Like muscle, poorer quality *scar tissue* fills the gap. This distributes force unevenly throughout the ligament and represents a weak site that is prone to failure with excessive joint motion. Because scar tissue is not as strong or capable as the ligament, it is weakened and more likely to be re-injured in the future.

■ SIGNS AND SYMPTOMS

The differences between a back *strain* and a back *sprain* become obvious when we compare the differences in how the injury occurred and what it felt like. The common denominator for both is pain, and localized swelling and tenderness when palpating the site of injury.

Ligament injuries are often accompanied by a snapping or popping sound, and there will be a specific area of pain that is readily accessible to the probing finger. Pain is felt immediately and gets worse gradually. The area over the torn ligament will probably not be swollen because the ligaments of the back are very deeply located.

Pain occurs many hours later with muscular strain rather than at the time of injury. Typically, the person wakes up the next morning with legs so sore, stiff, and tender that he can barely walk. The pain and tenderness derived from muscular strain generally extends over a very wide area. Whereas, pain will be confined to a specific area when there is a ligament sprain.

■ CONDITIONS TO RULE OUT

■ **SPINAL STENOSIS:** This is a condition where the spinal cord or the nerve roots coming out of the spinal cord in the low back are pinched by arthritic outgrowths of spinal bone. The space surrounding the nerves of the spinal cord is diminished when this occurs, which causes pressure on the nerves. This often happens in older people. The resulting pain radiates to the thighs and calves. It is often relieved by bending forward slightly in a stooped posture.

■ **DEGENERATIVE DISC DISEASE:** This type of disease occurs when the degenerative changes that accompany increasing age or excessive activity cause a breakdown of the intervertebral disc. People with *degenerative disc disease* (DDD) avoid sitting in soft chairs, but often feel comfortable in hard chairs. Flexion is usually not restricted with DDD and symptoms gradually diminish with activity. In contrast, with muscle or ligament injury to the low back, all movements are restricted and sitting in any type of chair brings relief. It is only painful when trying to get up out of a chair.

■ **ACUTE ANNULAR TEAR:** The *annulus* is the tough covering of the intervertebral spinal disc, and it can become torn. The pain from an acute annular tear can be confused with a spinal ligamentous sprain. While an acute annular tear is deeply located and not provoked by pinpoint tenderness, localization is often possible on palpation with a ligamentous tear. With a ligamentous sprain, pain would have been constant from the outset, particularly during spinal movement. The pain may ease off for a short while, only to recur and persist unless the person lies down. In contrast, a person with an acute disc tear of the outer annulus (prolapse) cannot entirely alleviate pain by the recumbent position, especially if the inner nuclear gel within the disc oozes outward and presses on the posterior longitudinal ligament, in which case pain will be felt even while lying down.

■ **ACUTE LOCKED BACK SYNDROME:** There are two important joints at the back of every spinal level called *facet joints* that lock that level of the spine into the space and prevent it from moving in directions that would injure the spinal cord or nerves. Sometimes, bending over in one direction, especially when done quickly, can cause one of these facet joints to move out of alignment with the other, resulting in what is called "locking." This condition can be agonizingly painful because the joint capsule surrounding the facet joint is well innervated with pain receptors. It can happen from something as trivial as bending over to pick up a piece of paper or from an unguarded movement during sleep. Pain in the back rarely radiates below the knee, although it can be so intense as to prevent one from being able to stand up straight. Any movement will worsen symptoms. Walking is accomplished by taking small steps and stair climbing will be impossible. Muscle strength and reflexes in the legs will be normal. Raising the legs will be painful and x-rays will appear normal. Often, people report similar episodes in the past. While symptoms can slowly resolve over several days, manipulation—whether performed by a chiropractor, physical therapist, or osteopathic physician—can help speed up the process and often results in immediate relief.

■ PREVENTION AND TREATMENT

■ **COLD THERAPY:** Cold may be applied in the form of an ice compress or ice massage in order to decrease spasm, inflammation, pain, and capillary blood flow. It is particularly helpful in cases of acute ligament sprain. Although the skin cools quickly, the rate of muscle cooling is directly proportionate to the thickness of overlying fat and may range from 10 to 20 minutes. Because of this, pain stemming from muscle strain to a particular area may require more than 20 minutes of cold application.

- **HEAT:** It is appropriate during the sub-acute or chronic states to apply heat, which can be delivered by using a moist heating pad.

- **ULTRASOUND:** Ultrasound is another method of applying deep heat using electricity that passes through special crystals, which vibrate at high frequencies. This vibration penetrates deep into tissues as heat energy and may helps minimize spasm and pain.

- **IONTOPHORESIS:** This is a method of delivering medication through the skin into superficial areas that are painful and inflamed. Ionitophoresis may be used to deliver hydrocortisone, xylocaine, or salicitate for immediate temporary relief and it may help validate a suspected superficial ligamentous injury. Phonophoresis is another way to deliver these medications to the painful site using pulsed ultrasound.

- **MEDICATIONS:** Pharmacological treatments taken orally can be categorized into *analgesics* that relieve pain, *anti-inflammatory medications*, and *muscle relaxants*. Anti-inflammatory drugs have both an anti-inflammatory and analgesic effect that promotes healing by increasing circulation and bringing necessary nutrients into the inflamed area and eliminating toxic inflammatory substances. This allows the person to perform the activities of daily life and more fully participate in physical therapy. Anti-inflammatory medications appear to be effective for relieving back pain if started within two days of onset of acute low back pain. Muscle relaxants operate by relieving skeletal muscle spasm in the back without interfering with muscular function. In this manner, they promote the greater mobility that is essential to the healing process. *Opiate* analgesics are appropriate for severely acute back pain. There is little chance for addiction if they are used for a short period of time. However, using opiates for longer periods of time for chronic back pain is not a good idea.

- **ELECTRIC STIMULATION:** This may be done by transcutaneous electrical nerve stimulation (TENS). It may reduce acute muscle spasm, decrease edema, and relieve pain.

- **INJECTIONS:** Selective therapeutic short- or long-acting injection of steroids and anesthetics into the area in which ligament disruption occurred may provide relief. Administration may be performed by a doctor. Injections may help confirm a suspected ligament tear.

- **BRACING:** A lumbosacral support or corset can be used to minimize movement of the back, thereby decreasing pain. This can be helpful to the person with a muscle strain. Use of a corset made of elastic or a more rigid material will also prevent postural changes while the ligament attempts to repair itself.

- **STRENGTHENING:** People with postural strain syndrome should exercise those weakened muscles that are excessively flexible. For example, people with excessive *hyperlordosis* (a posture of the low back that is excessively concave) should strengthen the abdominal and hamstrings muscles, and stretch the tight psoas and paraspinal musculature. Performing sit-ups with the hips and knees flexed activates the abdominal muscles. However, exercises should not be performed through a large range of motion as this will increase pressure on the lumbar disc. *Trunk curls* are best performed in a limited range of motion so that the shoulder blade just clears the floor, thereby minimizing strain to the lumbar spine while still successfully recruiting the abdominal muscles. A *reverse trunk-curl* is performed with the hips and knees flexed in such a way that the knees are brought up to the chest. This position also strengthens the abdominal muscles, while limiting stress to the lumbar spine. Spinal flexion exercises should not be done when there is ligament sprain because they will stress the injured ligaments. Instead, spinal extension exercises may be performed in the prone position. For example, lying on your stomach with a pillow placed under the abdomen to avoid stress on the spinal discs. Spinal extension exercises should not be performed when there is muscular strain because they might stress the injured muscle(s).

■ **STRETCHING:** Many large muscles span the trunk and legs and affect the low back because of their insertion at the pelvis. Stretching of all the muscles of the trunk (both stomach and back) should begin slowly. Avoid motions that provoke pain.

The stretch may be held for longer periods as symptoms recede and can compass a gradually enlarging range of motion. The hip flexors and extensors, in particular, should be stretched, because tightness of these muscles will rotate the pelvis excessively and may negatively impact on both posture and the magnitude of lumbar lordosis. *Hyperlordosis* is associated with anterior pelvic tilt, which causes the pelvis to rotate forward due to tightened hip flexors. Tight hamstrings cause a pull on the pelvis and rotate it backwards, increasing the shear forces in the low back and resulting in a "flat back." Stretching helps to offset the effects of these improper postures by gaining extensibility of these large and important muscles.

■ **ENDURANCE TRAINING:** Keeping the heart and lungs fit (known as cardiopulmonary fitness) is extremely important and may include brisk walking, jogging, swimming, tennis, and stationary bicycle activities. Many people find that brisk walking eases discomfort. Aerobic fitness exercise should emphasize activities that avoid high-impact and ballistic-type spinal movements.

21 Postural Back Strain

A 45-year-old housewife has had three children in the last 4 years, two of whom were fraternal twin boys. She is about 30 lbs. overweight and complains of chronic low back pain that cannot be traced to a specific event. Her pain has increased to the point of interfering with daily activities over the last several months. These episodes last for several days and then settle down. Her back pain, which is never felt in her thigh or legs, gets worse when she tries to bend over while washing the dishes, ironing clothes, or performing other similar movements. Standing, sitting, or walking for more than an hour and a half exacerbates her symptoms. Carrying heavy packages worsens her pain. She exercised regularly prior to getting married 7 years ago, although now she admits to feeling overwhelmed by her domestic responsibilities and no longer has time to participate in any sports-related activities. She has poor posture, including a rounded upper back and protruding abdomen and buttocks. She can walk on the sides of her feet as well as on her heels and toes, and can easily bend over and touch her toes. The source of this woman's back pain is postural back strain *syndrome, which is a very frequently encountered condition that occurs in people who are chronically inactive, overweight, and who have faulty posture.*

■ THE EFFECTS OF POSTURE

Good posture is the body position that minimally stresses the joints. Posture is something that is affected by many factors, including genetics, body type, and emotional state. Emotions certainly have an effect on head and neck posture. The individual who feels defeated by life will slump his shoulders and allow his head to sag down in depression. This posture is also assumed by a person who is embarrassed and experiences "loss of face." The classic image of a truck driver is someone who sits high in a 22-wheeler with both shoulders arched high, gripping a big steering wheel. Holding these and similar postures habitually can cause the muscles of the shoulder and neck to become accustomed to these positions. Even when the truck driver stops driving, or when the sad person feels happy, they may assume their accustomed positions.

Posture is dependent on the condition of the muscles spanning the limbs and surrounding the joints. Muscles that surround a joint should ideally pull equally across that joint. If one muscle is tighter, the opposite muscle will be lax and an imbalanced force will occur at the joint, causing abnormal posturing of that joint. The accumulated stress to the joint may stretch and weaken the ligaments that bind the joint together. It may even cause arthritic changes between the bony surfaces making up the joint. These factors play a very important role when we consider the muscles of the thigh and trunk that attach onto the pelvis.

PELVIC TILT

In order to understand the concept of *pelvic tilt*, we must understand what the pelvis is and how we use it. Many people think of the pelvis in terms of the gyrating movements of the late, great Elvis Presley. Belly dancers captivate audiences by rapidly tilting their pelvis to and fro in seductive ways. You have undoubtedly learned to perform these pelvic tilt exercises if you have been to a La Maze training class on natural childbirth. The pelvis can be tilted or rotated, although we do not usually do this during the regular course of the day. Cattle ranchers regularly undergo pelvic tilt, however, because riding a horse imparts a gyration to the upper body that is best tol-

erated by having the upper body rotate via the pelvis on the relatively immobile hips and buttocks. Pelvic tilting is accomplished by a synergy or cooperation of the two sets of muscles that attach onto the pelvis: the muscles of the trunk and upper leg.

■ THE PELVIS

The *pelvis* is the strong bony bowl that holds many of our internal organs. From a musculoskeletal point of view, it is the site of attachment of many of the powerful muscles of the thigh and hip, including the hamstrings, quadriceps, and adductors. It is also the attachment site for many of the trunk and back muscles. Changes in the length of the leg muscles caused by tight muscles may cause problems at the low back because the pelvis serves as the common attachment site for the trunk and upper leg muscles.

■ THE PELVIS AND POSTURE

Excessive sitting, lack of stretching or strengthening exercises, and being overweight can cause harmful posture in several ways. Several things happen when we tilt our pelvis forward in an *anterior pelvic tilt*: our quadriceps contract and shorten, our abdomen protrudes, and our low back becomes more concave, which is a condition called *lordosis*. This is known as the *sway back posture*. It is typical of the couch potato or the woman who has recently given birth. A person who overeats will develop an unflattering, protruding abdomen, which can cause pelvic tilting. The back will become sway backed and the quadriceps muscles at the front of the thigh will adapt to a shortened position. The problem with this posture is that the available space for the nerve roots to exit the spinal cord is made smaller, making them more likely to become compressed. Lack of

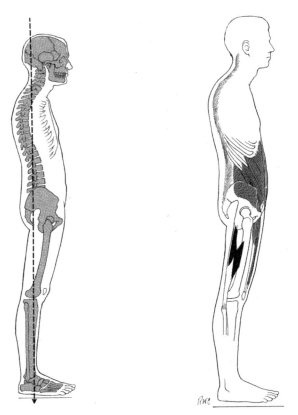

Sway back posture.
Kendall FP, McCreary EK, Provance PG: *Muscles: Testing and Function,*
4th Edition. Baltimore: Williams & Wilkins, 1993.

exercise can also weaken the abdominal muscles and cause tightness of either the hamstrings or quadriceps muscles.

Other problems can also occur. For example, when we tilt our pelvis backwards the hamstring muscles in the back of the thigh shorten and the lower back and abdomen flatten out in a military type of posture.

It is very easy to have these postures dominate the way we stand, sit, and move when we do not take care of ourselves. These harmful postures develop over time and can cause pain in certain areas of the body. For example, the joints of the spine do not like either the sway or straight back posture, and can develop arthritic changes that compress the nerve roots coming out to the limbs. Paying attention to your posture, taking care of yourself by stretching and strengthening regularly, and thinking positive can all impact positively on posture.

Shortened Quads vs. Hams

The armchair executive who sits all day and personifies the attitude of "all work—no play" eventually develops tight hamstrings because the hamstrings will assume a new shortened length in what is known as *tightness* or a *muscle contracture* after sitting for long periods. When this person eventually stands up to go home or go to the bathroom, his tight hamstrings will pull on his pelvis in such a way that the pelvis will tilt the low back into a more flattened than normal position known as *flat back*. This has the effect of increasing the shear forces at the lower back.

Most important, developing tightness or weakness in either the trunk or the muscles spanning the hip and thigh can reinforce postural imbalance in such a way that a vicious cycle is set up in which tightness or laxity of either the thigh or trunk muscles will cause problems by way of the pelvis. For example, a shortened thigh muscle will cause changes in the abdomen and low back that in turn reinforce the shortened thigh muscles. Identifying these problems and breaking out of this cycle is essential. A physical therapy evaluation is recommended.

Postural Strain

There are many causes of faulty posture. Wearing high-heeled shoes throws the chest outward and the buttocks backward, causing increased lumbar lordosis, shortened quadriceps muscles, and shortened calf muscles and Achilles tendons. Women who

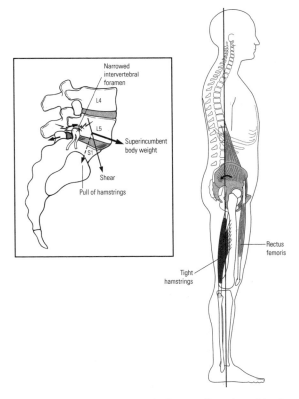

Tight hamstring muscles in the thigh can pull on the pelvis, thereby lessening the space available for the nerve root to emerge from the spine. Saidoff DC, McDonough AL: *Critical Pathways in Therapeutic Intervention: Extremities and Spine.* St. Louis: Mosby, 2002.

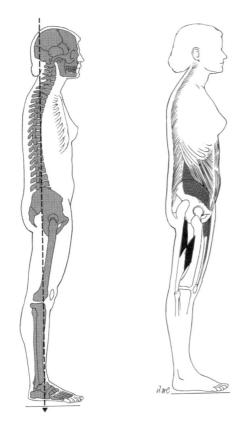

Flat back posture.
Kendall FP, McCreary EK, Provance PG: *Muscles: Testing and Function*, 4th Edition. Baltimore: Williams & Wilkins, 1993.

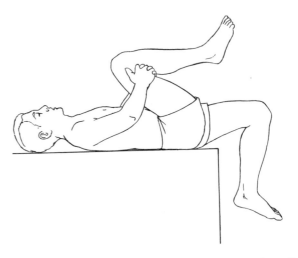

A positive Thomas test is indicated by the left leg that remains on the table. The left hip rises up instead of remaining on the table, indicating tightness of the hip flexor muscles located in the front of the thigh and pelvis. Kendall FP, McCreary EK, Provance PG: *Muscles: Testing and Function*, 4th Edition. Baltimore: Williams & Wilkins, 1993.

have several children in successive years may experience a sagging abdomen as well as back pain from residual lordosis of the back from the many months of pregnancy. These changes in posture will weaken the muscles and ligaments protecting the joints of the spine if the problem is not addressed. The chronic pulling on many of the ligaments and tendons attaching to the spine, which are well innervated by pain receptors, is experienced as *postural strain*. Although patients with postural pain are often free of pain after a good night's rest, maintaining faulty posture throughout the day may lead to backaches during the day that get worse with each passing year. Eventually, the strain on the ligaments and muscles causes them to fatigue, so that

they are more liable to experience an acute injury such as a herniated disc. Alternately, strain accumulates in the form of arthritic changes to the low back, which increases low back pain.

■ SIGNS AND SYMPTOMS

The person with postural back strain typically complains of chronic, mild low back pain that is aggravated by prolonged sitting, walking, and especially standing. Relief is experienced when lying down and when sitting for short periods of time. All spinal motions are typically within functional limits. Frequently, chores such as washing dishes, doing the laundry, and vacuuming aggravate discomfort. Although chronic degenerative disc disease with mild facet arthrosis may mimic this condition, x-rays will reveal no abnormalities, with the exception of an increased lumbosacral angle. The person often demonstrates a *positive Thomas test*, indicating tight hip flexor muscles. Symptoms in these people generally result from chronically poor posture secondary to inadequate musculature. The abdomen is prominent when standing and the lumbar lordosis is increased, which can strain the pain-sensitive soft tissues of the low back.

■ CONDITIONS TO RULE OUT

■ Herniated disc refers to a tear or rupture of the intervertebral disc at one of the levels of the spine in the low back area. The torn disc often pushes on the nerve root, causing pain to be felt in the buttocks, or even the thigh, leg, or foot. Often, there is weakness of the muscles of one leg as well as changes in reflexes.

■ Back sprain refers to a stretched or torn ligament that causes immediate back pain that does not radiate into the buttocks or legs. Instead, pain is localized to one area after bending over and suddenly lifting something heavy. A popping sound may be heard. The strength in the leg muscles or reflexes is not affected with this condition.

■ Back strain refers to a muscular ache or tear that occurs from excessive sudden and unusual activity—for example, shoveling an entire driveway of snow. Symptoms are usually not felt the day of the excessive activity, but the next morning there will be stiffness and pain. The strength in the leg muscles and reflexes are not affected with this condition.

■ PREVENTION AND TREATMENT

Regular stretching of the trunk and legs is the most important strategy in maintaining good posture. It is especially important to stretch the large muscles groups of the thigh and legs, including the quadriceps, hamstrings, adductors, iliotibial band, calf muscles, and Achilles tendon complex. Do not stretch to the point of pain. Work up to your individual tolerance level slowly and stop just short of pain.

■ **START SLOWLY:** Do not rush into an exercise program. Ease into it at a relaxed pace and build up tolerance. Increase your activity over time and stop short of pain. Do not stretch to the point of pain the very first time you stretch. Do not improve your extensibility at the price of sore or strained muscles.

■ **WARM UP:** Warm up before beginning any exercise. Not warming up is like turning on your car engine on a cold day and driving off without allowing the engine to properly warm up. Stretching is a great way to warm up before moving on to other activities.

■ **APPLYING HEAT:** Soft tissue is more easily stretched when warm than when cold. Therefore, taking a hot shower or bath prior to stretching helps soften up muscles, making stretching exercises more comfortable.

■ **HOLD THE STRETCH:** Hold stretches for 30 to 60 seconds and count 1,000, 1,001, 1,002, 1,003, etc. to ensure that you do not speed up too quickly. Holding a stretch helps preserve any extensibility gained from the stretch.

■ **BOUNCING:** Do not bounce into a stretch because it can cause microtrauma within muscle tissue, which will be filled in with scar tissue. This weakens the muscle and predisposes it to further injury.

■ **COOL DOWN:** Do not stop stretching, strengthening, or aerobic exercise abruptly. Instead, slow down gradually.

- **AEROBIC EXERCISES:** Strengthening and stretching exercises should be performed for 20 to 25 minutes at least three times per week in order to have a significant physiological impact.

- **KNOW YOUR LIMITS:** Do not overdo it. Pace yourself. Do a little bit the first day, a little more the next, and so on. In this way, your body can reap the benefits of exercise in a safe manner. Back off for a day or two if a muscle starts to get sore and then return to exercise after the pain eases up.

- **USE THE RIGHT EQUIPMENT:** Wearing the correct shoes and using the correct sports equipment can go a long way in preserving safety and avoiding injury.

- **ASK QUESTIONS:** Do not be afraid to ask if you are unsure about something. Be sure to ask an athletic trainer or physical therapist, no matter how trivial you think your question is.

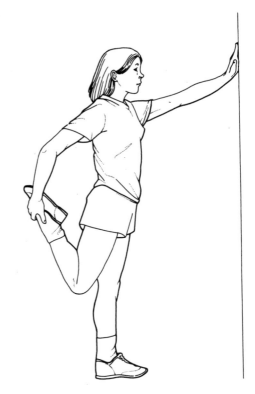

Stretching the hip flexor muscles.
Levy AM, Fuerst ML: *Sport Injury Handbook: Professional Advice for Amateur Athletes.* New York: John Wiley & Sons, Inc., 1993.

STRETCHING DIFFERENT MUSCLE GROUPS

- **HIP FLEXORS:** The hip flexor muscles are the *psoas* and *quadriceps muscles.* They contract when you flex your hip in order to bring your knee upward toward your face. These muscles can be stretched by lying on your back on a table or bed with your leg and hip as near the edge as possible and then letting your leg hang over the side in a relaxed position for at least 30 seconds before repeating. Alternately, you can grab your ankle behind you and pull upward. You will feel a definite stretch over the front of your thigh.

- **HIP EXTENSORS:** The hip extensors are primarily the *hamstring muscles.* They bring your leg behind you when you contract them. A good way to stretch these muscles is by lying on the floor next to a doorway and raising one leg against the door until you feel a slight stretch behind your knee. Hold for 30 seconds and repeat, and then do the same for the other leg. Lift your leg farther up the wall as your feel your hamstrings stretch during subsequent stretches.

- **HIP ADDUCTORS:** These thigh muscles are active when you cross one leg over the other. A good way to stretch them is to lie on your back on a firm surface with your hips and knee bent, holding your feet flat against the surface. Gently allow your knees to fall apart, while keeping the soles of

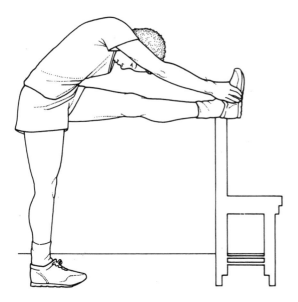

While standing, put one foot on a chair in front of you. Now bend your forehead forward and try to touch it with your knee. Use the same number of repetitions as for the toe-touch exercises. Repeat with the other leg. Levy AM, Fuerst ML: *Sport Injury Handbook: Professional Advice for Amateur Athletes*. New York: John Wiley & Sons, Inc., 1993.

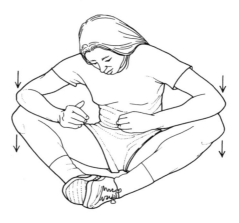

While sitting down, bend your knees so that the soles of your feet are touching each other. Now put your elbows on your knees and gradually push them outwards. Hold for 20 to 30 seconds. Levy AM, Fuerst ML: *Sport Injury Handbook: Professional Advice for Amateur Athletes*. New York: John Wiley & Sons, Inc., 1993.

your feet together, until you feel a stretch to your inner thighs. Hold for 30 seconds and then repeat.

- **HIP ABDUCTORS:** The hip abductors move the hip and thigh away from the body. Stretching the iliotibial band is a good way to stretch the hip abductors. See the illustration in Chapter 16 on page 143 for a good way to stretch the iliotibial band without any help from someone else. Count to 30 and then repeat the stretch.

- **CALF AND ACHILLES TENDON:** Stretching the calf muscle and Achilles tendon may be accomplished by way of a wall lean stretch with the knee in full extension. Stretches are best performed gently and slowly, and without bouncing. Passive gentle stretching via a wall *push-up* is one of the most important strategies in management of

Achilles tendon disease. Stretching by way of a wall lean stretch with the knee in full extension is shown in Chapter 21 on page 178.

- **LOW BACK STRETCH:** There are two very good stretching exercises known as Williams flexion exercises that should only be done if you do not have a history of back pain or problems. Otherwise, consult your doctor first. Pull your right knee toward your chest and shoulder with both hands and hold for 30 seconds before returning to the starting position. Do the same for the other knee. In the second exercise, pull up both knees to your shoulders, curl up into a ball, and hold for three seconds.

- **CAT STRETCH:** This is a good stretch for the low back. Get down on your hands and knees and let your back slowly sag down toward the floor. Then slowly arch your back away from the floor.

22 Pinched Back Nerve

A 35-year-old man came home from work, and just as he walked through the door he was greeted by his wife with a request to take out the garbage. He put down his briefcase and immediately walked out to the back of the house where the garbage cans were kept. He bent over at the waist to lift the first can, unaware that his wife had placed about 50 lbs. of old books and magazines in the can earlier in the day. He lifted the can quickly and almost immediately he felt an intense, stabbing pain in his lower back, followed by another sharp pain shooting down the back of his right leg into his foot. He dropped the garbage can and tried to straighten up, but the pain remained intense in both his lower back and his right leg. He also noticed that parts of his leg felt a little numb. He cried out for help and his wife came to help him get inside. He tried lying down on the couch and noticed that certain positions were more comfortable than others, but the pain was continuous and exacerbated by any movement of his right leg. This man has just experienced a pinched back nerve from a herniated *(slipped)* disc *in his lumbar spine.*

■ LOW BACK PAIN IS A COMMON EXPERIENCE

Low back pain is a problem that afflicts people of all ages, although the cause of the pain might differ based on age. Low back pain is estimated to affect at least 90% of all adults in the U.S. at some time during their lives. It is second only to upper respiratory problems as a reason to visit a doctor. More than $5 billion is spent on diagnosis and treatment of low back pain every year. Disability associated with low back pain is the most common cause of activity limitation in adults less than 45 years old, and it is second only to arthritis in those aged greater than 45 years old. As we will see, the term *low back pain* is used to describe virtually any type of pain originating in the lower back. However, it has numerous causes that differ greatly in each case. Not every cause of low back pain originates in the spine, although the majority does.

Ninety-three percent of all pain that originates from the spine comes from the five vertebrae in the lower portion of the spine (lumbosacral region), as compared with 7% from the seven vertebrae in the cervical spine (the neck region), and only 0.2% from the twelve vertebrae of the thoracic spine.

■ RISK FACTORS

Risk factors for low back pain include obesity, smoking, poor posture, menopause, osteoporosis, long-term steroid use, and age. Some of these risk factors cannot be changed (age, for example, although admittedly it would be nice). The water content of the intervertebral disc is about 85% in the preadolescent, but it diminishes to approximately 70% in middle-aged adults because the chemistry within the disc changes with age. Less water translates into less resiliency and a diminished ability to withstand stress, making the low back more vulnerable to a disc-related injury. Other age-related changes include arthritic changes in the bones near the disc, which cause arthritic outgrowths of bone that are more likely to aggravate a nerve.

Other risk factors including smoking are fairly obvious, and though there may not yet be absolute convincing scientific evidence that smoking is as important a risk factor as it now appears to be, there are numerous other good reasons to stop smoking. Cigarette smoking is thought to contribute to back problems because it robs the vertebrae of nutrients and lowers the available oxygen supply needed for proper fusion and healing. Estrogen replacement and alternatives to steroid therapy may help prevent serious back conditions.

Occupations that involve heavy lifting obviously place the low back at greater risk for injury. Vibration is common to truck drivers and jackhammer operators, and it is believed to increase the risk of back pain because of diminished disc nutrition secondary to spasm of the arteries that provide nutrients to the disc. High-risk groups for low back pain are those who spend much of their time sitting and bending forward—for example, office executives, clerks, secretaries and other computer operators, and truck drivers. This is because the greatest amounts of force are applied to the vertebral disc in the sitting position.

■ THE LUMBAR SPINE— ALSO KNOWN AS THE LOW BACK

The anatomic purpose of the lower back is to support the entire torso, shoulders, and head, and maintain the body in an upright posture. For the typical adult, this constitutes more than half of the body weight. The entire mass force from the weight of the upper portion of the body is focused down-wards onto the *lumbar spine*, that portion of the spine known as the *low back*. The spine supports this weight while standing, walking, running, and even while sitting. For the most part, the spine is built powerfully enough to accommodate the incredible stress associated with providing this type of support. At times, however, changes in body weight, the weight of objects held or carried, or other types of activities in which the body is engaged, may stress the lower spine, resulting in pain and sometimes other problems. To properly understand the nature of this stress and how best to prevent possible injury, it is necessary to review the basic anatomy of the lower back.

■ SPINE

The *spine* is a long, bony structure that begins just below the skull and ends at the *coccyx* (tailbone), which is a tiny bone at the very end of the sacrum that is the vestigial remnant of a tail left over from our biological ancestors. The functional center of the lower back is the *lumbar spinal column*.

The spine consists of twenty-four bones that are stacked one upon another and rest upon the fused bones of the sacrum. The primary purpose of the spine is to provide a bony armor to protect that delicate, whitish-looking, half-inch cable known as the *spinal cord*. We would not be able to turn and bend if the spine were one massive body column. The virtue of this multiple, small, stacked bones arrangement is that it allows the trunk to bend in different directions, even as much as 180 degrees of rotation, such as when you turn around to look over your shoulder.

The smallest spinal bones are located at the top of the spine. They support the head. These are called the *cervical vertebrae*, and they are found in the neck. The next twelve bones below the cervical vertebrae are connected to the bones of the rib cage and are called the *thoracic vertebrae,* and they are found in the chest. These vertebrae are hooked to the ribs and do not have a wide range of movement. These thoracic vertebrae are larger than the cervical spine bones, but smaller than the very large bones that lie below them. The largest bones are the vertebrae of the lumbar spine: the *lumbar vertebrae.* All of the other bones rest upon them; they form the heart of the lower back. In addition to the complex structure of the bony portions of the spine, the lower back also contains numerous muscles, ligaments, joints, and membranes. This highly complicated structure is subject to injury and stress-related pain at virtually every level.

Coming off the sides of the vertebral body and going towards the back of the spine (posteriorly) are two small bones called the *pedicles.* They form a bridge of sorts between the vertebral body in front and the posterior portions of the vertebrae in the back. They attach to a piece of bone that runs on the side of the vertebrae called a *lamina.* Bony horns grow out of the lamina on the side of the vertebrae. They are called the *transverse processes.* A large horn protrudes from the back-most portion of the vertebrae and is called the *spinous process.* The ring formed by the vertebral body in front, the pedicles and lamina on the side, and the spinous process in the back contains and protects the spinal canal where the spinal cord and nerve roots are located. The spinal cord itself does not continue all the way to the end of the spinal column. It generally ends about the level of the first or second lumbar vertebrae. Only nerve roots proceed further down the spine in a stringy tangle called a *cauda equina,* which means "horse's tail" because it resembles a horse's tail.

The vertebrae are stacked upon one another, leaving a small tunnel running from the spinal canal, through the ring of bone, and then outside the spine to the rest of the body. At each spinal level, two nerves exit the spinal canal (one on each side)

that go to the skin (in the case of *sensory nerves*), to muscles (in the case of *motor nerves*), or to organs (in the case of sensory, motor, and *autonomic nerves*). Severe pain and loss of normal function of the nerve results when the nerves running through these narrow tunnels become compressed. This will be discussed in more detail in the following section.

▓ SPINAL CURVES

The 33 vertebrae, 23 discs, 31 pairs of emerging spinal nerves, 400 muscles, and 1,000 ligaments are arranged into four gentle curves. In quadrupeds, the spine acts as a nicely balanced suspension bridge. However, the human spine is not well designed for our two-legged structure. The bones of the spinal column rest upon one another in a vertical line that is subject to damage by gravity. The

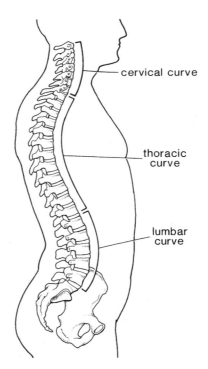

The curves of the spine. Siegel IM: *All About Bone: An Owner's Manual.* Demos, 1998.

spine curves noticeably at both the cervical level and the lumbar level due to the weight of the body. These curvatures are important for the task of supporting the upper half of the body weight, particularly when engaged in physical activity. These arches also act like a spring to absorb the jarring forces passed up and down the spine with each step.

THE INTERVERTEBRAL DISC

Each bone of the lumbar spine consists of a very large cylindrical portion called the *vertebral body.* This portion of the vertebrae lies in the front (anterior region) of the spine and provides most of the actual structural support.

Between each vertebral body lies a soft sac called an *intervertebral disc,* and the combined total of them adds an extra 6 inches of height to the spinal column. These discs were first described by the great Belgian anatomist Andreas Vesalius in 1555. They are almost entirely filled with fluid and resemble a balloon filled with water. Erect posture during the daytime causes compressive force, which results in loss of height. Sleeping for as little as 5 hours per night allows the discs to assume their normally full, rounded condition. Indeed, astronauts who returned to Earth after almost 80 days in space were found to be almost 2 inches taller than they were at liftoff because of the absence of the compressive force of gravity on the spinal discs.

Each of the twenty-three vertebral discs allows the two vertebral bodies that lie above it and below it to move against one another, permitting some degree of flexibility to the spine. The sac consists of a soft, gelatinous center called the *nucleus pulposus* and a peripheral fibrous ring called the *annulus fibrosus.* It cushions some of the forces transmitted along the vertical spine. If the fibrous ring ruptures, the soft gelatinous core can squeeze out like toothpaste coming out of a tube. This is a condition commonly called a *herniated* or *slipped disc* and often results in severe low back pain.

COMMON CAUSES OF LOW BACK PAIN

Diagnosis of low back pain is difficult, given the complexity of the structure of the low back and the numerous parts that can be injured. It is estimated

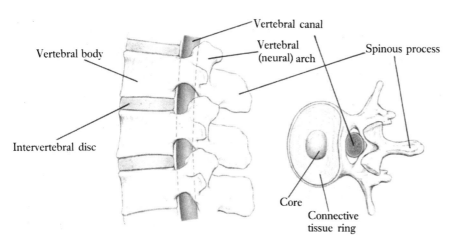

The bones of the spine and the intervertebral disc.
Peterson L, Renstrom P: *Sports Injuries: Their Prevention and Treatment,* Yearbook Medical Publishers INC, Chicago, 1986.

that as much as 85% of the time it is impossible to accurately associate localized low back pain with a precise anatomic cause. Frequently these problems are characterized as *back sprains* or *back strains*, without being more specific. If you receive such a diagnosis from your doctor, understand that it means the following: "You probably have some inflammation affecting the muscles, ligaments, membranes, or nerves in the lower back. We do not really know exactly what is inflamed or why." Specialists whose clinical focus covers ailments of the back utilize the terms *sprain* and *strain* of the back to refer to specific problems that are dealt with in detail in Chapter 20. Here we will briefly review some of the important points to consider when confronting low back pain, particularly in the context of *lumbar radiculopathy* due to a slipped disc or arthritic changes in the low back.

■ LUMBAR RADICULOPATHY

Lumbar radiculopathy is probably the most common cause of lower back pain, other than the nonspecific condition known as *back strain*. Lumbar radiculopathy is commonly referred to as a *pinched nerve* or *sciatica*. It occurs when the nerve root that exits the spinal cord is compressed (pinched) by some other structure. The nerve root contains the sensory nerves that convey sensation from the skin. Consequently, when the sensory nerves are compressed, the person commonly complains of pain and/or numbness along the stretch of skin that is supplied by the sensory nerve. The pain is not restricted to the back alone. In fact, it may not even be felt in the back at all.

Nerve root compression of the lower back causes pain that usually travels down the leg on the side where the compressed nerve root is located. The sciatic nerve is often the nerve that becomes entrapped by the disc or arthritic bone spur, although other nerve roots can also become pinched. Depending on the precise level of compression, the person will feel the pain:

- Across the front of the leg towards the groin (compression of the 3rd lumbar nerve root).

- Down the front of the leg, across the knee, and around the inside of the lower leg (compression of the 4th lumbar nerve root).

- Down the side of the leg then across the ankle into the great toe (compression of the 5th lumbar nerve root).

- Down the back of the leg into the heel (compression of the 1st sacral nerve root).

Motor nerves that enable us to move our muscles also run through the nerve root. Consequently, the person may complain of weakness in one leg if the motor nerves are injured. Often the reflexes that are tested during a neurological examination are diminished or absent entirely. Motor nerve compression is much less common than sensory nerve compression, but potentially more serious. There are two common causes of radiculopathy: a slipped disc and an arthritic spine.

■ THE SLIPPED DISC

There are many possible causes of lumbar radiculopathy. The most common cause in younger people is a *slipped* or *herniated disc*. The likelihood of disc-related backache is greatest between the ages of 40 and 50, diminishes between 50 and 60, and is rather unlikely after age 60.

As discussed above, the disc is a sac of gelatinous material that provides some cushioning between vertebral bodies, allowing for flexibility of the spinal column. It also provides cushioning that absorbs forces transmitted through the spine. The disc is soft, moist, and full of a gelatinous nucleus in young people. However, the discs become less moist, thinner, and a little tougher as we age, so that they are less likely to rupture when pressed. It is similar to the difference between squeezing a fresh grape versus a dried raisin.

Discs are susceptible to several kinds of injury. A really severe jolt such as a serious fall or auto accident can crush a disc often located at the bottom of the spine, requiring surgery to remove disc remnants and fuse two vertebrae together. The famous actress Liz Taylor, struggled with back problems all her life after being thrown from a horse at age 12 while filming *National Velvet*.

A less severe injury can rupture the tough outer envelope of a disc, causing the inner jelly-like substance to bulge outward (protrusion) or ooze out (extrusion) and press against a nerve root. The gelatinous material inside a disc frequently goes to one side of the vertebrae or the other when it gets squeezed out. There it encounters the nerve root exiting the spinal cord in a narrow, little space called a *foramen*. The foramen does not have space for the nerve root, the herniated disc, and the swelling and inflammation that usually accompanies this process. The compressed nerve, which is usually the sciatic nerve, causes severe pain and sometimes numbness and weakness down the length of the leg muscle it innervates. In addition, the back muscles are often thrown into a protective spasm that bend the person forward and may cause their torso to twist over the pelvis into what is called a stiff *trunk list*. These spasms of the back muscles are actually a protective effort that results because the muscles sense trouble and try to splint the low back in order to prevent motion that might cause additional damage.

If a person lifts a heavy object suddenly or even gradually in some cases, the force of that object is transmitted down the entire spine and is focused on the lumbar spine. The forces on the lumbar spine can be quite intense. The large, sturdy bones handle it well enough, but the soft, sack-like discs get compressed. The discs are particularly vulnerable to rotational forces—for example, when a person lifts something heavy while simultaneously twisting to one side in an unguarded movement. The force is multiplied if performed quickly. Such forces may tear the tough outer cartilaginous envelope, allowing the gelatinous core of the disc to be squeezed out of the fibrous ring that surrounds it. This is referred to as a *herniated nucleus pulposus* (HNP) in medical terms, but it is commonly called a *slipped disc*.

If the herniation is small, or if the extruded material goes to the front or back of the spine rather than to the side, the person will not feel anything. They may not know that the disc herniated unless an MRI is done for some other reason. Occasion-

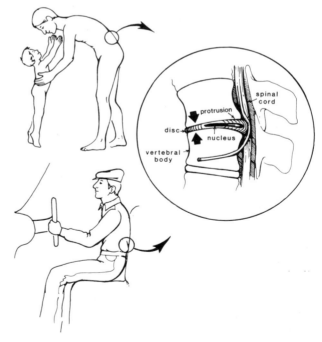

Disc herniation with protrusion because of the bent forward position of the low back, which causes the backward bulge to press on the nerve root. Saunders HD: *Evaluation, Treatment and Prevention of Musculoskeletal Disorders*, Minneapolis, Minnesota, Viking Press, 1985.

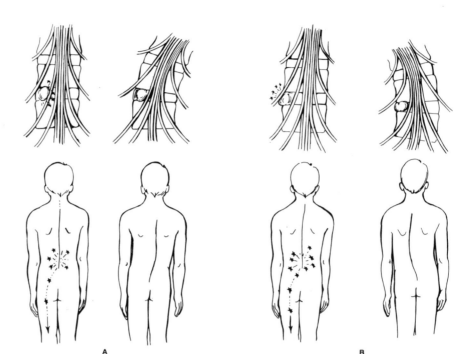

Trunk list contorts the back to avoid nerve compression, depending on where the bulge compresses the nerve. Saunders HD: *Evaluation, Treatment and Prevention of Musculoskeletal Disorders,* Minneapolis, Minnesota, Viking Press, 1985.

A   B

ally, if the disc is very large and goes straight back, it can compress the nerve roots on both sides of the spine, resulting in symptoms in both legs and pain across the entire back.

THE ARTHRITIC SPINE

The most common cause of chronic low back pain due to radiculopathy, especially in those over the age of 50, is arthritis of the spine. It may take two forms: *spinal stenosis* and *degenerative disc disease of the spine.*

The bones and joints of the spine may degenerate and be afflicted by arthritis as we age, just as the other bones and joints of the body do. Frequently, this results in local inflammation, bony spicules known as *osteophytes* that overgrow the normal limits of the bone, and narrowing of the spaces between the bones. These osteophyes have an appearance similar to the sharp stalactites located on the inside of limestone caves. The narrowing of the foramen

(tunnel) where the nerve roots leave the spine is of particular concern.

As discussed above, the intervertebral discs lose water with age and, therefore, height. As a result, the total length of the spine shrinks, leaving less space for the emerging nerve roots. Another possibility is that the weakened discs may bulge beyond their normal confines or tear and ooze the inner material. The nearby nerve roots may be painfully compressed in both of these situations.

The two conditions of slipped disc and an arthritic spine may be differentiated from one another through a variety of clinical clues. Frequently, pain from a herniated disc is sudden in onset and follows heavy lifting or some other strenuous activity. Pain from degenerative disease of the spine is usually gradual in onset and chronic in nature. Frequently, there is no precise start time and no association with any particular activity. That being said, there are many exceptions to these rules, and it is not uncommon to lack a precise trigger for a herniated disc. The surest way of determining the

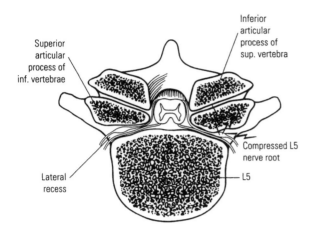

Superior
articular
process of
inf. vertebrae

Inferior
articular
process of
sup. vertebra

Compressed L5
nerve root

L5

Lateral
recess

Spinal stenosis ultimately results in the compression of the nerve root and similar symptoms such as those seen with a herniated disc. *Complete Guide to Pain Relief,* The Reader's Digest Association, INC. Pleasantville, New York, 2000.

buttock area or into the hips. Movement of nearly any kind frequently exacerbates the pain. Raising the leg straight upward in a *straight leg raise test* is often limited and painful. This test stretches the already pinched sciatic nerve and reproduces pain. X-rays are rarely helpful because abnormalities are frequently seen in many people who do not experience low back pain. These abnormalities may have little or no relationship to the actual cause of the problem. It is not uncommon for the onset of pain to be associated with some particular action such as bending down or lifting an object. Frequently, however, there is no known reason for the onset of the pain. There is no need for an extensive diagnostic work-up in most instances of uncomplicated low back pain without radiation that resolve with a few days of conservative therapy.

cause is to do radiological imaging with an MRI. If an MRI cannot be done, the next best test is a myelogram. This procedure involves a spinal tap and the injection of a contrast agent into the fluid surrounding the spinal cord. Then x-rays or a CT scan is done to visualize the area of the nerve root compression. Sometimes a CT scan without the injection of the contrast agent is sufficient to visualize the problem. Keep in mind that disc herniation and degenerative disease of the spine are so common that they are likely to be present on an MRI or CT scan, regardless of whether they are truly responsible for the low back pain. Consequently, the final diagnosis is primarily dependent upon the good clinical judgment of your doctor rather than the results of the imaging procedure alone.

■ SIGNS AND SYMPTOMS

The pain associated with back sprain is usually local. However, sometimes it may spread down to the

■ CONDITIONS TO RULE OUT

While herniated discs and bony degenerative disease account for the vast majority of nerve root compressions, sometimes there may be other more serious causes. For example, tumors or infections may result in compression of the nerve root in rare cases. Trauma can lead to compression, and congenital problems and pre-existing systemic diseases can predispose a person towards nerve root compression. It is for this reason that an imaging procedure is often recommended whenever someone has a new complaint of nerve root-related pain. An MRI or CT scan may not always provide a definitive diagnosis, but they are generally useful for ruling out other potentially very serious possibilities.

There are times when a more rigorous work-up is necessary in order to appropriately address low back pain. In these situations, the effort of the doctor to make a more specific diagnosis is done primarily to rule out certain specific syndromes that are managed differently from back sprain or pose a particular danger to the person. Some of these conditions are as follows:

- **SPINAL STENOSIS:** Overall, spinal stenosis accounts for about 3% of low back pain cases. Normally, the adult spinal canal containing the spinal cord is only about 7-9 inches wide. The spinal cord itself ends at the level of the second vertebral body, and only nerve roots run through the remainder of the lumbar spine. The bony and ligamentous structures that surround the canal and its exit points undergo degenerative changes as the body ages. These changes include arthritic changes, bony overgrowth, swelling of soft tissue, and thickening of the ligaments. All of these degenerative changes serve to narrow the spaces available for the nerve roots and may cause mild compression for prolonged periods of time. The blood supply to the nerve roots runs along the outer portions of the nerves, and when the nerves are chronically compressed, the blood supply may be diminished. The blood supply may be acutely compromised if anything should happen that further narrows the space around the nerve.

  Restriction of blood supply results in loss of oxygen to the nerve, which leads to pain and impaired functioning. The medical term applied to this condition is *neurogenic claudication*. This should be distinguished from another similar condition called: *vascular* or *intermittent* claudication. *Claudication* is a term that literally means *limping*. It implies difficulty in using the legs due to lack of blood flow. Intermittent or vascular claudication is a condition where severe atherosclerotic disease (cholesterol build-up in the arteries) blocks the major arteries supplying blood to the legs. A person with intermittent claudication experiences pain and difficulty walking long distances because the lack of blood flow to the muscles in the leg causes them to fatigue and become painful with minor exertion. A person

who has spinal stenosis experiences similar symptoms, but in this case the cause is lack of blood supply to the nerve that supplies the muscles in the legs. Typically, the person with spinal stenosis feels relatively comfortable when at rest. Pain usually begins after walking a short distance and is felt in the lower back radiating down the legs along the portion innervated (supplied) by the affected nerve roots. The pain causes the person to limp (neurogenic claudication). It is relieved only when the person stops to rest. Other symptoms include numbness and weakness in the legs. Both legs are often affected, although it may be asymmetrical. The person frequently learns to compensate by bending forward when walking because this maximizes the space in the canal, allowing more blood to flow into the compromised nerve root.

  Lumbar spinal stenosis may affect both men and women at nearly any adult age, but it is more common in men than women and much more commonly seen in the elderly and middle-aged than in the young. The diagnosis is usually a clinical one, but CT or MRI imaging is helpful in confirming the diagnosis. Sometimes, electrophysiological testing (EMG and NCV testing) is helpful as well.

  It is possible that the person may respond to conservative therapy if the symptoms associated with lumbar stenosis are relatively mild and of recent duration. Conservative therapy includes: bracing the lumbar spine, short-term bed rest, pain management, and physical therapy. Some experts recommend a light exercise program of bicycle riding or walking with brief periods of rest when pain occurs. The conservative approach is not always successful, and it may become necessary to consider surgery. The classical surgical procedure is called a *decompressive laminectomy*, during which the surgeon removes a portion of the bone covering the nerve root, allowing more room for blood to flow into the nerve. It may be necessary to perform this procedure at multiple spinal levels. The more levels involved, the poorer the prognosis of a full recovery. If multiple levels are involved, an alternative technique may be performed in which the surgeon removes small pieces of bone at each level rather than the entire laminar bone. This procedure creates small windows for the nerve root, which aid in improving blood flow but do not compromise the stability of the lumbar spine. Symptoms frequently recur after a few years, even with successful surgery, regardless of the procedure performed.

- **COMPRESSION FRACTURE:** The large vertebrae of the lumbar spine (lower back) are the primary supports for the weight of the upper body. They are solid, resilient cubes in young, healthy people that can tolerate a large amount of stress. In older people, particularly in post-menopausal women, the bones may thin or waste away due to the loss of estrogen that accompanies menopause. This process is called osteoporosis. It may also occur in people who take steroids for long periods of time. Compromised bone is not structurally fit to tolerate the stress that accompanies normal daily activities such as walking, standing, lifting objects, and falling, in particular, and it may collapse under the weight of the body when it is stressed too far. This is called a *compression fracture*.

A person with a compression fracture experiences severe, localized back pain in a restricted area of the spine. As a general rule, the pain does not travel far from the site of the fracture. There is usually also some tenderness over the fractured spine as well. The severity of the pain and its localization over one vertebra in a person having risk factors generally makes diagnosis easy for the astute doctor. The diagnosis may be confirmed by an ordinary x-ray of the back, which will show

that the vertebral body is shorter than it should be. Often the fracture line crossing the bone may be seen. If a compression fracture occurs in someone who is not elderly, post-menopausal, or using steroids long-term, then a tumor or an infection should be suspected, and the person will need an extensive medical work-up to determine the cause of the fracture. Infection and tumors also occur in older people, so the doctor may decide to do an additional work-up with them as well.

Treatment for an uncomplicated compression fracture is usually conservative. Analgesics are prescribed and bed rest is frequently recommended during the acute period. The underlying cause of any osteoporosis should also be addressed by the doctor. Sometimes the doctor may elect to recommend hormone replacement therapy or other medication to treat osteoporosis. The pain associated with vertebral compression fractures usually resolves over time, but sometimes it may result in a chronic pain syndrome. The orthopedist may recommend a procedure called *vertebroplasty* if the pain persists or if the fracture is severe. This procedure involves the injection of mineral preparations or cement mixtures into the vertebral body itself to provide more support. This procedure is frequently helpful, but not always. Recently, some doctors have begun to inject an anesthetic locally, with significant success in difficult cases.

MALIGNANT CAUSES OF LOW BACK PAIN

The causes of low back pain discussed above are all benign in nature. This means there is nothing potentially life-threatening about any of these conditions, although they may cause significant discomfort. However, not all of the causes of low back pain are benign. Malignant causes of low back pain are not related to the mechanical problem of a nerve being pinched, a slipped disc, or arthritis of the spine. Sometimes serious and even life-threatening conditions may present with low back pain, and it is important for the doctor evaluating someone with low back pain to ascertain whether or not a malignant condition is responsible. The most common and worrisome malignant causes of low back pain are:

- **KIDNEY DISEASE:** The kidneys are located in what is called the *retroperitoneal* region of the torso. This means that the kidneys are located in the back of the body, on either side of the spine, and just below the rib cage. When the kidneys become infected there is an associated inflammation; this condition is called *pyelonephritis*. The flank region on the side of the infected kidney becomes very painful. Sometimes the pain may radiate to the groin region. Pain may occasionally be exacerbated with urination, and there is usually evidence of infection in the urine. The diagnosis is usually a clinical one that can be made with confidence by your doctor. If not treated appropriately with antibiotics, pyelonephritis may become a very serious, even life-threatening infection.

- **INFECTION OF THE SPINE:** It is possible for infections to involve the spine itself and cause back pain, although this is rare. This may include meningitis, which is an illness where the tissues covering the spinal cord become infected, resulting in a high fever, neck stiffness, headaches, avoidance of bright light, and in severe cases, an altered mental status. Sometimes an infection of the spine may present as an abscess, a pocket of infection that is closed off within a capsule-like membrane, which presses on the spinal cord, nerve roots, or bones and ligaments. The abscess may be located within the tissues surrounding the spinal cord, in the bones of the spinal column, or

in the muscles and tissues outside the spinal column. The abscess might mimic in presentation a vertebral body fracture, a herniated disc (or any type of radiculopathy), or back sprain, depending on its exact location. It is much more dangerous than any of these possibilities, however. Abscesses of the spine may spread to the blood and cause sepsis, or to the spinal cord and brain, where they cause meningitis or encephalitis. An abscess may result in paralysis below the level of compression if it is allowed to grow and compress the spinal cord.

Spine abscesses are differentiated from these other possibilities on the basis of medical history, examination, and laboratory testing. People with a history of intravenous drug abuse, immunosuppression (malfunctioning immune system), tuberculosis, or other chronic infectious disease are more likely to get a spinal abscess. The diagnosis is highly unlikely without such a history. Abscesses will often be accompanied by a fever and severe local back pain with a great deal of local tenderness. There may also be radiating pain if the abscess compresses a nerve root. A spinal tap will usually show abnormal numbers of white blood cells and protein. The general white count from the venous blood will also show an increase in the number of white blood cells. Imaging with an MRI or CT scan is likely to show a mass lesion in the spine. Even ordinary x-rays may show signs of the abscess if it is in the vertebra itself.

- **CANCER:** It is rare for a primary cancer to arise in the spine or that general region. However, many varieties of cancer routinely spread to the spine when they metastasize. Frequently, cancer is first discovered when it spreads to the spine because it becomes symptomatic at that point. Cancer may mimic the pain associated with vertebral body fracture, radiculopathy, or back sprain, depending on where it is located in the spine. Symptoms generally come on gradually and get progressively worse. Pain is not always a feature, and sometimes the metastasis is discovered because of weakness or numbness in the legs resulting from compression of the spinal cord. Compression of the spinal cord is the greatest concern in these instances because it can potentially leave a person paralyzed below the level of the lesion, unable to feel his body below the level of the lesion, incontinent, and unable to perform sexually. There is a risk of spinal cord compression whenever a tumor spreads to the spine. This situation is a medical emergency.

It is critical to diagnose a spinal metastasis as soon as possible, before it has an opportunity to compress the cord. Diagnosis is primarily based on the history and physical examination. However, imaging with an MRI or myelogram is the most definitive way of confirming a diagnosis. Imaging is also necessary because treatment with radiation therapy requires that the full extent of the tumor be defined. Back pain associated with significant unexplained weight loss should raise specific concerns that cancer may be involved. Back pain associated with neurological signs of weakness or loss of sensation in both legs may be a red flag that something serious is going on. Often, the doctor will start therapy with steroids in order to reduce swelling around the tumor if there are symptoms of spinal cord compression at the time the tumor is discovered. This serves to decrease the amount of compression due to the tumor. The doctor will do a more extensive workup in order to identify the source of the tumor if one is found in order to determine the most effective form of therapy. Sometimes this will necessitate a biopsy.

■ MANAGING LOW BACK PAIN

The vague diagnosis of "back sprain" is adequate for most people because management of the problem would not change even if a more precise diagnosis could be made. Radiculopathy (a pinched nerve) may be treated conservatively in the vast majority of cases. Rest, non-steroidal anti-inflammatory medications, and time will often reduce the pain and allow a complete recovery. (This does not mean that the disc problem has necessarily disappeared. Rather, it means that the inflammation and swelling have resolved, taking pressure off the nerve root.) Conservative therapy is successful in at least 90% of cases involving herniated disc disease.

- **BED REST:** Many doctors recommend a brief period of bed rest and prescribe non-steroidal anti-inflammatory drugs (NSAIDS). Some also recommend the use of muscle relaxants, but it is not proven that they are of any significant value. Back exercises and weight loss regimens may be of benefit in preventing another attack once the acute pain has resolved.

  In the past, extended bed rest was recommended, but scientific studies suggest that prolonged bed rest probably does not help, and it may actually be harmful to recovery. It may even pose risks of developing additional complications, including blood clots in the legs. Some doctors recommend a brief period of bed rest—rarely more than two days are necessary—followed by moderate levels of activity with limits on lifting or exertion. Sitting for prolonged periods of time should also be avoided because sitting tends to put pressure on the lower spine and may exacerbate the problem. Relief may be obtained during sleeping by using pillows to relieve stress on the back. A pillow under the knees may help people who lie on their backs, whereas side-sleepers may benefit from a pillow under the waist and

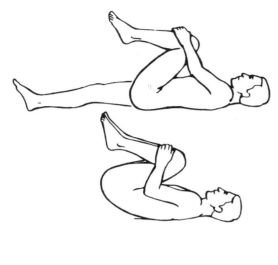

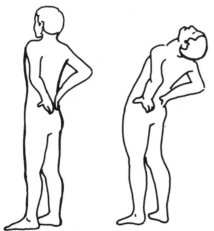

Top: Single and double knee-to-chest Williams flexion exercises. Saunders HD: *Evaluation, Treatment and Prevention of Musculoskeletal Disorders*, Minneapolis, Minnesota, Viking Press, 1985.

Above: Extension exercises. Saunders HD: *Evaluation, Treatment and Prevention of Musculoskeletal Disorders*, Minneapolis, Minnesota, Viking Press, 1985.

another under the shoulder to help level the spine.

- **MEDICATIONS:** Oral non-steroidal analgesics are helpful in alleviating pain and reducing inflammation. Narcotic analgesics may be used in cases of severe pain for brief periods of time. Long-term narcotic use can result in addiction and can cause constipation. Straining due to constipation is likely to exacerbate the underlying reason for the back pain, whatever the cause. Use of laxatives or stool softeners recommended by a doctor may be helpful in cases where there is underlying constipation.

- **INJECTIONS:** An epidural liquid steroid injection into the area of nerve irritation may sometimes be used in combination with morphine; this may cool down an inflamed nerve and avoid the need for surgery. The injection may be repeated once or twice, as needed. Some doctors may inject Novocain® or other local anesthetic.

- **EXERCISE:** Your doctor may recommend exercises such as swimming, walking, pool walking, or specific back exercises when the pain is under control. Paul Williams developed a series of exercises known as *Williams flexion exercises* in the 1930s that emphasize bending or curling forward while lying on your back with the legs in various positions. However, these postures increase the pressure within the intervertebral disc and may not be appropriate for people with disc problems. People with disc problems may experience more relief from *Mackenzie exercises*, which emphasize back extension while lying on your stomach and arching the back upward.

- **TRACTION:** Using spinal traction may be beneficial in dealing with low back pain due to a disc problem. Traction delivered quickly and with sufficient force may create a suction effect in the area of the disc that encourages the disc to slip back into its correct position, thereby easing pressure on the pressed nerve root. The negative pressure realized by vertebral distraction may also stretch the back muscles. At least 80% of total body weight must be exerted along the length of the spine for traction to be successful in the area of the low back because the spinal ligaments holding it together preclude most forces from distracting the back. This method of manual traction was advocated by the famed orthopaedic surgeon Dr. James Cyriax and should only be applied by medical personnel who have been trained in the technique.

■ **MANIPULATION THERAPY:** Manipulation is used by osteopathic doctors and chiropractors. It involves a high-velocity thrust to the low back so as to move the disc away from the nerve root. Physical therapists utilize a less forceful, low-velocity technique known as *mobilization.*

■ **ICING:** Ice can be used to cool down the back if there is acute pain. A commercial ice pack or package of frozen vegetable from the freezer can be applied to the painful spot for up to 15 minutes at a time, two or three times a day. Moist heat is more penetrating than dry heat, such as that of an electric heating pad, and showers, baths, and whirlpools should be used to help relieve pain and promote relaxation once the acute phase has passed. Using TENS (transcutaneous electric nerve stimulation) has been found to help relieve low back pain in some cases.

■ **CREATIVE VISUALIZATION:** Visualizing yourself to better health has been advocated by some in order to reduce pain. Creating a mental image in which the back is free of pain and injury may make pain less of a problem for some people.

Tapping into the power of suggestion may positively affect low back pain through a psycho-immunologic mechanism.

■ **EDUCATION:** Back Schools are structured intervention programs that involve education regarding the spine and how to prevent low back injury. This type of program was developed in Scandinavia and has spread across the industrialized world. They have been shown to reduce work absenteeism by at least five days per year per employee. These programs are cost effective and have been embraced by some industries as a legitimate option for keeping employees on the job and getting them back to work in the event of a back injury.

■ **COUNSELING:** Many people with low back pain may suffer from an inability to cope with adversity, which magnifies their back pain. This is borne out by a high association of chronic low back pain and psychological disturbance. Cognitive therapy negates the ineffective coping strategies that accompany pain and emphasizes positive thinking and self-affirmation. Counseling offers some relief to people who suffer from chronic pain.

WHEN IS SURGERY NECESSARY?

More aggressive means of therapy may need to be considered if pain fails to resolve within 4 to 6 weeks. This may include local injections of steroids and/or analgesics, and surgery. More than 300,000 people undergo surgery to relieve back pain every year. Doctors may recommend surgery for people who have loss of function due to unremitting intense pain, muscle weakness in the area affected by the damaged nerve, or in those who experience loss of bowel or bladder function. The type of surgery performed is usually a *discectomy*. During this procedure, the pieces of herniated disc are removed and/or a laminectomy is performed, wherein the surrounding bone is removed to make more room for the compressed nerve root. This may be performed as an open procedure or as an arthroscopically guided procedure. The advantage of using an arthroscope is that the area of surgery is more restricted, resulting in improved recovery time and fewer post-operative complications. This procedure has become increasingly popular over the last few years. There is a longstanding debate among doctors as to the most appropriate time to refer a person for surgery. Most doctors will consider surgery only as an option of last resort because surgery does not always alleviate the problem completely and sometimes not at all.

A new type of operation known as *intradiscal eletrothermal annuloplasty* (IDET) takes 15 to 20 minutes under local anesthesia. This procedure seals the hole in the outer portion of the disc and destroys any nerve fibers that are causing pain because they have invaded the disc. An additional advantage to this procedure is that it allows people to walk out of the operating room.

▧ PREVENTING BACK PAIN

The prevention of recurrent low back pain primarily involves the reduction of risk factors and firming up support for the spine. Some of the risk factors and activities that might improve low back support are as follows:

- **WEIGHT LOSS:** The lower spine supports the entire upper portion of the body and the weight of the body is literally focused on this single supportive structure. The greater the weight, the more pressure and stress are focused on the lower spine and the greater the risk of injury. This is

true for back sprains and strains as well as slipped discs and vertebral body fractures. Excessive weight does not directly cause spinal degenerative disease or spinal stenosis. However, these conditions may be exacerbated if the person is overweight. Obesity is one of the most important risk factors in both acute and chronic low back pain, and many people report a dramatic improvement in their condition after significant weight loss. It is time to consider a rapid weight loss program if you are overweight and experience back pain. If you are obese and do not yet have back pain, you should take special precautions to avoid activities such as heavy lifting that may precipitate low back pain. The best advice even then, of course, is to lose the excess weight.

- **POSTURAL ISSUES:** There are ways of minimizing the stress on your lower back by taking care as to how you perform your routine daily activities. Maintaining correct posture is one important way you can reduce your risk of developing low back pain. Slouching while walking or sitting places added curvature and greater stress on the spine. Walk with your shoulders back and your head up high. Slouching in a chair is a common practice because most people relax when sitting. Good posture is possibly even more important when sitting than when standing. It is very important to sit in a chair that supports your back and helps you maintain a healthy posture. Sometimes, placing a small pillow behind your lower back will provide added support. It is helpful to have a comfortable mattress that provides support. You should roll to one side first when getting out of bed and then swing your legs over the edge of the bed.

- **SITTING AND SLEEPING:** The best chairs are firm recliners with contoured support and an adjustable lumbar (low back) cushion. The most harmful are soft chairs that cannot be adjusted.

Japanese and Swedish car seat models are best because they usually support the curve of the spine as well as the head and neck. The seats in American cars often lack contoured support. The best bed is an adjustable waterbed that does not make too many waves or an adjustable airbed. Soft, saggy mattresses may cause you to wake up with a sore back. An extra firm mattress will do for most people. Using plywood board cut to size and inserted between the mattress and box spring will firm up an overly soft bed.

- **LIFTING AND CARRYING:** Be careful when lifting and carrying heavy objects. Bending at the waist and lifting straight up poses a risk for straining the back or causing a slipped disk. It is better to squat down and shift some of the burden to the knees and upper thighs. Avoid lifting objects that you feel may be too heavy. Holding a heavy object close to the body while carrying it minimizes the risk of an acute back injury.

- **BRACING:** Braces and corsets have long been used to provide additional support for the back. The abdominal and back muscles of the trunk provide a rigid girdle to support the trunk. However, an overly large stomach can upset this balance and cause the abdominal muscles to become weak. The back muscles will try to compensate by working harder to carry the additional load. This is why pregnant women often experience backaches. The rationale for the use of braces in low back pain is to unload some of the weight stress from the muscles of the back. Individuals have reported some benefit from their use, but there has been no scientific verification of the value of braces.

- **EXERCISES:** The low back consists of numerous muscles, in addition to the bones, ligaments, and nerves described above. These muscles play a major role in contributing to the support for the spine and other structures. As with other body parts, the muscles of the lower back perform their function best when they are strong and well developed. Numerous exercises have been proposed to strengthen the back muscles, reduce the risk of injury, and aid in the healing process following an injury. There is little scientific data to support this, but the accumulation of longstanding clinical experience suggests that for the most part they are beneficial.

Recommendations vary as to which exercise programs are most useful. Many recommend swimming laps or walking through water because the buoyancy of the water takes much of the stress off the lower spine, and at the same time the back muscles are strengthened. Swimming is particularly helpful following the acute phase of an attack of low back pain, regardless of the underlying cause.

Others recommend daily flexion and extension cycles. These exercises should be performed with the intention of building stamina and endurance rather than increasing strength as the primary objective. The normal curvature of the spine should be preserved in the course of the exercise. Specific exercises should be determined in consultation with an orthopedist or a physical therapist so that the most appropriate ones for the individual situation are prescribed.

- **STRETCHING:** Sciatica may be prevented by exercises that stretch the large muscles of the thighs. The sciatic nerve runs through the large muscles of the leg. From its origin point as a nerve root to its distal nerve in the lower leg, it moves in minute increments in relation to limb and muscle movement. If these muscles are tight and inflexible, the sciatic nerve contained within them is less likely to tolerate movement. On the other hand, muscle flexibility helps the sciatic nerve move more easily along its tract, and it may be less likely to become bound down if compressed at the level of the nerve root.

- **TOPICAL RELIEF:** Topical painkillers such as oil of wintergreen, Ben-Gay®, Ice Hot®, and Tiger Balm® offer relief because they stimulate blood circulation. However, be sure to generously ventilate your skin when using them, and do not cover the applied area with anything other than normal clothing. Heating skin that is covered with these helpful ointments with a heating pad or excessive clothing can cause an unhealthy increase in absorption of these products.

- **FOOTWEAR:** Shoes absorb energy imparted from the ground that is jarringly passed up to the spine with every step. Therefore, it is important to protect the back by wearing cushioned shoes or by inserting a cushioned insert into your shoes. Wear shoes that have moderate heels.

- **WORK HARDENING:** This is a program that introduces work-related activities under the guidance of a physical therapist so that proper body mechanics and posture are maintained. Different occupations have different tasks, which are analyzed. Then performance of those tasks is taught in the safest possible way so as to avoid the likelihood of back injury.

Hand and Wrist

THE HAND is a versatile and bewildering array of levers and hinges that move the finger joints millions of times during a lifetime of use. The hands are comprised of eight wrist bones, five palm bones and fourteen finger bones—a total of twenty-seven bones in each hand. The wrist is often the site of overuse injuries because of the structure of these bones and the nerves that pass through them. The hands account for more than one-fourth of all the bones in the skeletal system. Humans are differentiated from all other primates in that we are capable of precisely opposing our thumb and forefinger in what is known as the "precision grip."

23 de Quervain's Disease

A 46-year-old widow decided fix her son's tree house that had been wrecked by a recent storm. First, she lay down precut 2" by 4" planks parallel to each other to form the floor and hammered them into the numerous thick tree branches that extended outward like a wide canopy. Next, she hammered in 3½ inch nails every 2 inches around the periphery of each plank in a regular pattern. She took a week off from work and worked 5 to 6 hours each day on the tree house.
She had completed nailing in the slanted roof planks by the end of the third day. That night, she was awakened by a searing hot pain at the base of her right thumb. It felt a little better when she squeezed it. She took some aspirin and eventually went back to bed. The pain returned the next day after hammering for 2 hours and it intensified when she ignored it. Any movement of her right thumb was painful by the end of the fourth day, and the base of her right thumb was painful to touch. She found that she could not grasp the hammer tightly on the fifth day. This woman has tenosynovitis of the tendons at the base of the thumb, a condition known as de Quervain's disease.

WHO WAS "DE QUERVAIN?"

FRITZ DE QUERVAIN (1868-1940) was a French surgeon who first described this inflammatory condition of the tendons at the base of the thumb that cause pain. de Quervain's disease is one of the classic repetitive injuries that occur when tendons undergo more than 1,500 to 2,000 manipulations per hour. The force necessary to excessively hammer nails or perform any similar manual activity using the hands may result in more stress than the tendons can tolerate, resulting in an overuse injury.

APL AND EPB

The superficial tendons located just under the skin that are involved in de Quervain's disease are known as the *abductor pollicis longus* and *extensor pollicis brevis* ("APL" and "EPB"), terms derived from Latin. *Abductor pollicis longus* means "the long tendon of the thumb that abducts or moves away from" and *extensor pollicis brevis* means "the short tendon of the thumb that extends or moves upward." In this way, the technical names for the tendons explain their function.

CAUSES OF DE QUERVAIN'S DISEASE

The APL and EPB tendons pass through a shallow bony groove between the wrist and the thumb known as the "anatomic snuffbox." This name derives from the fact that the small, shallow indentation near the base of the thumb conveniently holds a smidgen of snuff, a habit common to the eighteenth century. These two tendons touch each other at precisely this spot, where they lie against

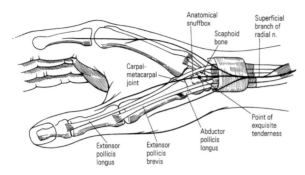

Anatomy of de Quervain's disease.
Saidoff D, McDonough AL: *Critical Pathways in Therapeutic Intervention: Upper Extremity.* St. Louis: Mosby, 1997.

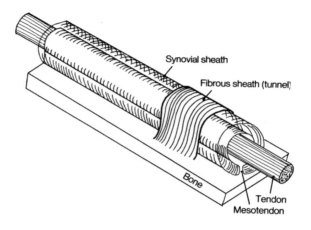

Anatomy of the synovial sheath. Goldberg S: *Clinical Anatomy Made Ridiculously Simple.* Miami: MedMaster, Inc., 1984.

the bony tunnel. They may succumb to friction from rubbing against bone as well as from rubbing against each other during excessive repetitive use of the wrist and hand.

WHO IS MOST LIKELY TO HAVE DE QUERVAIN'S DISEASE?

These tendons tend to lose extensibility and become more likely to break down and sustain injury when they begin to age in midlife. Manual laborers who combine wrist motion with forearm rotation are particularly vulnerable to developing de Quervain's disease. This condition classically affects carpenters who repetitively hammer nails, an activity that involves forceful ulnar deviation and wrist flexion. Jackhammer operators are also vulnerable to developing de Quervain's in both hands simultaneously. de Quervain's disease is also more common in diabetics, people with hypothyroidism, and people with rheumatoid arthritis.

The old term for de Quervain's disease was "washerwoman's hands" because prior to the invention of the washing machine women who spent many hours per day washing clothes by hand were more likely to develop problems due to the difficult and repetitive nature of this type of chore. In fact, de

Quervain's disease is anywhere between 3 to 10 times more common in women, especially those between 30 and 50 years of age. The reason for this gender difference has to do with differences in wrist motion between men and women. The tendons passing from the wrist to the hand undergo between 110 and 105 degrees of angulation during wrist motions. These angulations are greatest in females and women are more likely to develop de Quervain's disease because angulation places more stress on a tendon. It is also more common during pregnancy and may persist until breastfeeding ends.

SYNOVIAL SHEATH

Many tendons have a poor blood supply and therefore they are enveloped in a supportive *synovial sheath* that provides them with nutrients. A synovial sheath is very similar to a bursa. (See Chapter 18 for a discussion regarding bursae.) The synovial sheath is actually a two-layered membrane that keeps the tendons from rubbing against other tendons or nearby bone. Instead, the two layers rub against each other, thereby reducing the amount of

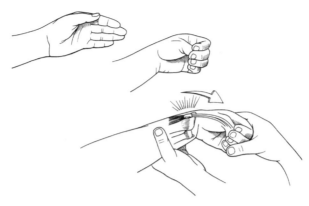

Finkelstein's test for de Quervain's disease.
Saidoff D, McDonough AL: *Critical Pathways in Therapeutic Intervention: Upper Extremity.* St. Louis: Mosby, 1997.

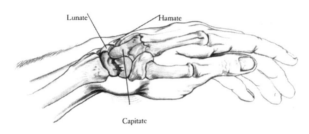

Fracture of the scaphoid bone in the wrist.
Peterson L, Renstrom P: *Sports Injuries: Their Prevention and Treatment.* Chicago: Yearbook Medical Publishers Inc., 1986.

friction to the tendon. Synovial sheaths are mostly found in the hands and feet because these parts of the body have many long tendons that enable us to perform fine motor work such as writing and painting. They also help distribute weight over the forefoot when pushing off to the next step with the toes during walking.

The walls of the synovial sheath may undergo injury or wear down if motion is excessive enough, precipitating swelling and inflammation of the synovial walls that make up the sheath; this condition is

known as *tenosynovitis*. It is the body's way of telling us to slow down and rest.

■ SIGNS AND SYMPTOMS

You might feel a searing hot pain at the thumb side of the wrist radiating up the forearm or down to the fingers. All thumb motions will be difficult and painful. The site of the anatomic snuffbox may feel thickened and may be tender to the touch. There may also be a crackling sound when moving the thumb, which is a condition known as *crepitus*. Mimicking the motion that caused pain in the first place helps confirm suspected de Quervain's disease. This is accomplished by the Finkelstein test, in which the EPB and APL tendons are passively stretched. This is accomplished by the examiner suddenly moving the wrist gently in the direction of the pinky (ulnar side). Trying to move the thumb move upward in the direction of the nail bed will also elicit pain.

■ CONDITIONS TO RULE OUT

- **SCAPHOID FRACTURE:** The *scaphoid* is a small bone located at the base of the wrist close to the thumb in the area of the anatomic snuffbox. A fracture of the scaphoid is often misdiagnosed as a sprained wrist or thumb. A scaphoid fracture should be suspected if pain is felt at the snuffbox following a fall onto outstretched hands.

- **BASAL JOINT ARTHRITIS:** This is a type of osteoarthritis that develops at the base of the thumb. This condition is quite common and symptoms may resemble de Quervain's disease in that there is painful motion of the thumb as well as a positive *Finklestein test.* Pain will be felt about ½ inch closer to the wrist rather than at the snuffbox. Also, unlike true de Quervain's disease, the pain of basal joint arthritis is not elicited when the thumb is forcefully moved backward.

- **RADIAL NERVE NEURITIS**: The *radial nerve* has a superficial branch close to the skin that runs along the thumb. It provides sensation to parts of the thumb and the thick flesh known as the *thenar eminence* located just beneath the thumb. This nerve supplies sensation to the top side of the other fingers. In some people, the movement of pronating the forearm, which means to rotate it in such a way that the top side of the hand faces upward, compresses this nerve and causes numbness.

PREVENTION AND TREATMENT

Ninety percent of those with de Quervain's disease can expect relief with either physical or occupational therapy. An eclectic management approach is best and may include:

- **REST:** It is important to rest and not work so hard that the tendons of your thumb get stressed. Purchase a bent hammer if you are doing carpentry work because this type of hammer bypasses the need to flick your wrist forward every time you aim the hammer at the nail head. This will spare your tendons.

- **ICE MASSAGE:** Massage with ice can decrease inflammation and alleviate other symptoms that may occur after exercise or other overuse activities. Ice massage may be used 4 to 5 times per day for up to 10 minutes at a time for the first 2 days. It is important to try to avoid the bony protrusions near the thumb and hand as these areas may become painfully overcooled. Ice is very helpful during the acute state when used in conjunction with elevation.

- **MEDICATIONS:** Oral non-steroidal anti-inflammatory drugs are very helpful in controlling the pain and inflammation associated with de Quervain's disease. Over-the-counter medications include ibuprofen (Motrin®, Advil®, Nuprin®, and Medipren®) and prescription medications (Naprosyn®, Indocin®, Feldene®, and Relafen®). All medications should be used under the direction of a doctor because of potential side effects. Local steroid injections may be performed by a doctor, although no more than two or three are recommended.

- **IONTOPHORESIS:** This is a method involving the use of a mild, battery-operated electric current to deliver medication such as hydrocortisone, xylocaine, or salicitate thru the skin to painful, inflamed tendons. It may help validate suspected de Quervain's disease.

- **PHONOPHORESIS:** This method uses pulsed ultrasonic waves to move medicine through the thin layer of skin overlying the tendons in the anatomic snuffbox. This may bring relief of symptoms.

- **SPLINTING:** Wearing a splint along the forearm, wrist, and thumb immobilizes the wrist and hand joints, and rests the involved tendons. The splint may be worn throughout the day and may provide relief from painful symptoms. It may also be worn at night, depending on instructions from your physician or therapist.

- **RANGE OF MOTION EXERCISES:** These exercises can be performed for 10 to 15 minutes at a time. This type of exercise enhances circulation, prevents sticky adhesions from forming between the tendon and the inflamed sheath, and minimizes joint stiffness. This should be done when pain is at a minimum.

WHEN IS SURGERY NECESSARY?

Surgical decompression known as *tenosynovectomy* may be performed when conservative measures do not bring relief. During this outpatient procedure, the surgeon opens the fibrous sheath covering the tendon and allows more space, which relieves much of the pressure. A splint is worn for several days following this minor operation, after which time range of motion exercises and physical therapy can begin.

24 Carpal and Cubital Tunnel Syndromes

A middle-aged female piano teacher complains of waking up in the middle of the night with painful tingling in her left hand. She can get back to sleep by wringing her hand for several minutes and running cold water over it. She experiences the same symptoms during the day while playing the piano or holding the steering wheel of her car when driving. She entered menopause 2 years ago and recently gained so much weight that she was diagnosed with non-insulin dependent diabetes. She also complains of increasing numbness during the daytime in the palm side of her thumb, index, and middle finger. This woman has carpal tunnel syndrome *of her left hand.*

■ MY HAND FEELS FUNNY!

THE HAND is one of the most remarkable parts of the body. A concert pianist, a skilled surgeon, a major leaguer pitcher, and many others all make use of their hands to create a special type of magic. The value they place on the use of their hands is immeasurable. Most of the rest of us have a tendency to take our hands for granted until we damage them in some way. Then we begin to appreciate the magic that our own hands are capable of creating.

Carpal tunnel syndrome is one of the most common types of hand injuries. It has been estimated that 10% of the population will develop this syndrome at some time in their lives. With the advent of frequent computer use, most experts believe that this estimate will prove to be too low. Close to 90% of all of the people who are wheelchair-bound develop carpal tunnel syndrome because they constantly use their hands to propel their wheelchairs forward. The number of cases of carpal tunnel syndrome reported in 1980 was approximately 0.1% of the adult population. It is now estimated that this syndrome affects approximately 0.6% of men and about 5.8% of women. The direct medical costs associated with it are greater than $1 billion a year. Carpal tunnel syndrome is now recognized as a serious occupational hazard and employers must conform to standards set by OSHA to protect workers from this form of repetitive strain injury.

Carpal tunnel syndrome often goes unrecognized because the symptoms associated with it begin very nonspecifically. Some people may complain that their hands "feel funny." They may have some numbness, tingling, or a dull ache in the thumb and first two fingers of their hands, and sometimes in the ring finger as well. These symptoms tend to come and go. They might also notice that their hands seem less capable of doing the complicated tasks they were previously able to do. Their hands may seem clumsier than before the symptoms started. They may have difficulty grasping objects and may drop things easily. Significant weakness of the hands may set in as the condition progresses, and ultimately they may be unable to use them for fine manipulations. There may be either a burning sensation or sharp, shooting pains in the hands at times. These symptoms might be exacerbated during sleep and improve on awakening by shaking the hands out or rubbing them vigorously. The intermittent nature of the symptoms, their subtlety, and their relatively nonspecific nature cause many people to ignore the symptoms or attribute them to something else during the early stages of the syndrome. For most people, a delay in seeking treatment will not have any serious consequences. For some, however, particularly diabetics and others predisposed to serious nerve compression injuries, a prolonged delay in the recognition and appropriate treatment of this condition could result in permanent injury to the hands.

■ THE CARPAL TUNNEL DEFINED

The wrist is an anatomically interesting and fairly complex structure. It contains a group of eight small bones called carpal bones that are arranged in two rows of four. *Carpal* is derived from *karpus,* a Greek word meaning "wrist." Each bone has a unique cube-like structure that resembles an irregularly-shaped dice. These bones give form and structure to the wrist. The carpal bones are arranged so

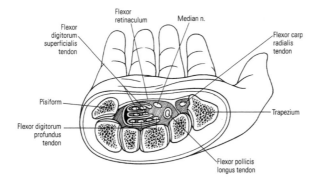

The components of the carpal tunnel.
Saidoff DC, McDonough AL: *Critical Pathways in Therapeutic Intervention: Upper Extremity.* St. Louis: Mosby, 1997.

that they form a deep groove on the side facing the palm of the hand. This groove and a ligament called the *transverse carpal ligament* form the carpal tunnel. The eight carpal bones are at the bottom of the carpal tunnel and the stout *carpal ligament,* known as the *flexor retinaculum,* is at the top. The carpal tunnel is a fairly narrow space, and it is crowded with a number of important structures. Nine tendons that attach the muscles in the forearm to the finger bones pass through this small space pass. They enable you to move your fingers and grasp objects. The median nerve, which is one of the three nerves that control the hand, also passes through the carpal tunnel. The median nerve enables you to feel with your thumb, index finger, middle finger, and a portion of your ring finger. It also enables you to bend your thumb inwards and bring your thumb and little finger together.

■ SIGNS AND SYMPTOMS

There is barely enough room in the carpal tunnel for the ten structures that pass through it, and all of them would get squeezed if anything else tried to fill the space. The tendons within the tunnel are covered by a slippery membrane called the *tenosynovium,* which lubricates the tendons under normal circumstances and allows them to slide easily against one another when the fingers are being moved. However, these tendons can become irritated or inflamed with excessive repetitive use of the hand and the tenosynovium can thicken, crowding the space even further. This is the most common type of repetitive strain injury. These tendons are tough structures that tolerate compression fairly well. The median nerve, however, is very sensitive to compression, and it begins to function abnormally when it is slowly strangled of its precious blood and oxygen supply by the swollen tendons. This process is similar to what happens when your hand or foot "falls asleep" from nerve compression. You experience numbness, tingling, and sometimes even weakness. The nerve will gradually resume its normal function and the symptoms will go away once you adjust your position and relieve the compression.

CAUSES OF CARPAL TUNNEL SYNDROME

The most common cause of carpal tunnel syndrome is repetitive strain of the flexor tendons, which control finger movements. This is usually caused by any activity that calls for repetitive hand movements, such as repeatedly grasping, twisting, or turning objects with the hand. These types of activities account for the fact that carpal tunnel syndrome is found twice as often in blue-collar workers who do heavy manual labor with their hands rather than in white-collar workers. Nevertheless, the incidence of carpal tunnel syndrome is increasing in the white-collar work force. Long hours working at computer terminals account for a new type of repetitive strain to the flexor tendons of the hands. Interestingly, working under the tension of a deadline, anxiety associated with having a supervisor looking over your shoulder, or other psychological stress may exacerbate the tendency to develop carpal tunnel syndrome. It is hypothesized that increased muscle tension in the hand constricts blood flow to the carpal tunnel, further compromising the median nerve and adding to the irritation around the muscle tendons.

WHO IS MOST LIKELY TO DEVELOP CARPAL TUNNEL SYNDROME?

Although anyone can develop carpal tunnel syndrome at any point in their lives, there are groups of individuals who are at particularly high risk. Some of the major risk factors are associated with body characteristics; others are associated with certain types of activities:

■ **AGE:** Carpal tunnel syndrome may occur at almost any age. However, it occurs most frequently in middle-aged adults having an average age of about 50 years. The higher incidence during middle age probably represents a combination of the fact that at this age most people have been actively participating in repetitive hand activities for years, and their muscles and tendons are beginning to show signs of age and can no longer tolerate repetitive strain as well as they once did. It is also a time when body weight and fluid retention patterns are shifting. These may also add to the tightness of the space in the carpal tunnel.

■ **GENDER:** Carpal tunnel syndrome is about three times more common in middle-aged women than in men, suggesting that hormonal fluctuations relating to menopause are a contributing factor. The ratio of women to men with carpal tunnel syndrome gets even larger as the population gets older. Older women are four times more likely to develop carpal tunnel than older men. Pregnant women may be particularly predisposed to developing carpal tunnel syndrome. This is most likely due to the fact that pregnant women retain large amounts of fluid, which may contribute to swelling in the carpal tunnel and other restrictive body spaces. It is estimated that 20% of pregnant women have symptoms suggestive of carpal tunnel syndrome. Only about 1%, however, go on to fill the diagnostic criteria for carpal tunnel syndrome, which is based on examination and electrophysiological recordings. Symptoms usually begin in the third trimester when swelling is at a maximum and are often relieved following delivery of the baby. Contraceptive pills, premenstrual syndrome, and other conditions that increase fluid retention may also predispose a person to the development of carpal tunnel syndrome.

- **OBESITY:** One of the strongest risk factors for the development of carpal tunnel syndrome is obesity. In one study, 46% of random cases had an abnormally high body mass index (a measure of obesity), compared with only 18% in a matched control population. Seventeen percent of those with carpal tunnel syndrome in this study were morbidly obese as compared with only 5% in the control population.

- **WRIST SHAPE:** The shape of the wrist is also an important risk factor. Short, square-shaped wrists are predisposed to developing carpal tunnel syndrome, probably due to the tighter confines of the compartment.

- **MEDICAL CONDITIONS:** A number of medical conditions are associated with a significantly increased risk of developing carpal tunnel syndrome. The most important of these is diabetes. Both juvenile and adult onset (type I and type II) diabetics are predisposed to developing compressed nerve syndromes of various types, including carpal tunnel syndrome. This may be due to the fact that the small blood vessels that supply the median nerve with nutrients are damaged by diabetes, and the lower grade of compression could result in impaired function than in an individual with healthy blood vessels. Other diseases associated with an increased risk of carpal tunnel syndrome include: thyroid disease, connective tissue disorders, gout, lupus, rheumatoid arthritis, and osteoarthritis. Carpal tunnel syndrome is also a common complication of chronic renal failure for those undergoing regular renal dialysis. There is a rise in fluid in the arm through which dialysis occurs and deposits are often found that thicken the flexor retinaculum.

- **OCCUPATIONS:** Work that necessitates extended periods of repetitive hand activity is likely to cause the development carpal tunnel syndrome. This is particularly true of jobs that require forceful use of the hand such as carpentry, construction work, plumbing, jackhammer operation, and other blue-collar jobs. Secretaries, stenographers, data entry personnel, computer programmers, and others who spend long periods of time typing at a keyboard are also at increased risk. There has been some debate in the literature as to how important these activities are in predisposing a person to carpal tunnel syndrome. While virtually everyone would agree that repetitive activity of the hand could lead to carpal tunnel syndrome, some studies suggest that age, gender, obesity, and the shape of the wrist are more important risk factors.

- **ATHLETIC AND RECREATIONAL ACTIVITIES:** Activities that involve repetitive hand movements may also increase the risk of carpal tunnel syndrome. Activities with a particularly high risk factor include: tennis, golf, mountain climbing, rowing, archery, and basketball.

DIAGNOSIS OF CARPAL TUNNEL SYNDROME

Your doctor will diagnose carpal tunnel syndrome by asking you questions about your symptoms and by conducting a thorough examination.

- **HISTORY:** Your doctor will ask you to describe your symptoms. The presence of symptoms such as numbness, tingling, or pain in the thumb and first two fingers of your hand is suggestive of carpal tunnel syndrome, but these symptoms do not support a definitive diagnosis. Some people report being awakened from sleep with burning pain in their hands that goes away when they

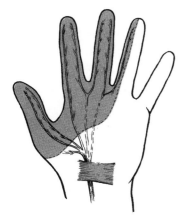

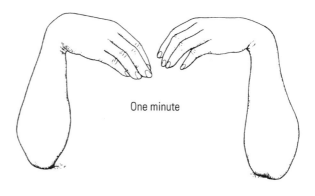

One minute

The medial nerve is compressed where it runs beneath the carpal ligament, causing altered sensation in the darkened area.
Dandy DJ: *Essential Orthopaedics and Trauma*, Edinburgh: Churchill Livingstone, 1989.

Phalen's test: Holding both hands.
Saidoff DC, McDonough AL. *Critical Pathways in Therapeutic Intervention: Extremities and Spine*, Mosby, St. Louis, 2002.

wring their hands or run cold water over them. There may be complaints of burning and tingling during waking hours that are precipitated by activities involving repetitive wrist motions such as sewing or hammering. Sometimes compression of nerve roots in the neck may result in these same types of symptoms. Weakness of the fingers, an inability to bend the thumb perpendicular to the palm, or touch your thumb and little finger together against resistance are also strongly suggestive of carpal tunnel syndrome, but they are not diagnostic.

- **PHYSICAL EXAMINATION:** The physical examination will focus on determining which muscles in your hand or arm might be weak; you should not have weakness if you have carpal tunnel syndrome. Your doctor will check to see if you have developed abnormal reflexes and attempt to determine any pattern of loss of sensation. Loss of sensation on the palm side of your thumb and first two fingers, but not the palm itself, is also strongly suggestive of carpal tunnel syndrome. In addition, the doctor may tap over the carpal tunnel itself with either a reflex hammer or finger. If

this elicits tingling or pain in the thumb and first two fingers, it is supportive of a carpal tunnel syndrome diagnosis. This is called a *Tinel's sign*. Your doctor may have you place your wrists in complete flexion for about a minute, and if you develop numbness or other discomfort, this is known as *Phalen's sign*. It also suggests the presence of carpal tunnel syndrome. Phalen's sign reproduces symptoms because bending the wrist to 90 degrees and holding it in that position maximally increases pressure within the carpal tunnel. These tests do not definitively prove the presence of carpal tunnel syndrome. However, carpal tunnel syndrome is not ruled out by their absence.

- **ANCILLARY TESTS:** Your doctor might choose to have you undergo electrophysiological testing called *nerve conduction velocity* measurements, in addition to taking a history and performing a physical examination. Electrodes will be placed a specific distance apart on either side of your wrist and on your forearm. The electrodes on your forearm will deliver a small electrical impulse that will feel like a small shock. It is not pleasant, but it is not really painful either. The electrodes at the base of the thumb will record the electrical impulse when it reaches them. By measuring the time it takes for the impulse to travel between the two sets of electrodes, the examiner can tell how quickly the median nerve is conducting electrical signals. This is known as *conduction velocity*. Nerve conduction velocity is slowed when a nerve is compressed, in comparison to normal nerves. This is probably the most objective and definitive test for carpal tunnel syndrome, but even this test is not always indicative of the presence or absence of carpal tunnel syndrome.

Of note is the fact that the more difficult it is to make a definitive diagnosis of carpal tunnel syndrome, the better the prognosis for a complete recovery.

▨ PREVENTION OF CARPAL TUNNEL SYNDROME

Whether you fall into a high risk factor category or not, there is still a significant possibility that at some point in your life you may develop carpal tunnel syndrome. As with any medical condition, the best way to prevent carpal tunnel syndrome is to avoid those things that may cause it. The strongest risk factors appear to be age, gender, and obesity. There is not much you can do about age and gender, but obesity may lend itself to corrective measures. Being aware of these risk factors could help avoid problems later on, even if correcting obesity is not currently practical. For example, if you are an obese, older woman it would be inadvisable to engage in an occupation involving repetitive hand movements for prolonged periods of time.

Some doctors suggest wearing a prophylactic wrist splint that maintains the wrist in a neutral position may prevent carpal tunnel syndrome when engaging in repetitive activities, because flexion or extension of the wrist increases the pressure within

the carpal tunnel. The logic of this approach is compelling, but in one clinical study it was shown that wearing a splint prophylactically actually increased the risk of developing carpal tunnel syndrome. This may be due to the pressure over the carpal tunnel from the splint itself.

Simpler and probably more effective approaches make use of improved ergonomics in the workplace. For example, your chair should be adjusted to a comfortable height with arm rests on the sides when you sit at a computer. The mouse should be directly in front of you on the desk and when you use it, you should keep your elbows close to your body. Use your entire arm to move the mouse, not just the wrist. The keyboard should be tilted downwards so that you can maintain your wrist in a neutral position. Commercially available ergonomic keyboards help maintain the wrist, hand, and fingers in a nearly ideal position during typing, thus eliminating or reducing the stress on the tendons in the carpal tunnel.

Schedule numerous rest periods throughout the day, no matter what type of repetitive activity you engage in. It is also wise to vary your activity as much as possible so that you are not engaged in the same repetitive hand activity for greater than an hour or two at a time. Shifting from one activity to another will allow individual muscles and tendons to rest.

▨ CONDITIONS TO RULE OUT

- **C6 NERVE ROOT COMPRESSION:** Pinching of the *sixth cervical nerve root*, which is located in the neck, usually occurs in middle-aged or elderly people and causes symptoms nearly identical to carpal tunnel syndrome. Symptoms are primarily felt when awakening from sleep, but will not wake a person who is sleeping. This condition differs from carpal tunnel syndrome in that the pain may radiate down the shoulder blade and may be more intense when sneezing, coughing, or bearing down during a bowel movement. Also, there is no relief from wringing the hands.

- **PRONATOR SYNDROME:** This condition is caused by compression of the *median nerve*, which is the same nerve that is compressed during carpal tunnel syndrome, although constriction occurs at the level of the *pronator muscle* in the forearm. Symptoms will vary slightly because the site of nerve injury differs. There will no pain at night. Uncorking a bottle or using a screwdriver with force will increase the pain. Moreover, both the Phalen and Tinel signs will be negative.

TREATMENT OF CARPAL TUNNEL SYNDROME

The treatment for carpal tunnel syndrome varies from simple noninvasive approaches to surgery. In general, one should begin with the least invasive approach and use more invasive treatments only if conservative measures fail. However, sometimes it might be necessary to begin with the most aggressive types of therapy, depending on the severity of the initial symptoms.

- **REST:** It is very important to identify the activity that is causing stress to the median nerve at the wrist and modify how that activity is performed, or simply stop doing it until symptoms improve.

- **EXERCISES:** A variety of different exercises have been recommended for those suffering from mild carpal tunnel syndrome. These maneuvers are designed to stretch the transverse carpal ligament, which forms the roof of the carpal tunnel, providing more room within the compartment and enabling the compressed tendons to move easily. They also help diminish the amount of accumulated fluid within the tunnel by isolating the movement of each tendon.

Stretching the flexor retinaculum involves placing the forearm between the thighs and pulling the thumb backwards with your opposite hand while pressing the thighs together to force the hand into an extension position.

Nerve-gliding or sliding exercises are essential in preventing the scar tissue that may form as a result of the inflammation accompanying carpal tunnel syndrome, especially after surgery. The hands are held straight out in front of the body in these exercises and the wrists are bent upward in extension for about 5 seconds. Then, straighten the wrists and relax. Next, bend the wrists downward in a flexion position for 5 seconds. Repeat this pattern about ten times.

- **SPLINTING:** The use of wrist splints to maintain the wrist in slight dorsiflexion, which will maximize the space in the carpal tunnel, is the most common therapy used to treat mild to moderate carpal tunnel syndrome. Splints should be worn continuously during the acute phase of the illness, especially at night when sleeping and whenever engaged in repetitive hand activities. Splinting is highly effective, but there is a significant likelihood that symptoms may return after use of the splint has been discontinued for awhile.

- **MEDICATIONS:** Few medications have proven very effective in relieving the symptoms of carpal tunnel syndrome. Steroids and non-steroidal anti-inflammatory medications that reduce swelling and inflammation within the carpal tunnel have been tried. These drugs may relieve pain and some of the tingling sensations in mild cases, but they do not significantly alter the course of the illness.

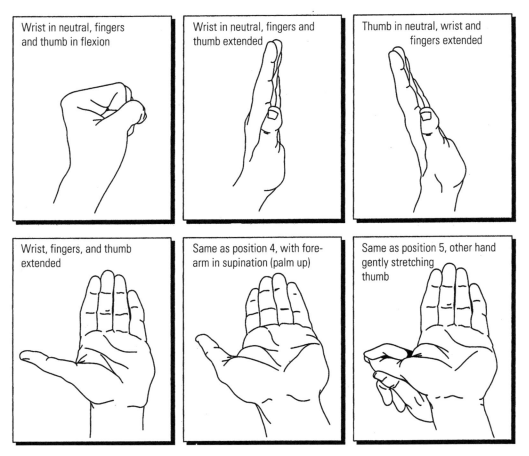

Nerve-gliding exercises.
Hunter JM, Schneider LH, Mackin EJ (eds.): *Rehabilitation of the Hand: Surgery and Therapy*, 3rd Ed. St. Louis: Mosby, 1990.

■ **VITAMINS:** Although evidence regarding vitamin therapy is inconclusive, several studies have shown that 50 mg of vitamin B6 (pyroxidine) three times per day is beneficial to nerves and may help the recovery of the compressed median nerve at the wrist. Some people have reported relief from bromelain, an anti-inflammatory enzyme found in pineapples. The usual dose of 1,000 mg taken twice per day between meals seems most effective when taken together with vitamin B6.

Do not take more than 200 mg per day of vita-min B6 because high dosages may actually cause nerve damage. Vitamin E in dosages between 800 and 1,000 IU per day may relieve inflammation and prevent swelling.

■ **INJECTIONS:** Steroid injections directly into the carpal tunnel, but not into the nerve itself, are somewhat more effective than oral medications and may help avoid the need for surgery in moderately severe cases. Often, however, relief is short-lived with symptoms returning within 6 months of the procedure approximately 50% of the time. No more than three to four injections should ever be permitted for the same wrist because steroids weaken the tendons within the carpal tunnel.

WHEN IS SURGERY NECESSARY?

Surgery is appropriate if physical therapy does not improve symptoms or if loss of sensation persists. The traditional surgical approach to treating carpal tunnel syndrome involves making a two-inch incision over the palm side of the wrist and exposing the transverse carpal ligament that forms the roof of the tunnel. The ligament is cut open and left that way, and the skin above the site is sutured closed. This relatively quick and simple surgical procedure is known as a *transverse carpal release*. It releases the pressure on the median nerve within the carpal tunnel.

There is a newer, less invasive approach called *endoscopic carpal tunnel release*, which involves making a ½ inch incision over the palm side of the wrist and inserting a small arthroscopic tube under the transverse carpal ligament. A small knife attached to the arthroscope cuts open the transverse carpal ligament. The result is the same as with the traditional approach. However, with a smaller incision there is usually less post-operative pain and scarring, and a quicker return to normal functioning. Often, either surgical approach results in immediate and gratifying relief.

DOUBLE CRUSH

Surgery does not always relieve symptoms of carpal tunnel syndrome because the nerve may be compressed somewhere else, although it may be partly compressed at the wrist. Typically, a second site of nerve constriction can occur anywhere in the arm between the neck and the wrist. The nerve is said to undergo a "double crush" when this happens. A good analogy is when you are trying to water your lawn and someone inadvertently stands on the hose. This would be the "first crush." Then, someone else also stands on the hose. This would be the "double crush." Only a dribble of water can manage to come out of the spout when there are two "crushes." With pressure in two places (the neck and wrist) the likelihood of transmission of effective nerve impulse becomes—like the garden hose analogy—even less likely. Management involves increasing the range of motion and flexibility of the muscles and soft tissue throughout the forearm, upper arm, shoulder, and neck in order to gain increased extensibility.

CUBITAL TUNNEL SYNDROME

Although compression of the median nerve at the carpal tunnel is the most common nerve compression syndrome, there are many others. The second most common type of nerve compression in the arm and hand involves compression of the ulnar nerve near the elbow. The ulnar nerve is the nerve

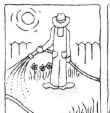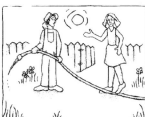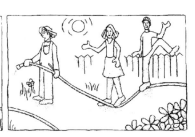

Double crush syndrome can be likened to a garden hose being stepped on in two places.
Fried SM: *The Carpal Tunnel Helpbook*. Cambridge Massachusetts: Perseus Publishing, 2001.

that tingles when you hit your "funny bone." It is responsible for feeling things along the outer part of the ring finger and the little finger. This nerve travels from the spinal cord to the hand, passing along a small groove in the middle, outer portion of the elbow. From there it passes through a narrow area called the *cubital tunnel* before entering the forearm. Like the carpal tunnel, the cubital tunnel has very little room for additional structures, and the ulnar nerve is easily compressed within it.

The ulnar nerve may be compressed within the *condylar groove* before it reaches the cubital tunnel. The condylar groove is a very shallow area and the ulnar nerve may be easily injured by forces external to the body—for example, by falling asleep while leaning on your elbow, especially when it is bent. The ulnar nerve is especially prone to being compressed when the elbow is flexed because this elbow position narrows the diameter of the cubital tunnel. The ulnar nerve may be compressed within the cubital tunnel due to arthritis of the joint, tumors, bony abnormalities, or by degenerative changes in the muscles that border the cubital tunnel. Most often, however, an exact cause cannot be identified, and we refer to it as *idiopathic ulnar compression*, which basically means: "We do not know the cause." In most instances where the cause of ulnar nerve compression is unknown, it is due to a problem in the cubital tunnel. However, there is no clinical means of differentiating compression of the ulnar nerve at the condylar groove from compression within the cubital tunnel. Both of these conditions feel the same and will appear the same to the doctor. A good way to provoke symptoms and confirm that the ulnar nerve is, indeed, compressed at the elbow region is to perform the elbow flexion test to stretch the nerve.

People with cubital tunnel syndrome will often report feeling numbness, tingling, or pain in the distribution of the ulnar nerve, meaning in the ring and little finger. Some may simply report that their "funny bone" is unusually sensitive. They may have hand weakness and even some thinning out (atrophy) of the hand muscles when cubital tunnel syndrome is severe. The doctor should carefully examine the arm along the entire course of the nerve to determine if there is some abnormal growth that might be compressing the ulnar nerve and causing symptoms.

■ TREATMENT OF CUBITAL TUNNEL SYNDROME

The object of conservative therapy is to minimize pressure at the condylar groove and the cubital tunnel in cases where there is no obvious growth compressing the nerve. The elbows should be leaned on as little as possible. Arms of chairs that are frequently used may be covered with padding. Elbow pads should also be worn to limit external compression and also to limit bending of the elbow, because compression and bending increase the pressure within the cubital tunnel and over the condylar groove. The elbow pad should be worn around the clock when the cubital tunnel syndrome is severe, but it is especially important to wear it at night when most of the natural compression occurs. There is a very limited role, if any, for medications and injections in the treatment of cubital tunnel syndrome.

■ WHEN IS SURGERY NECESSARY?

It may be necessary to consider surgery if conservative approaches do not work. The procedure usually involves splitting the *flexor carpi ulnaris* muscle, which borders the cubital tunnel, thereby releasing the pressure within the tunnel. Some surgeons advocate removing the nerve from the cubital tunnel and condylar groove, and placing it within a different portion of the forearm. This is a more complicated type of surgery that is usually reserved for situations where the nerve is injured from severe bony or joint abnormalities, those situations where the nerve cannot be decompressed simply by opening the cubital tunnel. The danger of this proce- dure, however, is that the surgeon may compromise the normal blood supply to the nerve by moving it, thereby predisposing the nerve to more permanent injury.

Elbow

THE ELBOW is particularly vulnerable to sports injuries involving the use of the whole arm. Overuse of the forearm muscles during sports such as tennis and golf can result in overloading of the tendons and muscles that connect the hand and wrist to the elbow, often resulting in fatigue, injury, and inflammation. This section discusses proper technique and use of equipment in order to avoid injuries of the elbow.

25 Tennis Elbow

A recently divorced 44-year-old dentist began playing tennis with gusto after a 2-year hiatus. After about 2 weeks of playing just about every day, he complained of left elbow pain toward the end of each game. Lately, he is beginning to feel symptoms at work while holding his dental instruments. Bending his wrist toward his pinky and bending his hand upward against resistance reproduces symptoms. This man has tennis elbow.

ELBOW PAIN

Tennis elbow does not usually occur from playing tennis, but typically follows a weekend of hedge clipping, excessive use of a screwdriver or hammer, or other activities that require constant squeezing or gripping. You may be susceptible to getting tennis elbow if you do not rest adequately, and if you have already come down with tennis elbow, it may become severely painful, leading to temporary loss of function and motion of the elbow. Pain is experienced when rotating the hand in a clockwise direction—for example, as when screwing in a light bulb. Long-term disability rarely occurs.

Several of the muscles that move the wrist and fingers, and form the bulk of muscles beneath the top side of the forearm blend into a shared tendon known as the *common extensor tendon*. This tendon attaches onto the *humerus* at a bump of bone known as the *lateral epicondyle*, which is located on the outer (lateral) side of the elbow. These muscles travel across the wrist and attach onto the hand as tendons. They extend the top of the wrist and hand when they contract along their bulk near the elbow. They are called *forearm extensors*.

TENNIS ELBOW DEFINED

The technical name for tennis elbow is *lateral epicondylitis*. It is the most common overuse type injury of an upper limb. *Overuse injuries* are also known as *repetitive stress injuries*. They are due to excessive use and the fact that the tissues of the body are less capable of dealing with stress with each advancing year. People between the ages of 30 and 50 are particularly prone to tennis elbow, especially if they use

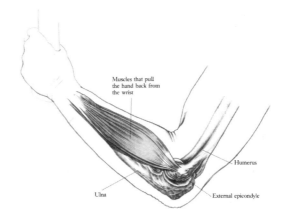

Muscles that pull the hand back from the wrist

Humerus

Ulna

External epicondyle

Peterson L, Renstrom P: *Sports Injuries: Their Prevention and Treatment.* Chicago: Year Book Medical Publishers Inc., 1986.

their forearm and wrist extensively or play tennis three or more times per week. This leads to excessive stress of the wrist extensor muscles and focuses a high load per area on the common tendon attachment on the *lateral epicondyle,* located near the elbow. Overuse of the forearm muscles results in overloading of the *common extensor tendon* beyond its ability to tolerate stress. As a result, the tendon becomes fatigued, injured, and inflamed. The *-itis* suffix refers to inflammation of the common extensor tendon at the epicondylar bump.

WHO IS MOST LIKELY TO HAVE TENNIS ELBOW?

Approximately one-third of America's tennis players suffer from tennis elbow at some point. Tennis elbow occurs in both elbows over 50% of the time and most commonly occurs in the dominant elbow, particularly 1 month or so after playing with a new racquet. It is more common in women, due to the variability of hormones from gynecologic factors such as menopause and hysterectomy. However, the majority of people do not develop tennis elbow from playing tennis, but from daily activities such as gardening, carpentry, scouring pots, or simply carrying an attaché case to and from work every day. The common denominator of these activities involves repetitive forearm use while gripping an object. Excessive overuse of the *extensor* muscles, which are the muscles that bend the top side of your hand toward your face, may also occur from needlework or playing squash. Professionals who are particularly prone to developing tennis elbow are politicians (from shaking hands) and dentists, who grip precision instruments for extended periods of time. Golfers can also suffer from tennis elbow, but usually on the nondominant side. A left-handed golfer may experience pain in the right elbow if she pulls the club through the swing with the right wrist.

The risk of tennis elbow is even greater for middle-aged players because the tendons lose some of their resiliency after age 30 and are less capable of withstanding the constant repetitive stress that accompanies a spirited, frequent game of tennis that can last up to 2 hours. This loss of resiliency is normal to all people as they age. It is known as the *degenerative process,* in which the body is incapable of recovering fast enough from the stress caused by sustained activity or overuse. Hence the term "overuse syndrome."

WHY TENNIS ELBOW HURTS

The common extensor tendon can be injured because the extensor forearm muscles pull too strongly on the lateral epicondyle or because they become fatigued. Both processes result in microscopic tears of the tendon-bone junction where it attaches to the elbow. This initiates the inflammatory process, which is a natural response of the body to injury. With time, the body attempts to painlessly heal the tear by creating scar tissue. However, if activity continues without sufficient rest, continued tearing may occur before healing is complete, causing the repair cycle to start all over again. If this interruption of normal healing continues to reoccur, the torn tendon will not receive enough oxygen because of diminished blood flow. In response, the body may get defensive and overreact by treating the tear like a bone fracture. Bone crystal in the form of an irregular spicule develops within the cleft of tendon that gets larger with increased activity. It irritates the tendon further by rubbing against it.

CONTRIBUTING FACTORS: POOR TECHNIQUE

Tennis is a game of physical and mental challenges. Tennis elbow is not merely an elbow problem, just

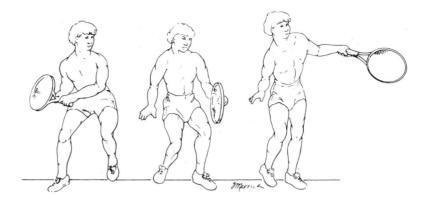

Phases of the tennis backhand. From left to right: preparation, acceleration, and follow-through.
Nicholas JA, Hershman EB: *The Upper Extremity in Sports Medicine*, 2nd Edition. St. Louis: Mosby, 1995.

as tennis is not exclusively an upper limb activity. Executing a good racquet swing requires a synchronized group of body movements, not just swinging the arm. Many people punch at the ball instead of using the whole body to sling through a backhand stroke. For most players, a successful backhand is an especially difficult stroke to master. Many players aggravate the elbow by hitting the ball late on a backhand swing. Stress to the forearm muscles can be diminished by using the torso and shoulder during a backhand swing stroke.

Faulty backhand technique often brings on tennis elbow in a majority of the tennis players who develop lateral epicondylitis. You are more likely to fatigue the forearm extensor muscles if you lead with your elbow on the backhand stroke. A correct backhand stroke involves adequate anticipation of the stroke so that the player's entire body, including the lower body, prepares for the oncoming ball. The force of impact should derive from the trunk and lower body, and not simply the forearm. The elbow and wrist must be held firm, with minimal motion. A backhand stroke is more difficult to perform than the forearm stroke. The player usually gets the racquet back too late or is too slow in getting to the ball on time, and then tries to compensate by using the forearm muscles as a primary power source, hitting the ball with excessive wrist motion. By incorrectly leading with the elbow on the backhand stroke, the

racket lags behind the elbow and then picks up speed as it moves in to meet the ball. The racket comes to an abrupt stop on impact. It is the force of this abrupt stop that moves up the arm to the lateral epicondyle. You may also get tennis elbow by turning your wrist to put more spin on the serve.

■ **CONTRIBUTING FACTORS: INAPPROPRIATE EQUIPMENT**

Equipment plays an important role in the development or prevention of tennis elbow:

- **HEAVY TENNIS BALLS:** Dead or wet balls require greater effort to serve or stop. Using new or recently used balls is easier on the arm and elbow.

- **HARD COURTS:** Concrete courts cause the ball to rebound faster, increasing the impact force against the racket and the arm. Clay, grass, wood, or asphalt courts are softer and much preferred.

- **HIGH STRING TENSION:** Tight strings are often recommended for their superior ability to strike a ball farther and faster. However, they absorb the shock of forceful impact less efficiently and increase stress transmitted to the elbow. It is best to stay on the lower end of the manufacturer's recommendation for string tension in order to reduce torque and vibration. The optimal stringing materials for non-tournament players is synthetic nylon (16" gauge) that is restrung every 6 months.

- **RACQUET SIZE:** A smaller racquet reduces the "sweet spot" available for optimal force contact between the racquet and ball. This mathematical center of percussion is located in the middle of the racquet face and is the ideal place for striking the ball. A smaller racquet has a smaller sweet spot and will correspondingly increase torsion, unwanted force, and vibration to the arm. The mid-size (95 to 110 square inches) to larger size racquet is preferable.

- **RACQUET MATERIAL:** Metal racquets, particularly aluminum ones, are considerably stiffer and vibrate at impact. They are more likely to aggravate the extensor forearm tendons. Graphite composites absorb vibration and minimize torsion most efficiently. They are recommended as the primary choice for racquet material. Wood or fiberglass racquets are preferred over metal rackets.

- **RACQUET WEIGHT:** A casual player is cautioned to use a light racquet because an oversized, heavier racquet causes the arm to experience greater loads. While a larger racquet allows for a larger sweet spot, it is self-defeating to use one if it is too heavy to easily position. Players are one and one-half times more prone to tennis elbow from a medium-weight racquet than a lightweight one. A large, graphite racquet is best because it is lightweight. It can more readily absorb torsion and allows the player wider access to striking an oncoming ball.

- **RACQUET GRIP SIZE:** A bigger grip helps reduce the possibility of tennis elbow because a racquet grip that is too small reduces hand control of the racquet, resulting in excessive wrist motion. A grip that is too large also compromises good racquet control because the player may find the racquet too unwieldy to swing. A reliable method of measuring your hand for the right type of grip is to measure the length between the upper tip of the ring finger and the first large crease on the palm (the one closest to the wrist) with a tape measure. (Note: some experts believe the middle finger should be used.) This is one way of determining the ideal diameter of the grip for each individual. Another popular way that is recommended by experts is to grip the racquet normally and measure a finger width in the gap between the fingers and the thick swelling of muscles on the palm of your hand between the base of the thumb and your wrist.

■ SIGNS AND SYMPTOMS

Tennis elbow evolves through several stages of injury, with each stage representing a higher-grade

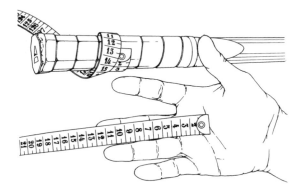

Measuring the right size racquet grip. The distance between the midline of the palm and the tip of the middle finger is equal to the correct size of the grip.
Peterson L, Renstrom P: *Sports Injuries: Their Prevention and Treatment*. Chicago: Year Book Medical Publishers Inc., 1986.

injury of the common extensor tendon at the lateral epicondyle. These stages are:

- **STAGE I:** In the early stage of injury, generalized elbow soreness is felt after activity. Unfortunately, while this should be a sign to players to rest and minimize athletic participation, most people simply ignore this feeling and continue the activity. This sets up a vicious cycle of irritation, inflammation, and inadequate healing. Listen to your body. Rest. This is the best time to recognize early warning signs and prevent tennis elbow.

- **STAGE II:** The outer side of the upper elbow area becomes sore to the touch in the next stage of tennis elbow. Continuing work or other activities even though experiencing pain disrupts the body's efforts to heal and worsens the original injury. Occasionally, the outer elbow may appear slightly swollen and feel warm to the touch. Pain will typically interfere with activity—for example, as when turning a doorknob—and the player may be unable to swing a backstroke. There will be no real muscle weakness, but rather a perception of weakness due to pain limitation. Confirmation of a suspicion of stage II tennis elbow involves resist-

ing wrist extension and simultaneously bending the wrist to the outer side (lateral deviation) while the elbow is extended. Suspected tennis elbow is confirmed if there is pain as a result of this test.

- **STAGE III:** This stage corresponds to a full-blown case of tennis elbow that has worsened to the point that even the simple activities of daily living become difficult or painful. Turning a doorknob, holding a pencil, shaking hands, or lifting a coffee mug to your mouth to drink are all examples of daily activities of living that may become difficult and precipitate pain. A tennis player may even experience sudden twinges of pain that cause him to drop his racket.

■ CONDITIONS TO RULE OUT

Several different conditions may mimic tennis elbow and should be ruled out by a health professional. Tennis elbow is diagnosed by history and clinical examination. X-rays are not helpful. Conditions to be ruled out include:

- **PINCHED NERVE:** A pinched nerve in the lower neck may cause pain at the elbow and possibly be mistaken for tennis elbow. This often occurs in middle-aged people with arthritis rather than from excessive use of the wrist and forearm. Different postures of the neck either worsen or improve elbow pain with a pinched nerve. Neck movements have no effect on how much pain you feel with tennis elbow. Instead, resisting the wrist from bending back into extension often worsens pain, whereas a pinched neck nerve will not be affected by wrist motion.

- **RADIAL TUNNEL SYNDROME:** This condition involves entrapment of the *radial nerve*. This

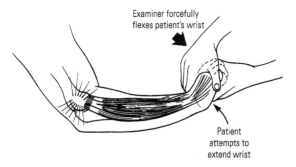

Examiner forcefully flexes patient's wrist

Patient attempts to extend wrist

Provocative test of tennis elbow, which involves trying to move the wrist upward while someone pushes your wrist downward forcefully. Pain is considered confirmation of tennis elbow.
Saidoff DC, McDonough AL: *Critical Pathways in Therapeutic Intervention: Extremities and Spine.* St. Louis: Mosby, 2002.

nerve enters the forearm near the extensor *carpi radialis brevis* muscle. This is the most commonly inflamed muscle during a bout of tennis elbow. The inflammation may spread to the nearby radial nerve and cause irritation, mimicking symptoms of tennis elbow.

- **ELBOW JOINT INFLAMMATION:** This condition involves inflammation of the joint near the elbow, which is made up of two bones: the *radius* and *humerus*. The radius is a long forearm bone along the thumb side of the arm that spans the space between the wrist and elbow, and the humerus is the long upper arm bone spanning between the elbow and shoulder. These two long bones meet at the elbow and form the *radiohumeral joint*. This joint may become inflamed in people with gout, although they usually know they have gout from previous gouty episodes in the big toe. Radio-humeral joint inflammation may also occur in people with rheumatoid arthritis, a condition that is accompanied by many other symptoms throughout the body. Inflammation may also occur from infection at this joint and is often accompanied by a red, swollen, and warm elbow; these are signs that do not occur with tennis elbow.

PREVENTION AND TREATMENT

The majority of cases of tennis elbow get better with a broad therapeutic approach rather than just focusing on one approach. Stretching and strengthening exercises are the main methods of prevention and treatment of this condition. If you are feeling pain in your elbow, forearm, or wrist during or after a game of tennis, do not panic. Do not try to keep playing, or you may make it worse. Simply use the following approaches to avoid a full-blown case of tennis elbow. Do not rush back to your previous level of activity using the forearm muscles once you start to feel better. Instead, increase your level of activity gradually. All treatment should be performed following an evaluation and under the direction of a healthcare professional.

- **REST:** As stated above, resting between games or other strenuous activities is critical. The old adage "no pain—no gain" can lead to overuse injuries in many people. Pain is the body's way of saying "Please rest!" So, be kind to your body and let it rest. A short time out between playing tennis or other activities involving the elbow may go a long way in preventing injury. Stretching the muscles prior to engaging in any activity is also very important in avoiding injury. Avoiding or cutting back on the activity that led to the injury is recommended. The best type of rest for tennis elbow is to use the elbow normally for all activities that do not aggravate the pain. Do not rest your arm in a sling. You can gradually increase the activities that were painful after your elbow begins to heal.

- **PROTECTION:** Protecting the elbow from injury and chilling is important (particularly chilling) because the elbow has little or no covering of subcutaneous fat and the resulting exposure can lead to injury. The sensation of pressure from wearing a protective sleeve may mask the pain during the initial healing process and remind the wearer to be careful. It also serves to keep the elbow warm.

- **ICE AND HEAT:** Cold therapy is very helpful during the acute inflammatory stage because it decreases inflammation and limits pain. Icing that includes the application of a barrier oil may be performed two to three times per day for approximately 10 to 15 minutes per icing after work or sports activities involving the affected elbow. It can be applied using an ice bag or by massage using an ice cube. Applying heat locally after the acute phase is over and the chronic phase has begun will continue to support heal-ing. Alternating hot and cold local applications may have the effect of "washing out" the accu-mulation of pain chemicals and bring in the needed repair substances.

If you have diabetes, peripheral neuropathies, or other conditions that make your body partially insensitive to temperature, consult your profes-sional medical provider before attempting to use hot and cold applications.

■ **MEDICATION:** Oral non-steroidal anti-inflamma-tory drugs are very helpful in controlling both the pain and inflammation associated with tennis elbow. Non-prescription medications include ibuprofen (Motrin®, Advil®, Nuprin®, and Medi-pren®) and prescription medications (Naprosyn®, Indocin®, Feldene®, and Relafen®). All medica-tions should be used under the direction of a doc-tor because of potential side effects.

■ **WARMING UP:** Adequate warm-ups should be performed for 10 minutes before engaging in physical activities. Warm-ups include stretching and gently moving the joints through the entire range of motion in a relaxed manner. Pay partic-ular attention to the elbow. Range of motion and stretching should always be performed after sports activities. This is known as "cooling-down."

■ **STRETCHING:** Be sure to stretch all of the major muscle groups before and after engaging in sports activities, paying particular attention to stretching the forearm extensors. It is easy to be misled by the common misconception that if your forearm looks good and strong and has bulging muscles, it will protect you from getting tennis elbow. Not so. A big, strong forearm may be so tight from pumping iron that it lacks adequate flexibility. It is essential to stretch muscles to keep them strong. You will be predisposed toward get-ting tennis elbow if the forearm wrist extensors are tight. The elbows may have to take on exces-sive or abnormal movement in compensation for a tight neck and shoulders. This can lead to faulty movement patterns and increase the likelihood of tennis elbow. So, be sure to stretch the fore-arm muscles and the muscles of the neck and shoulder girdle back to normal length.

Gaining flexibility and muscle length in the extensor muscles of the forearm through stretch-ing will take up some of the pull placed on the lat-eral epicondyle. Place the back of your hand on a flat surface while keeping the elbow straight in order to stretch the wrist extensors. Then, gently lean forward and feel the stretch in your forearm.

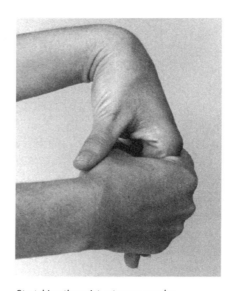

Stretching the wrist extensor muscles.
Brotzman SB, (ed.): *Clinical Orthopaedic Rehabilitation.* St. Louis: Mosby, 1996.

■ **STRENGTHENING:** Lack of adequate forearm strength can lead to tendonitis because lack of muscle strength means there will be less of the soft tissue necessary to diminish the stress deliv-ered up the arm. Strengthening of the forearm muscles should begin with the elbow halfway bent, followed by stretching with the elbow out straight. Exercise increases muscle bulk, which helps dissipate injurious forces. Exercises such as wrist curls should be increased gradually; begin with small weights and progress to greater weights slowly. Eccentric exercises involve lengthening of muscle fibers and are particularly helpful.

■ **BRACING:** A lateral counterforce brace is worn near the elbow both during work and when participating in sports. This strap may provide effective prevention for those who have recovered from previous tennis elbow and wish to prevent future recurrences. Apply the 4-inch strap snugly around the relaxed upper forearm in order to minimize stress at the lateral epicondyle. It is important to avoid putting these bands on too tightly and possibly cutting off circulation! Bear in mind how easy it is to fall into the false security that a brace can be used as a sole means of treatment. Rather, counterforce braces should supplement muscular stretching and strengthening exercises.

Wrist braces keep the wrist bent gently backwards and ease the tension on the common extensor tendon at the elbow, thereby relieving pain. This type of brace may be used during the day, but preferably not at night.

■ **THERAPEUTIC MASSAGE:** Massage of the forearm muscles is often helpful and pleasant. It can be performed while taking a shower or bath. Friction massage involves rubbing the injured area back and forth or in a circular motion with the thumb or fingers. This may actually increase pain at the time it is performed, but it will feel good afterwards. Massage promotes healing because it increases local blood flow. The local fluid collection known as *edema* is caused by inflammation. Massage presses this fluid and the accumulated pain chemicals out of the tissues. This deep form

of massage also stretches the healing fibers, thereby allowing them to heal in a stretched manner, which is more desirable.

■ **ULTRASOUND:** Ultrasound involves electricity passed though special crystals, which vibrate at ultrasonic (high) frequencies. This vibration penetrates deep into tissue as heat energy and may provide relief once tennis elbow passes beyond its acute stage. Ultrasound applied in the pulsed mode may deliver pain-relieving medications to the inflamed extensor tendon.

■ **INJECTIONS:** Steroid injections may be considered when the above-described measures have not been successful, or in the event that pain is severe. Typically, a shot of cortisone is injected into the area of the common extensor tendon in order to decrease inflammation. Occasionally, one shot is not enough and a second shot is necessary. No more than three shots should ever be administered because steroids are so strong they can weaken the tendon and cause it to rupture. Avoid cortisone shots until you have tried everything else. Consider it as a last resort, not an easy solution.

■ **POSTURE:** Good posture is an essential component of health, and it is necessary to prevent overuse injuries such as tennis elbow. Muscles that are tight do not allow the torso and limbs to move normally and place undue strain on muscles, tendons, and joints.

■ **EDUCATION:** Hiring a sports technique instructor for several visits is well worth the time and money because he can point out faulty form and teach better body mechanics and tennis technique. Faulty tennis strokes move the lower body minimally and use the arm as the primary power source, thus making the elbow more vulnerable to injury. Also, adopting a two-handed backhand considerably reduces the chance for injury. While this may seem more cumbersome, it may certainly be worth considering if it lessens the chance for injury.

■ WHEN IS SURGERY NECESSARY?

Surgery is indicated when a conservative course of action has failed over the course of several months, and the person is still complaining of significant pain and inability to use the arm. There are two types of surgeries for tennis elbow: (1) A small incision is made and the abnormal tendon is trimmed; and (2) a portion of tendon is released from the bone and then reattached. People who have either type of surgery return home the same day with the arm in a sling. Most of them cannot drive for a week. Surgery is quite successful in relieving pain and usually allows for a return to daily activity without pain in less than 6 months. However, returning to sports or heavy use of the arm may take several months.

26 Golfer's Elbow

*A 46-year-old man was recently able to retire because of financial success due to stock options
that he owned prior to his company's successful initial public offering. Now he spends most
of his time avidly playing golf. He is right-handed and complains of both right and left elbow pain.
He has spent the last 4 days out on the golf course, and his elbow pain is getting increasingly worse,
although taking aspirin seems to help. He experiences pain with both resisted left wrist
flexion and extension of his right wrist against resistance. This man has golfer's elbow
in his trailing arm and tennis elbow in his leading arm.*

GOLF

THE GAME OF GOLF has its origins in fourteenth
century Scotland. It gained popularity in the
sixteenth century when it was taken up by James IV,
the King of Scotland. The game later spread to the
European continent when his granddaughter, Mary
Queen of Scots played the game in France. Participation in golf has literally exploded since that time,
and it has been adopted throughout the world as a
sport that is as relaxing as it is focused. Today, some
24 million Americans of different ages and skill levels play golf at least once per year at approximately
14,000 golf courses scattered throughout the
United States.

A person who does not play golf might imagine
that it is less taxing than other sports. This is truly a
misconception because injuries involving the arms,
legs, and back are frequent. Most golf injuries are
related to the golf swing and, therefore, most golf
injuries occur to the hands, forearms, elbows, shoulders, and back. The most common mechanism of
injury is too much practice, which causes overuse
syndromes. These syndromes occur in the recre-

ational golfer because of a poorly executed swing.
They may occur from the repeated stress of practice by the professional golfer. Other common
causes of injury include unintentionally striking
trees, roots, or hard ground with the golf club. Two
of the most common injuries to the elbow region
are medial epicondylitis and lateral epicondylitis,
commonly known as golfer's elbow and tennis
elbow, respectively. Believe it or not, tennis elbow
occurs more commonly from playing golf than does
traditional golfer's elbow, especially in amateurs.

Golfer's elbow can occur with any activity that
involves using the hand and wrist in a particular way.
It can happen from gardening and carpentry just as
easily as it can happen from playing golf.

GOLFER'S ELBOW DEFINED

Several of the muscles that move the wrist and fingers, and form the bulk of muscles on the bottom
side of the forearm, blend into a shared tendon
known as the *common flexor tendon*. This tendon
attaches onto the *humerus* at a bump of bone known

as the *medial epicondyle* (literally, "side bump") located on the inner (medial) side of the elbow. These muscles travel across the wrist and attach onto the hand as tendons. They contract along their bulk near the elbow and pick up (flex) the underside of the wrist and hand. They are called *forearm flexors*.

The technical name for golfer's elbow is *medial epicondylitis*, and it is less common than tennis elbow. *Overuse injuries* are also known as *repetitive stress injuries*, which are due to excessive use and the fact that the tissues of the body are less capable of dealing with stress with each advancing year. People between the ages of 30 and 50 are particularly prone to golfer's elbow, especially if they use their forearm and wrist extensively, or play golf three or more times per week. This leads to excessive stress of the wrist flexor muscles and focuses a high load per area on the common tendon attachment at the *medial epicondyle,* located near the inner portion of the elbow. Overuse of the forearm muscles results in overloading of the *common flexor tendon* beyond its ability to tolerate stress. As a result, the tendon becomes fatigued, injured, and inflamed. The *-itis* suffix refers to inflammation of the common flexor tendon at the epicondylar bump. Golfer's elbow can also result from trauma—for example, when a golf club head hits a rock, tree root, or other object.

The most common mechanism of injury in the right-handed golfer is caused by hitting from the top. This means that instead of pulling the club through with the left side using the legs, back, shoulder, and other muscles, the golfer throws the club from the top of the backswing (take-away) down into the ball at impact. This is similar to hitting a forehand in tennis or "kill shot" in racquetball, and it can cause extreme stress on the flexor muscles, especially at the medial epicondyle. Golfer's elbow usually occurs in the left (lead) elbow because golfers are right-handed.

Ignoring golfer's elbow may cause it to become severely painful, leading to temporary loss of function and motion across the elbow. This may be avoided with adequate rest of the forearm, wrist, and fingers on the affected side. Long-term disability rarely occurs.

◼ WHO IS MOST LIKELY TO HAVE GOLFER'S ELBOW?

Golf is one of those activities that look easy until you try it. Golf is a strenuous game, and many frustrated

A. Golfer illustrating bent elbow and poor swinging mechanics. B. Golfer illustrating poor weight shift and poor swinging mechanics. C. Golfer illustrating correct swing position at top of take-away. Nicholas JA, Hershman EB: *The Upper Extremity in Sports Medicine,* Second edition, Mosby, St. Louis 1995.

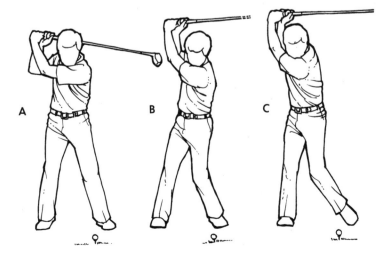

weekend golfers try to play when they are not in good shape. Many of these weekend golfers ruin the entire golf season by developing overuse injuries in the shoulder, elbow, wrist, and back—not to mention the pain, aggravating loss of function, and inconvenience. The likelihood for epicondylitis from playing golf increases in proportion to the number of rounds played, with more than two to three rounds per week as a threshold for increased incidence.

Gymnasts are also particularly prone to developing golfer's elbow. The upper extremities of humans are smaller and weaker than the legs, thighs, and feet because we did not evolve for the purpose of walking on the hands and arms. The upper extremities are designed for finer manipulation and movements. However, gymnasts who repetitively use the upper extremities for bearing full body weight subject the muscles and tendons of the hands and arms to heavy compression loads. This places chronic traction stress across the medial epicondyle. Baseball pitchers or other athletes who are required to throw are also more susceptible to developing medial epicondylitis because of the repetitive stress applied to the flexor-pronator muscle mass with each throw.

Golfer's elbow may develop in recreational tennis players who use faulty forehand technique. It can also develop in top-level players who serve a ball with the wrist flexed and *radially* deviated inwardly (tilted toward the thumb side) at the same time that the forearm is pronated. Golfer's elbow can also happen to tennis players who *pronate* (rotate) their forearm too much while hitting an exaggerated topspin on the ball. A baseball pitcher imparting a spin to cause a curveball whips his arm forward with the wrist, forearm, and elbow postured in such a way that considerable traction is focused on the common flexor tendon and the medial epicondyle. Repetitive stress applied to the flexor-pronator muscle mass with each throw accumulates to the point of injury. Because of this, baseball pitchers are bet-

ter off using a pitch that spares injury to the elbow, such as a knuckle-ball pitch.

AGE AND STRENGTH

Golfer's elbow usually occurs in players between 35 and 55 years of age. The risk for golfer's elbow is greater in middle-aged players because the tendons lose some of their resiliency after age 30 and are less capable of withstanding the constant repetitive stress that accompanies a spirited game of golf that can last up to several hours. This loss of resiliency is normal to all people as they age. It is known as the *degenerative process,* wherein the body is incapable of recovering fast enough from the stress caused by sustained activity.

Muscles become weaker as people get older. Golf is a game that requires force to be expended throughout the body, not just the shoulders or trunk. For example, driving power involves the buttocks, quadriceps, hamstrings, and lower back muscles. The lower back muscles and hip flexors are involved in allowing for a good hip turn, and the impact velocity from swinging the club at the ball requires strong triceps and *latissimus dorsi muscles.* In the same vein, if a golfer has strong shoulder muscles but weak forearm flexors, she will be more likely to stress her medial epicondyle.

CONTRIBUTING FACTORS: POOR TECHNIQUE

Golf is a game of physical and mental challenges. Golfer's elbow is not merely an elbow problem, just as golf is not exclusively an upper limb activity. Executing a good golf club swing requires a synchronized group of body movements, not just swinging the arm. The correctly executed golf swing includes five separate components in a smooth chain of motion that involves all parts of the body. Force is transferred from the ankles to the legs and to the back, the shoulders, and right out through the wrist. Stress to the forearm muscles can be diminished by using all of these joints and posturing the limbs in the correct manner.

The force of impact should derive from the trunk and lower body, not simply the forearm. The elbow and wrist must be held firm and move with minimal motion. Some players try to compensate by using the forearm muscles as the primary source of power, and they hit the ball with excessive wrist motion. The force to drive the ball should come from the whole body.

■ CONTRIBUTING FACTORS: INAPPROPRIATE EQUIPMENT AND SWING

Equipment and swing mechanics play an important role in the prevention and treatment of golfer's elbow:

■ **SWEET SPOT:** Using cavity-backed irons that have larger sweet spots will dampen the vibrations transmitted to the wrists and forearms from off-center hits. The "sweet spot" is the mathematical center of percussion located in the middle of the clubface. It is the ideal site for striking the ball. A smaller club head has a smaller sweet spot that will correspondingly increase torsion and unwanted force and vibration to the arm.

■ **CLUB MATERIAL:** Metal clubs, particularly aluminum ones, are considerably stiffer and vibrate on impact. Thus, they are more likely to aggravate the flexor forearm tendons. Graphite composites absorb vibration and minimize torsion the best. They are recommended as the primary choice for golf clubs. Wood or fiberglass clubs are preferred over metal clubs.

■ **CLUB WEIGHT:** Casual players are cautioned to use lightweight golf clubs because a heavy club causes the arm to experience greater loads. A graphite club shaft is recommended because it is lightweight and can more readily absorb stress. In contrast, steel shafts are less flexible than graphite and result in increased vibrations from hitting fast shots.

■ **CLUB GRIP SIZE AND SHAPE:** The proper size and shape of the grip are important in order to ensure proper swing mechanics and to relieve torsional stress on impact. A larger club grip is eas-

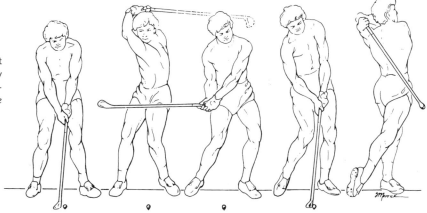

The five phases of the golf swing from left to right: take-away, forward swing, early acceleration, late acceleration, and follow-through. Nicholas JA, Hershman EB: *The Upper Extremity in Sports Medicine.*

ier to wield and delivers less tension to the medial epicondyle. The stiffness of the shafts and the length and weight of the club also play an important role. The swing right grip is the standard accepted golf grip, consisting of a vertical shaft. The newer Bio-Curve grip decreases torsional stress to the arm and hand by virtue of having a curved grip. Unfortunately, it is not in common use because it has not yet been approved by the United States Golf Association.

■ **SWING:** It is especially important to swing the golf club correctly. If the swing is too flat, meaning that it is too close to parallel to the ground, the elbow will be under too much stress. If the swing is too steep, meaning it is too close to perpendicular to the ground, the hands and wrists will overcompensate in order to position the head for ball impacts. This increases the risk of hitting a fat shot, which transmits decelerative forces to the hands, wrists, and elbows. Bending the left elbow on take-away causes the elbow to be extended sharply into the ball at impact, causing increased stress to the forearm that may lead to golfer's elbow.

■ SIGNS AND SYMPTOMS

Golfer's elbow evolves through several stages of injury, with each stage representing a higher-grade injury of the common extensor tendon at the medial epicondyle. These stages are:

■ **STAGE I:** In the early stage of injury, mild elbow soreness and discomfort is felt after activity, while bending or straightening the elbow, or when performing activities that involve counter-clockwise rotation of the hand such as screwing-out a light bulb or screwing a lid off a jar. Unfortunately, while this should be a sign to players to rest and

minimize athletic participation, most people simply ignore this feeling and continue activity. This sets up what is technically known as a vicious cycle of irritation, inflammation, and inadequate healing. Listen to your body. Rest. Recognize these early warning signs and prevent golfer's elbow.

■ **STAGE II:** The inner side of the upper elbow area becomes sore to touch in the next stage of golfer's elbow. Continuing work or other activities, even though experiencing pain, disrupts the body's efforts to heal and worsens the original injury. Occasionally, the inner elbow may appear slightly swollen and feel warm to the touch. Pain will typically interfere with activities such as turning a doorknob, and the player may be unable to swing a club during a round. There will be no real muscle weakness, but rather a perception of weakness and limitation due to pain. Confirmation of stage II golfer's elbow involves resisting wrist flexion and simultaneously bending the wrist to the inner side (medial deviation) while the elbow is extended. Suspected golfer's elbow is confirmed if there is pain during this test.

■ **STAGE III:** This stage corresponds to a full-blown case of golfer's elbow that has worsened to the point that even the simple activities of daily living become difficult or painful. Turning a doorknob, holding a pencil, shaking hands, or lifting up a coffee mug to your mouth to drink are all examples of daily activities that may become difficult and precipitate pain. A golfer may even experience sudden twinges of pain that cause her to drop her golf club.

■ PREVENTION AND TREATMENT

The majority of cases of golfer's elbow get better with a broad therapeutic approach rather than just focusing on one approach. Stretching and strengthening exercises are the mainstays of prevention and treatment of this condition. Do not panic if you feel pain in your elbow, forearm, or wrist during or after a game of golf. Do not try to keep playing, or you may make it worse. Simply use the following approaches to avoid developing a full-blown golfer's elbow, and do not rush back to your previous level of activity using the forearm muscles once you start to feel better. Instead, increase your level of activity gradually. Keep in mind that injuries, sore muscles, and frustrating days at the golf course may be offset by adhering to a pre-season, regular season, and off-season conditioning program. Gymnasts with medial epicondylitis do not need to take time out from gymnastics in order to heal. They can recover rapidly by using adequate icing, strengthening, stretching, and resting via technique adjustment.

- **REST:** Adequate rest between games is an important part of sports. The old adage "no pain—no gain" can lead to overuse and injury in many people. Pain is the body's way of saying "Please rest!" So, be kind to your body and let it rest. A short time out between playing golf and participating in other activities involving the elbow may go a long way in preventing injury. Stretching the muscles prior to engaging in any activity is also very important to avoiding injury. Avoiding or cutting back on the activity that led to injury is recommended. The best type of rest for golfer's elbow is to use the elbow normally for all activities that do not aggravate the pain. Do not rest your arm in a sling. You can gradually increase the activities that were painful after your elbow begins to heal.

- **PROTECTION:** Protecting the elbow from injury and chilling is important (particularly chilling) because the elbow has little or no covering of subcutaneous fat and the resulting exposure can lead to injury. The sensation of pressure from wearing a protective sleeve may mask the pain during the initial healing process and remind the wearer to be careful. It also serves to keep the elbow warm.

- **ICE AND HEAT:** Cold therapy is very helpful in the acute inflammatory stage because it decreases inflammation and limits pain. Icing that includes the application of a barrier oil may be performed two to three times per day for approximately 10 to 15 minutes per icing after work or sporting activity involving the affected elbow. It can be applied using an ice bag or via massage using an ice cube. Applying heat locally after the acute phase is over and the chronic phase has begun will continue to support healing. Alternating hot and cold local applications may have the effect of "washing out" the accumulation of pain chemicals and bring in the needed repair substances.

- **MEDICATION:** Oral non-steroidal anti-inflammatory drugs are very helpful in controlling both pain and inflammation associated with golfer's elbow. Non-prescription medications include ibuprofen (Motrin®, Advil®, Nuprin®, and Medipren®) and prescription medications (Naprosyn®, Indocin®, Feldene®, and Relafen®). All medications should be used under the direction of a doctor because of potential side effects.

- **WARMING UP:** Adequate warm-ups should be performed for 10 minutes before engaging in physical activities. Warm-ups include stretching and gently moving the joints through the entire range of motion in a relaxed manner. Pay particular attention to the elbow. Range of motion and stretching should always be performed after sports activities. This is known as "cooling down."

- **STRETCHING EXERCISES:** Exercises may be used to maintain good range of motion of the arms, legs, and back. Joints may be prone to injury without the maximal attainable flexibility. It is easy to be misled by the common misconception that if your forearm looks good and strong and has bulging muscles, it will protect you from getting tennis elbow. Not so. A big, strong forearm may be so tight from pumping iron that it lacks adequate flexibility. It is essential to stretch muscles to keep them strong. You will be predisposed toward getting golfer's elbow if the forearm wrist extensors are tight, so be sure to stretch all of the major muscle groups before and after engaging in sports activities, paying particular attention to the forearm extensors. Gaining flexibility and muscle length in the extensor muscles of the forearm through stretching will take up some of the pull placed on the lateral epicondyle. Place the back of your hand on a flat surface while keeping the elbow straight to stretch the wrist extensors. Then, gently lean forward and feel the stretch in your forearm.

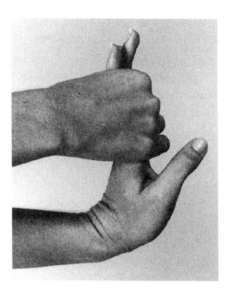

Stretching the wrist flexor muscles. Brotzman SB, ed: *Clinical orthopaedic Rehabilitation*, Mosby, St. Louis, 1996.

■ **STRENGTHENING:** Strength by itself will not enable a golfer to hit the ball better or longer, but it does allow the player to strike shots with more consistently explosive power over extended periods of time. A golfer with a weak area in the arm, such as at the elbow, is at risk for injury at one of the epicondyles. Lack of adequate forearm strength can lead to tendonitis because lack of muscle strength means there will be less of the soft tissue necessary to diminish the stress delivered up the arm. Strengthening of the forearm muscles should begin with the elbow halfway bent, followed by stretching with the elbow out straight. Exercise increases muscle bulk, which helps dissipate injurious forces. Exercises such as wrist curls should be increased gradually; begin with small weights and progress to greater weights slowly. (See illustration in Chapter 25 on page 222.) Eccentric exercises involve lengthening of muscle fibers and are particularly helpful.

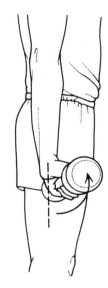

Resistive strengthening of the forearm muscles.

Sports Injury Handbook: *Professional Advice for Amateur Athletes*, by Allan M. Levy and Mark L. Fuerst, John Wiley & Sons, Inc. New York, 1993.

■ **CONCENTRIC EXERCISES:** When you pick up a gallon of milk, your biceps contract concentrically, which means the muscle fibers bunch up and move closer together. Concentric exercises can be accomplished by using gym exercise machines, dumbbells, elastic bands, or weighted cuffs.

■ **ECCENTRIC EXERCISES:** It is necessary for muscle fibers to work in a slow, graded, and controlled manner when attempting to lower an object such as a heavy gallon of milk to a table. Otherwise, you might drop it. In this case, the biceps muscle eccentrically absorbs the downward force of gravity on the gallon of milk. This type of muscle distracting is known as an eccentric contraction. (See Chapter 19 for a detailed discussion of eccentric contractions.) Eccentric exercises are valuable in strengthening the ability of muscles to distract. They are also valuable in protecting other tissues such as tendons and ligaments from injury. An eccentric exercise program should be designed by a physical therapist or exercise trainer. It can be part of an overall exercise program to remain strong and healthy. Eccentric contraction is extremely important because it absorbs energy.

■ **ENDURANCE TRAINING:** Playing golf requires you to climb hills and walk eighteen holes, often in hot, humid weather. It can be strenuous exercise for the heart and lungs and, therefore, exercising your heart and lungs is important prior to playing golf. In addition to regular endurance exercises to build up your stamina, it is helpful to avoid taking the easy way out by using the golf cart to get around during the game. Instead, build your endurance and walk on the golf course. Make sure you maintain your endurance by jogging, swimming, walking, and cycling regularly when you are not on the golf course.

■ **BRACING:** A lateral counterforce brace is worn near the elbow both during work and when participating in sports. This strap may provide effective prevention for those who have recovered from previous tennis elbow and wish to prevent future recurrences. Apply the 4-inch strap snugly around the relaxed upper forearm in order to minimize stress at the lateral epicondyle. It is important to avoid putting these bands on too tightly and possibly cutting off circulation! Bear in mind how easy it is to fall into the false security that a brace can be used as a sole means of treatment. Rather, counterforce braces should supplement muscular stretching and strengthening exercises.

■ **WRIST BRACES:** This type of brace may be worn to keep the wrist bent gently backwards and ease the tension on the common flexor tendon at the elbow, thereby relieving pain. This type of brace may be used during the day, but preferably not at night.

■ **THERAPEUTIC MASSAGE:** Massaging of the forearm muscles is often helpful and pleasant. It can be performed while taking a shower or bath. Friction massage involves rubbing the injured area back and forth or in a circular motion with the thumb or fingers. This may actually increase pain at the time it is performed, but it will feel good afterwards. Massage promotes healing because it increases local blood flow. The local fluid collection known as *edema* is caused by inflammation. Massage presses this fluid and the accumulated pain chemicals out of the tissues. This deep form of massage also stretches the healing fibers, thereby allowing them to heal in a stretched manner, which is more desirable.

■ **ULTRASOUND:** Ultrasound involves electricity passed though special crystals, which vibrate at ultrasonic (high) frequencies. This vibration penetrates deep into tissue as heat energy and may provide relief once golfer's elbow passes beyond its acute stage. Ultrasound applied in the pulsed mode may deliver pain-relieving medications to the inflamed extensor tendon.

- **INJECTIONS:** Steroid injections may be considered when the above-described measures have not been successful or in the event that pain is severe. Typically, a shot of cortisone is injected into the area of the common flexor tendon in order to decrease inflammation. Occasionally, one shot is not enough and a second shot is necessary. No more than three shots should ever be administered because steroids are so strong that they can weaken the tendon and cause it to rupture. Avoid cortisone shots until you have tried everything else. Consider it as a last resort, not an easy solution.

- **EDUCATION:** Hiring a sports technique instructor for several visits is well worth the time and money because she can point out faulty form and teach better body and golf swing mechanics. Faulty swings move the lower body minimally and use the arm as the primary power source, thus making the elbow more vulnerable to injury.

WHEN IS SURGERY NECESSARY?

Surgery is indicated when a conservative course of action has failed over the course of several months and the person is still complaining of significant pain and inability to use the arm. There are two types of surgeries for golfer's elbow: (1) a small incision is made and the abnormal tendon is trimmed; and (2) a portion of tendon is released from the bone and then reattached. People who have either type of surgery return home the same day with the arm in a sling. Most of them cannot drive for a week. Surgery is quite successful in relieving pain and usually allows for a return to daily activity without pain in less than 6 months. However, returning to playing golf may require waiting several months.

HELPFUL SAFETY TIPS WHEN PLAYING GOLF

- Do not jerk a heavy bag of golf clubs out of the car. Instead, keep your back straight, pull the clubs in close to your belly button (center of gravity), bend your knees, and then straighten them when attempting to lift. In this way, you can lift safely and avoid a back injury before getting to your first tee-time.

- Drink plenty of water to prevent dehydration, heat exhaustion, or heat stroke.

- Remember to wear a hat on the golf course because reflective sunlight can significantly increase sunlight exposure, raising the chances of getting skin cancer.

- Call it quits when skies look threatening because lightening kills golfers every year.

Neck and Shoulder

MANY PEOPLE have neck and shoulder pain at some point in their lives. Pain can be caused by many different conditions, and knowing exactly how the neck and shoulder function and how problems develop is a good way to learn how to avoid injury. In this section, the neck and shoulder are placed together because the pain in one area often radiates to the other.

27 Rotator Cuff Disorders

A 24-year-old school psychologist swims 100 laps per day, alternating between the crawl and butterfly strokes. Lately, she complains of pain when lifting her dominant left hand over her head and when carrying a briefcase in her left hand. She feels a slight grinding or crunching sensation when lifting her hand over her head and admits that she is beginning to feel pain in her left shoulder. There is no history of injury. She appears to be strong, and can position her hand and shoulder in any position. Resisting external rotation and abduction of her shoulder is painful. This woman is experiencing an impingement syndrome *of her left* rotator cuff muscles, *which specifically involves her left* supraspinatus tendon.

A 48-year-old housepainter spent the last 16 years of his working life specializing in painting the ceilings of mansions, museums, and government buildings. He reports a history of right shoulder tendonitis and a clicking sound when raising his right hand over his head. He lost his footing on a ladder about 2 weeks ago and fell onto his right shoulder. Although no bones were broken during the fall, he cannot use his shoulder the same way as before. His right shoulder feels weak and stiff, and he can just barely get his arm up over his head on his own, although someone else can lift his hand for him two-thirds of the way up without any pain. His right shoulder feels tender, but he can rotate his shoulder easily in either direction. He easily feels touch everywhere on his shoulder, hands, and arms. His deep tendon reflexes are normal, and aside from elevating his shoulder, his arm and hand are still strong. This man has completely torn the supraspinatus tendon *of his right* rotator cuff muscles.

■ THE SHOULDER JOINT

THE SHOULDER JOINT appears to be designed as a weight-bearing joint in creatures that ambulate on all four legs. However, once humans stood up on their hind legs, their forefeet—or rather the forearms—became freed up for manipulating objects, including reaching up overhead to pick fruit off the trees for eating. The shoulder became more versatile than the hip joint and assumed a virtually limitless number of options for movement in space.

The human shoulder is endowed with the ability to basically move every way the hip can, but it can do so over a much wider (360 degree) arc of motion. The shoulder is a ball-and-socket joint like the hip, although its greater mobility is allowed by a much shallower socket than the hip. The downside of this evolutionary change is that while it allows us to position our hands almost everywhere, we sacrifice stability for our newfound mobility. Because of this, the mobile shoulder joint is more likely to dislocate than the more stable hip joint.

▪ SUBACROMIAL ARCH

When humans began to stand erect, the bones, muscles, tendons, and ligaments of the upper extremity all became considerably smaller than their counterparts in the hip, leg, and foot because the bones of the shoulder were originally designed to bear weight. They later adapted for different functions. One of the important bones overhanging the shoulder is called the *acromion* (Greek for "shoulder"). Unfortunately, evolutionary adaptation of the shoulder was less than perfect, and the many tendons that raise the shoulder are all packed beneath this knob of bone together with a ligament, resulting in an unyielding arch known as the sub-acromial arch. The subacromial arch limits how much you can raise your shoulder.

The design of the subacromial arch varies from person to person. Some people have a rather flat arch, others have a curved arch, and some have an arch with an architectural design that resembles a hook. It is the hook type that projects downward into the space normally reserved for the shoulder tendons that lift up the shoulder. The space these tendons normally occupy is known as the *subacromial space.* Within this space is a series of tightly packed tendons that form the *rotator cuff.* Their muscle bellies attach to the upper back portion of the shoulder girdle.

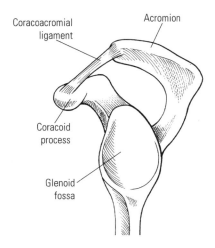

The subacromial arch.
Saidoff DC, McDonough AL: *Critical Pathways in Therapeutic Intervention: Upper Extremity.* St. Louis: Mosby, 1997.

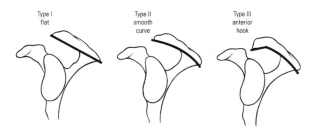

Type of subacromial arch. The hook variety shown on the right places the shoulder at maximum vulnerability for developing a rotator cuff problem.
Saidoff DC, McDonough AL: *Critical Pathways in Therapeutic Intervention: Upper Extremity.* St. Louis: Mosby, 1997.

▪ ROTATOR CUFF

The shoulder is a complex joint controlled by twenty-six muscles, four of which make up the rotator cuff. This group of four muscles connects your upper arm bone (*humerus*) to your shoulder blade (*scapula*), which is a triangular, large, flat bone located in your upper back. A good analogy to describe how the tendons of the rotator cuff muscles attach onto the head of the humerus is by com-

paring them to a *cowl* (a hooded cloak that covers the head) worn by monks of the sixth century St. Benedictine monastic order. The rotator cuff tendons encircle the humeral head in a manner similar to the way the cuff of a shirt sleeve encircles the wrist. They cause the shoulder to rotate upward, inward, or outward when they contract. Thus, they are called the "rotator cuff."

The rotator cuff muscles maintain stability of the shoulder throughout its remarkable range of motion. Muscles can function optimally within a very narrow range. A muscle cannot contract normally if it is slightly stretched or placed under excessive tension. How do the rotator cuff muscles maintain an ideal length through a wide range of motion? The secret is the amazing scapula (shoulder blade) to which they attach. A corresponding motion of the scapula accompanies every movement of the shoulder. The scapula works in synchrony with the shoulder, making sure the muscles are the ideal length necessary to contract most efficiently.

▇ IMPINGEMENT AND TENDONITIS

The tendons of the rotator cuff lie atop the ball-like head of the humerus bone, which is located at the shoulder just beneath the subacromial arch. The rotator cuff tendons contract to elevate the shoulder when the arm is lifted over the head. However, the tendons of the rotator cuff are in a very vulnerable position between two bones, and they may get squeezed or pinched. In occupations and activities that involve a lot of overhead work, such nursing, warehousing, longshoring, carpentry, painting a ceiling, picking fruit, or tree pruning, the rotator

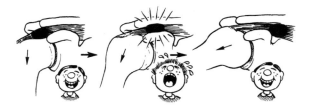

Painful impingement of the rotator cuff tendons, especially the supraspinatus tendon. Dandy DJ: Essential *Orthopaedics and Trauma.* Edinburgh: Churchill Livingstone, 1989.

cuff tendons may become inflamed, swell, and get pushed up against by the unyielding subacromial arch. The space inside the subacromial arch is limited and, because it is also filled with other structures such as bursae and the long tendon of the biceps muscle, one or more of the tendons may become pinched or impinged. The fact that the tendons of the rotator cuff have a rather poor blood supply does not help the situation. One or more of the tendons may become stretched or frayed near its attachment on the humerus bone if impingement continues without allowing the tendon to rest sufficiently. This condition is called *rotator cuff tendonitis.*

The most commonly injured tendon of the rotator cuff is the supraspinatus tendon. This all-important tendon assists in externally rotating the shoulder joint. When the supraspinatus tendon becomes inflamed, it is sensitive and painful when the person is asked to externally rotate the shoulder against resistance. Carrying a heavy object such as a briefcase or gallon of milk is quite painful because it stretches the already inflamed tendon.

A very important function of the supraspinatus tendon is to pull the humeral head downward (inferiorly) when you pick your hand up over your head. This action is known as the *humeral head depressor mechanism.* Shoulder elevation (flexion or abduction) allows the humeral head and the contents of the subacromial space to clear easily under the subacromial arch. The supraspinatus cannot perform this action properly if it is injured. In this situation, the supraspinatus, its co-tendons, and bursa become repeatedly jammed against the arch during shoulder elevation, setting into motion a vicious cycle of inflammation and degeneration. While this process may be accelerated in younger persons, such as swimmers, pitchers, or ceiling painters, progressive loss of the depressor mechanism occurs with the passage of time, causing the humeral head to migrate upwards with aging.

▪ ROTATOR CUFF TEAR

The tendon(s) experience rubbing, pinching, irritation, and wear and tear as more and more strain is applied to the rotator cuff. The underside of the acromion responds to repetitive rubbing by growing a spicule of bone that is similar to a stalactite or icicle hanging from the roof of a cave. This sharp spicule of bone is known as a *bone spur,* and it hastens the wearing down process of the rotator cuff. It may actually cut into the rotator cuff. The tendons may partially tear in what is known as a *partial (thickness) tear* of the rotator cuff muscles. A fully torn tendon is known as a *full-thickness tear.* This usually happens after age 40, where there is a history of longstanding impingement or tendonitis. The tendon finally succumbs after a fall onto the shoulder, or possibly while doing something as trivial as opening a stuck window. The tendon is unlikely to heal once a tear occurs. A partial tear heals with scar tissue and is inherently weaker than the original tendon, making it more likely to tear again and more completely.

▪ RISK FACTORS

- **AGE:** The normal wear and tear on your rotator cuff may result in a breakdown of the collagen that makes up muscle proteins after age 40. Also, tendons are less extensible and more likely to undergo attrition and injury with increasing age. Most rotator cuff tears occur after age 40 for this reason.

- **REPETITIVE STRESS:** Repetitive overhead movements of the shoulder can stress the rotator cuff muscles and tendons, causing them to become inflamed and eventually tear. This is common among laborers in the building trades such as carpentry and painting. It also occurs in baseball

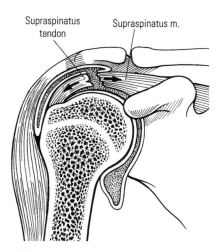

A full thickness tear of the supraspinatus tendon, one of the rotator cuff muscle-tendons.
Saidoff DC, McDonough: *Critical Pathways in Therapeutic Intervention: Extremities and Spine.* St. Louis: Mosby, 2002.

pitchers and tennis players, especially during an overhead shot. Overdevelopment of the chest wall in weight lifters may alter the biomechanics of the shoulder joint and stress the rotator cuff tendons. Lifting the arm above shoulder level is also implicated. Swimmers who use the Australian crawl or the butterfly stroke place excessive stress on the rotator cuff tendons and predispose them to injury. Baseball pitchers tend to stress the rotator cuff muscles more than any other athletes, especially considering the force and speed imparted to a ball that can travel as fast as 100 mph.

- **POSTURE:** People with poor posture who allow their head, neck, and shoulders to slouch may stretch the muscles of the rotator cuff and diminish its ability to move. This may indirectly affect the cuff tendons and predispose them to injury.

- **LIFTING:** Improper lifting or lifting something that is too heavy, especially overhead, can strain or tear a tendon or muscle.

■ SIGNS AND SYMPTOMS

The most common symptom of rotator cuff injury is pain that is primarily experienced when reaching upward. However, some of the symptoms of impingement syndrome may vary from that of tendonitis tendon tear (rupture).

■ **IMPINGEMENT SYNDROME:** This condition often occurs in people under 25 years of age, although it may happen at any age. People with this type of early stage of rotator cuff problem usually try to work it out themselves and only go to the doctor or therapist after their symptoms fail to resolve. There may be pain, stiffness, shoulder weakness, or a feeling of "catching" when the arm is moved through various motions. It may hurt to sleep on the injured shoulder. Routine activities such as lifting a gallon of milk out of the refrigerator may be difficult. There may be a crunching noise when raising the arm overhead. A good way to detect whether impingement has occurred is by using a test called the *positive impingement sign* in which the shoulder is elevated with the arm rotated so that the thumb points inward. Impingement is indicated if there is pain during this test. This early stage of rotator cuff disorder is reversible, but it sets the stage for the next stage: tendonitis.

■ **TENDONITIS:** If shoulder activity continues unabated and early symptoms are ignored, the tendon will become inflamed, resulting in swelling (edema). This, in turn, will result in even less space within the already cramped subacromial space. The thickened tendons may also inflame the subacromial bursa, which will have to work harder to try to decrease the friction caused by continuous movement. Microtears may occur within the substance of one or more of the cuff tendons. These microtears will eventually be replaced by scar tissue. This type of injury most commonly occurs between the ages of 25 to 40. People complain about pain similar to a toothache that is most frequently felt in the shoulder after athletic or vigorous activity, or while sleeping at night. It may be harder to move the shoulder due to stiffness and thickening. The pathologic process is set in motion once tendonitis has set in, and a vicious cycle eventually leads to tearing of the tendon.

■ **ROTATOR CUFF TEAR:** This stage of rotator cuff injury involves a partial or full thickness tear of one of the tendons of the rotator cuff, usually the supraspinatus tendon. A partial tear must be identified and treated because if it is ignored, it will continue to tear, similar to a rip in nylon fabric. This usually happens after a history of impingement or tendonitis, although it can happen with no previous history—for example, when a person falls onto the shoulder, causing an acute rupture of the rotator cuff. *Acute tears* can occur in persons under 35 years of age who engage in rigorous athletics. *Chronic degenerative tears* often occur to people in their 70s and 80s. This age group may have a partial rotator cuff tear but may not know it because they have been symptom-free for years. Seniors may report gradually increasing difficulty in performing mundane daily activities such as trying to trim a tall bush, reaching for dishes on the top shelf of a kitchen cupboard, or combing their hair. However, any new stress to the rotator cuff can cause a painful flare-up or even an *acute tear*—for example, from a fall onto the shoulder or an activity as trivial as opening up a stuck window sash. There may be complaints of pain and stiffness that interferes with sleep. Many people with a complete rotator cuff tear have significant shoulder weakness that prevents them from lifting their arm away from their side. Someone with a partial tear may be able to elevate her shoulder about halfway. However, she will not be able to sustain it when someone pushes down on the arm, nor will she be able to slowly lower their arm to their side. This is known as the *positive drop arm test*, and it indicates a tear of the rotator cuff. A person with a full thickness tear will not be able to lift her hand overhead, not even with a steroid shot into the subacromial space to relieve pain. The *glenoid* head appears on x-ray to migrate upward and indeed, it subluxates superiorly so that the humeral head rams up into the arch. This is due to the lost effect of the supraspinatus pulling downward on the humeral head.

■ DIAGNOSIS AND CONDITIONS TO RULE OUT

Rotator cuff disorders occur along a continuum of conditions, each one more debilitating than the next. Diagnosis is made by taking a careful history and physical examination, and often helped by x-rays. Magnetic resonance imaging (MRI) can reveal the spectrum of rotator cuff disease from tendon degeneration, which is associated with impingement or tendonitis, to partial or complete tears. A torn rotator cuff can be seen on x-ray. It results in upward migration of the entire humeral head because one of the functions of an intact cuff is to

pull downward on the humeral head to allow it to clear the subacromial arch during the motion of lifting the hand over the head. Some other conditions that might cause similar symptoms include:

- **BURSITIS:** As discussed in previous chapters, a *bursa* is a fluid-filled sac. The sac itself is made up of synovial membrane, which is the same material that lines the inside of many joints. Bursae are situated at sites of high friction and work to minimize friction between moving parts. There are about twelve bursae in and around the shoulder joint, but the one most commonly inflamed is the subacromial bursae, which is located in the subacromial space. The bursae are located in this space because they are needed to minimize friction. They may become overworked with excessive motion, which results in the inflammation of the bursa known as *bursitis*. Bursitis is differentiated from impingement or tendonitis of the rotator cuff because it involves severe pain that has a very swift onset. A good treatment for bursitis is diathermy (deep heat treatment) and ultrasound, both of which should be applied by a physical therapist or under the guidance of a doctor.

- **CERVICAL SPONDYLOSIS:** This is a condition in which a nerve is pinched in the cervical (neck)

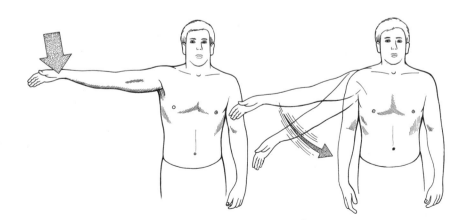

Positive drop arm test reveals a complete tear of the rotator cuff. Saidoff DC, McDonough: *Critical Pathways in Therapeutic Intervention: Upper Extremity*, Mosby, St. Louis, 1997.

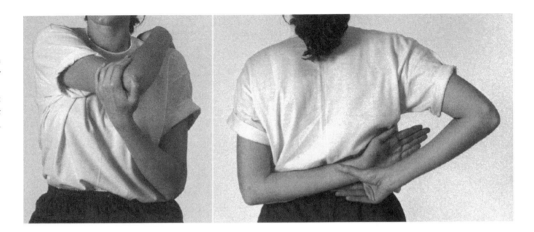

Two ways to stretch the posterior shoulder capsule.
Brotzman SB, (ed): *Clinical Orthopaedic Rehabilitation.* St. Louis: Mosby, 1996.

region at the level of the C5 or C6 spinal vertebra. Pain and weakness similar to rotator cuff disorders may occur as a result. Cervical spondylosis is differentiated from impingement or tendonitis of the rotator cuff because it includes loss of sensation and weak or absent reflexes.

■ PREVENTION AND TREATMENT

Unfortunately, the body's ability to heal rotator cuff disorders is limited because the tendons of the rotator cuff have a poor blood supply. Therefore, it is essential to begin treating rotator cuff injuries as soon as possible before irreversible changes set in.

■ **REST:** Avoid lifting weights and hitting tennis serves. Do not put your hand up over your head too quickly or forcefully. If you must put your hand up high, do it slowly with your thumb pointed outward in external shoulder rotation. Take frequent breaks to reduce the risk of impingement if your job requires frequent overhead movements such as lifting or working on a ceiling.

■ **ACTIVITY MODIFICATION:** It is important to avoid painful reaching overhead until inflamma-

tion has subsided because it can pinch the already irritated rotator cuff further.

■ **ICE AND HEAT:** Application of ice or a bag of frozen vegetables several times per day for 15 minutes is helpful during the acute stage. Once symptoms settle down, heat may be applied, provided that enough padding is interposed between the hot pack and skin to avoid a burn. Limit heat applications to 20 minutes.

■ **MEDICATIONS:** Oral non-steroidal anti-inflammatory medications such as aspirin, ibuprofen, and naproxen may control pain and reduce soreness and swelling. Follow the label directions and stop taking these drugs when the level of pain improves.

■ **INJECTIONS:** Steroid injections may be administered by an orthopedic surgeon, rheumatologist, physiatrist, or a doctor specializing in sports medicine. The injection is usually directly into the bursa that is located above the rotator cuff tendon. It will help relieve both the pain and inflammation. Too many injections should not be given because they can do more harm than good to the tendon and its surrounding structures. Injections relieve pain but do not improve function.

- **RANGE OF MOTION:** Total inactivity may result in a stiff, frozen shoulder. Therefore, gentle exercises within the painless arc of shoulder motion are essential to keeping the shoulder joint limber. A good way to start is with *pendulum exercises* in which the shoulder is moved by bending over and swaying the trunk, not by effort at the arm or shoulder. (See illustration in Chapter 28 on page 250.) In this way, the shoulder and arm follow the movement of the trunk and may be moved less painfully to and fro, back and forth, and in circular motions. Overhead motions may be introduced using an overhead pulley when the person becomes more tolerant of different motions. There should be an emphasis on slow, relaxed, nonpainful exercises.

- **JOINT MOBILIZATION:** This involves moving a joint to ensure proper flexibility. Many joints, such as the shoulder joint, are enveloped by a tight, ligamentous shoulder capsule enveloping the joint. Once the supraspinatus tendon becomes inflamed, portions of the capsule, and particularly the posterior capsule in back of or behind the shoulder joint, become stiff and inter-

fere with normal shoulder motion. Because of this, it is essential to have the posterior shoulder (*glenohumeral*) joint capsule stretched regularly. Maintaining scapular mobility is also essential in normal motion of the shoulder.

- **STRENGTHENING:** It is important to strengthen the rotator cuff muscles and the surrounding musculature of the shoulder girdle. This type of exercise should only be performed in the nonpainful range of motion. This may be accomplished by using wall weights or elastic bands.

- **TENS UNITS:** A TENS device delivers transcutaneous electrical stimulation that helps decrease pain. This modality may be helpful in relieving some of the pain associated with rotator cuff pathology.

- **STRETCHING:** It is very helpful to stretch the rotator cuff muscles, provided it does not provoke pain. Many muscles of the upper extremity, especially the pectoralis major, may be too tight and may contribute to the likelihood of abnormal biomechanics of the shoulder joint. These muscles

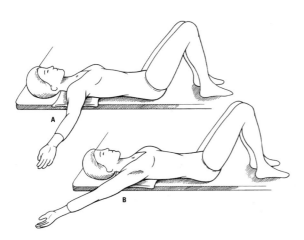

Stretching of the upper and lower fibers of the pectoralis major muscles. Saidoff DC, McDonough: *Critical Pathways in Therapeutic Intervention: Extremities and Spine.* St. Louis: Mosby, 2002.

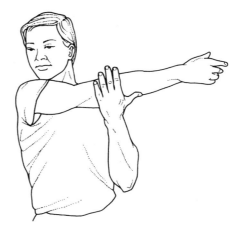

Stretching the posterior capsule. Levy AM, Fuerst ML: *Sport Injury Handbook: Professional Advice for Amateur Athletes.* New York: John Wiley & Sons, Inc., 1993.

should be regularly stretched. The posterior joint capsule may also be self-stretched.

- **SHOULDER SHRUGGING:** This type of movement may be very helpful in loosening up a painful shoulder and in dealing with some of the fear and anxiety associated with a problem shoulder. The *Feldenkreis Technique* may be helpful. This approach includes shrugging the shoulder up and down, forward and backward, and rotating it in circles in all directions. (See illustrations in Chapter 31 on page 271.)

- **MASSAGE:** Transverse friction massage can be applied by a physical therapist to inflamed tendons to help disrupt scar tissue formation and adhesions within the tendon by broadening its insertion at the bone. General massage to the muscles of the shoulder girdle may be relaxing and restore extensibility to tight muscles such as the upper *trapezius* and *pectoralis major* muscles. Soft tissue massage also promotes increased circulation.

■ SURGERY

Surgery may be considered for recalcitrant impingement syndrome or tendonitis if a rigorous course of physical therapy for about 6 weeks is unsuccessful in relieving pain and weakness. A partial or full tear in a professional athlete or a full tear at any age is sufficient reason to operate. If an x-ray shows a thickened acromion or acromial bone spur causing impingement, it can be removed with a burr using an arthroscope. Success in terms of return of function is greater in a younger person. A torn rotator cuff tendon can be repaired using one of several techniques. After outpatient surgery is completed, the shoulder is supported in a sling or brace for a short period of healing, followed by range of motion, strengthening, and stretching for anywhere from 2 to 6 months before the shoulder resumes normal function and range of motion.

28 Frozen Shoulder Syndrome

A 49-year-old woman was released from the emergency room with her arm in a sling after breaking her pinky in an accident. She was told to see her doctor in 2 weeks. For the next 10 days she kept her arm in the sling. When she went to the doctor's office for her follow-up appointment, she removed the sling and found that her shoulder was very stiff and painful. She was able to shrug her shoulder, but she could not raise her hand to her chin without considerable difficulty. This woman has a frozen shoulder, *a condition also known as* adhesive capsulitis.

THE CLASSIC TALE of frozen shoulder is of someone who breaks her pinky and then leaves the emergency room with her shoulder and arm in a sling, and no instructions from the doctor to move the shoulder or elbow regularly. The shoulder will start to freeze up almost immediately with disuse, and she will begin to feel a throbbing pain that may even keep her up at night. She will be more and more unable to move her shoulder and eventually she will learn that just keeping it as still as possible is the most comfortable thing to do. After her pinky heals, she will realize that her shoulder has grown stiff and useless, much like a water-soaked towel left in the freezer, except that her shoulder may stay *frozen* in this manner for up to a year and a half. What happened here?

■FROZEN SHOULDER DEFINED

Frozen shoulder is a painful condition that commonly follows injury to the shoulder joint. It is often caused by minor trauma such as a fall or bump.

Curiously, whereas other large and small body joints also become stiff when injured, the shoulder will become frozen stiff even when the injury does not involve the shoulder directly. The reason for this is unknown. It may be the result of a nearby injury such as a broken wrist. Although this may be attributed to a lack of motion in many people, the shoulder may nevertheless become painful and stiff despite normal usage in others. Thus, while the shoulder is the joint with the greatest movement capability of the body, it is an extremely sensitive barometer of other abnormalities or injuries in the upper portion of the body.

Frozen shoulder may be precipitated by a mastectomy, a pinched nerve, a broken rib, a fractured bone, surgery anywhere along the arm, or even by the arm pain that often accompanies angina. The common thread tying these various conditions together is that they all cause a person to use his shoulder less. In fact, it is often most comfortable to just let the shoulder hang down by the side and ignore it. Unfortunately, this is where the problem often begins!

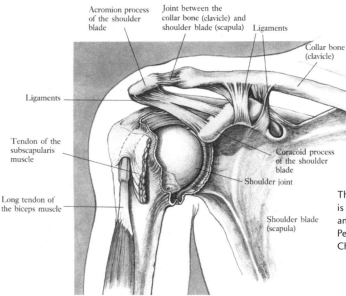

Anatomical representation of the shoulder region.

The shoulder joint is a ball-and-socket joint. The ball (*humeral head*) is kept within the socket (*glenoid fossa*) by the surrounding muscles and ligaments.
Peterson L, Renstrom P: *Sports Injuries: Their Prevention and Treatment.* Chicago: Year Book Medical Publishers Inc., Chicago, 1986.

INTERESTING FACTS ABOUT FROZEN SHOULDER:

- Frozen shoulder is rarely seen before the age of 40 or after 70 years of age

- Frozen shoulder is more likely in the nondominant arm

- Frozen shoulder usually involves one arm, but may occur in both shoulders

- Women are twice as likely to develop frozen shoulder

- Most women who develop frozen shoulder are simultaneously undergoing or have just completed menopause

- People with diabetes are much more likely to develop frozen shoulder

BASIC BIOMECHANICS OF FROZEN SHOULDER AND THE ROLE OF THE INFERIOR CAPSULE

Your shoulder is a ball-and-socket joint. The "ball" is the *humeral head* that fits into the *glenoid fossa* (Greek for socket), which is on the side of the shoulder blade (scapula). Note how the humeral head is kept within the glenoid by the surrounding muscles and ligaments. The round end (humeral head) of your upper arm bone (humerus) rests precariously within the glenoid on the shoulder blade much like a golf ball rests on a golf tee. This concave bowl is much smaller than the bulbous humeral head, but it serves as a horizontal shelf for the humeral head to rest upon during most of the movements of the shoulder. This shelf becomes increasingly vertical as you raise your arm straight up to the ceiling. In fact, the humeral head would roll right off and slip downward in what is known as a *shoulder dislocation*, if not for the ligamentous thickenings of the shoulder joint capsule located beneath the shoulder joint, which tense up in order to hold the shoulder in place. The ligamentous thickenings have wide spaces between them similar to pleats. These ligaments have a drawback.

Imagine holding a medium-sized water balloon in your open hand with your fingers spread apart. The balloon is similar to the humeral head and your fingers are similar to the shoulder ligaments beneath the joint. The balloon can more easily be pushed through the pleats formed by your cupped hand with the fingers spread than if your fingers were held together. These restraining ligaments form a floor to the shoulder joint and therefore are called the *inferior capsule*. They have a built-in design flaw in that they are pleated and, therefore, they may allow the glenoid head to slip beneath the shoulder, an event which is called a subluxation or dislocation. The degree to which this may happen varies from person to person, depending on how pleated (crenated) the inferior capsule is.

The glenoid acts as a basin when the arm hangs down at the side. It balances the humeral head, so that the inferior capsule becomes slack. The inferior capsule becomes more and more taut as you raise your arm until it becomes a tense hammock when your hand is pointing directly upward. This tense inferior capsule ensures that the glenoid head stays centered within the shoulder.

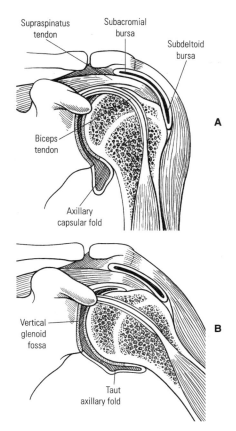

The shoulder joint is enveloped by capsular folds of tissue, the bottom portion of which is known as the *axillary fold* because it is located in the *axilla* (Latin for "armpit"). A. This inferior capsule becomes slack when the shoulder is at rest and the arm is at the side. B. The inferior capsule is drawn taut when you raise up your arm.
Saidoff DC, McDonough AL: *Critical Pathways in Therapeutic Intervention: Extremities and Spine.* St. Louis: Mosby, 2001.

◼ THE PROTECTIVE POSTURE OF THE SHOULDER

The usual reaction after injury directly to the shoulder or somewhere on the arm is to protect the arm by cradling it close to the body. This is actually good because this position is the least painful and protects the arm from further injury. However, if this position is held too long, three problems will occur:

◼ The shoulder will rapidly lose the ability to move. The shoulder capsule will shrink, dry out, and become less resilient without the benefit of the stretching that occurs during motion. The fluid within the shoulder, which is normally present and helps lubricate the joint during movement, also dries up. Over time, the capsule wraps tightly around the humeral head, like tight adhesive tape, and does not allow for any motion.

- The shoulder joint capsule has multiple pain receptors and any attempt to move an injured shoulder may aggravate the joint capsule, precipitating an inflammatory reaction. This makes the tissue in the shoulder capsule sticky and movement becomes even more difficult. It is similar to what happens when you have an eye infection—you might wake up in the morning to find your eyelid is stuck shut with mucus. It is for this reason that frozen shoulder is also called a *adhesive capsulitis*, which means "inflamed and sticky capsule."

- When the inferior capsule is in a slackened position, its two ends come closer together, which blocks movement, especially when reaching up or outward. This situation may degenerate, and whereas the inferior capsule normally helps movement, it will restrain movement once frozen shoulder sets in, similar a tight leash on an active puppy.

SIGNS AND SYMPTOMS

Frozen shoulder goes through three stages that together may last up to 18 months:

- **PHASE I:** There is gradually increasing pain and an inability to move the shoulder during the *freezing phase*. Attempts to raise the arm over the head are frustratingly met with shoulder-hiking. This stiffness is felt more and more, to the point of interfering with combing your hair, washing your face in the morning, putting on a shirt or blouse, or simply lifting a spoon to your mouth. It is hard to pinpoint the pain, which often keeps you up at night and hurts if you roll onto your shoulder.

- **PHASE II:** In contrast to the first phase, the most outstanding feature of the *frozen phase* is stiffness.

The level of pain actually lessens, especially if you do not move your shoulder, and so your natural inclination is to move your arm less and less. This sort of behavior actually helps the shoulder become even stiffer. The quality of the pain is less excruciating in nature and is more like a dull ache.

- **PHASE III:** The shoulder capsule returns to its normal state during the *thawing phase* when both stiffness and pain begin go away. Movement and function gradually return during this phase.

CONDITIONS TO RULE OUT

Several different conditions mimic frozen shoulder and should be ruled out. Frozen shoulder is diagnosed by history and clinical examination. An arthrogram, while helpful, is not necessary in most cases. Conditions to be ruled out might include:

- **POSTERIOR JOINT DISLOCATION:** This is a painful injury in which the humeral head comes out of its socket and moves backward. This does not happen very often and when it does, it usually happens to elderly people from either a blow to the front of the shoulder or from falling onto an outstretched hand. It may also occur if someone's purse is snatched from behind and the owner refuses to let go. Posterior dislocation is easy to miss because it lacks a striking deformity. It differs from frozen shoulder in that the person has a history of a specific fall or injury, which is not the case with frozen shoulder. An x-ray will rule out joint dislocation.

- **JOINT MICE:** As previously discussed, some people have small pieces of bone fragments loose within the shoulder joint. They move about, hence, the analogy to mice. They may occasionally cause the shoulder to lock or catch, causing a block or slowing of motion as the arm is held high. Joint mice can often be seen on x-ray.

- **TENDONITIS:** Tendonitis of the rotator cuff or biceps tendon may occur following excessive activity. For example, someone who decides to paint the ceilings in one weekend may overdo it and aggravate these tendons, resulting in inflammation. It will be painful to rotate the shoulder outward or raise it. This diminished motion is also present in frozen shoulder, but all directions of movement are limited. Also, the history of tendonitis is different in that it is preceded by a specific activity such as overhead painting in which excess activity precipitated the inflammation.

- **CALCIFIED TENDONITIS:** A portion of the rotator cuff has a poor blood supply, and overuse over many years may trick the body into thinking that the tendon is injured. As a result, the body attempts to repair the tendon by treating it like a broken bone and laying down bone, which makes the tendon bony. This strategy actually works in a way because it prevents movement, especially since excessive shoulder movement provoked the problem in the first place. The calcified tendon is usually visible on x-ray.

- **ROTATOR CUFF RUPTURE:** This may occur suddenly from falling onto the tip of the shoulder. If the rotator cuff tendons are already damaged from a past history of tendonitis or other condition, they may rupture from something as trivial as lifting a stuck window sash. Tears of the rotator cuff usually occur in those over 40 years of age. Stiffness is not present early on, and attempts to pick up the arm with a torn rotator cuff result in mere shrugging of the shoulder. Once again, frozen shoulder has a different history and is characterized by stiffness early on.

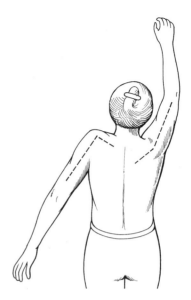

Shoulder-hiking of the left shoulder results from trying to lift a stiff and painful frozen shoulder.
Saidoff DC, McDonough AL: *Critical Pathways in Therapeutic Intervention: Extremities and Spine.* St. Louis: Mosby, 2001.

- **SHOULDER BURSITIS:** As discussed in previous chapters, a bursa is a small fluid-filled sac similar to a balloon filled with water that facilitates motion. The fluid inside the bursa may heat up and expand when there is excessive activity. The swollen bursa may endure rubbing from adjacent structures in the shoulder. If the excessive activity continues without adequate rest, the bursa may become painfully inflamed. This condition may be confused with frozen shoulder. As with other conditions, shoulder bursitis differs from frozen shoulder in that excessive activity often provokes it. When in doubt, an injection into the bursa will quickly relieve pain, although it will not help with frozen shoulder.

- **SHOULDER ARTHRITIS:** This form of osteoarthritis is similar to frozen shoulder in that it occurs gradually and is also accompanied by stiffness and pain. However, arthritic symptoms usually occur slowly over many years and are rarely excruciating. In addition, arthritis is often accompanied by creaking joints, especially when bracing weight through the arm. Finally, arthritis is often worsened by inclement weather and relieved by a hot bath or shower. This is not so for frozen shoulder.

■ **TUMORS:** A tumor at the shoulder is suspected in the elderly, especially when pain occurs at rest and when sleeping at night. This is highly suspect in someone who has a previous history of cancer that may have metastasized from the breast or prostate. Malignancy can be ruled out by x-ray, bone scans, and blood tests.

■ PREVENTION AND TREATMENT

Prevention is an important part of managing frozen shoulder because as many as 70% of those who get frozen shoulder have some residual loss of motion

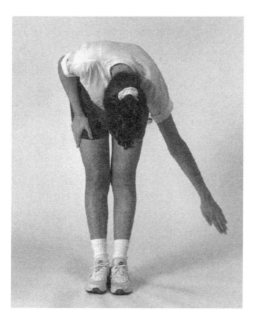

Pendulum Exercises. Brotzman SB: *Clinical Orthopaedic Rehabilitation.* St. Louis: Mosby, 1996.

after the condition goes away. If any part of the arm, except for the shoulder, needs to be kept immobilized in a sling, make sure that the shoulder is regularly rotated in both clockwise and counterclockwise directions. If direct shoulder injury has not occurred, a good way to practice raising your hand is to let your fingers walk up and down the wall in the shower while hot water pours over the shoulder.

An eclectic management approach is best in the event that the shoulder begins to stiffen. Treatment may include:

■ **MEDICATIONS:** Oral non-steroidal analgesics are helpful in alleviating pain and reducing inflammation and may include aspirin (Anacin®, Bayer®, and Bufferin®) ibuprophen (Motrin®, Advil®, and Nuprin®) naproxen sodium (Aleve®) and ketoprofen (Orudis KT®).

■ **MOIST HEAT:** Superficially heat the shoulder with a heating pad, using several layers of towels between the pad and skin to prevent a burn. The advantage of heat is that it feels good; it is relaxing, and it makes the soft tissue more stretchable so you will be able to move your shoulder more easily.

■ **PENDULUM EXERCISES:** This type of exercise is performed with your trunk bent over so that the painful arm hangs limply beneath you toward the floor. Swing the arm from side to side or in a circular movement by leaning your body forward. Because the movement of the shoulder does not come directly *from* the shoulder, but rather from the momentum of the body movement, the pain felt is less than if you tried to move the shoulder itself. This motion allows for a slow gain of motion, and the motion itself promotes healing. A cuff weight is sometimes added to further stretch the joint capsule.

- **RANGE OF MOTION (ROM):** These exercises can be initiated by a therapist. They should be gentle and should not stress the limits of pain. The frozen shoulder may be able to move without assistance once some improved motion occurs.

The second stage of treatment begins approximately 2 weeks after treatment begins, after the pain begins to subside:

- **JOINT MOBILIZATION:** A physical or occupational therapist may perform joint mobilization by essentially wiggling the joint. This gentle motion stretches the joint capsule and allows it to return to its normal elastic state. Those portions of the joint capsule that are particularly tight will be stretched so that motion may occur. Joint mobilization is a very effective therapeutic tool that often provides immediate improvement. Special care must be taken, however, when mobilizing the shoulder of someone with osteoporosis.

- **ULTRASOUND:** Ultrasound is one of the forms of treatments that helps the joint capsule regain elasticity. It involves electricity passed though special crystals, which vibrate at ultrasonic (high) frequencies. This vibration penetrates deep into tissue as heat energy, which may provide relief. Ultrasound breaks down the molecular binding that causes the criss-crossed collagen fibers within the joint capsule to adhere to each other. This deep heating modality penetrates to the soft tissue-bone interface. It may be applied with the arm in positions that best reach those taut portions of the joint capsule. Ultrasound is also helpful prior to manual techniques, such as range of motion and joint mobilization, as it promotes elasticity of the soft tissue of the joint capsule.

- **STRENGTHENING:** Combat the muscle foreshortening and weakness that often accompanies frozen shoulder with strengthening exercises. This will also ward off pain and the reflex inhibition to motion. Exercise should begin as soon as movement begins to return. Isometric exercises precede isotonic exercises, which may be followed by resistive exercises with free weights or an elastic band.

- **MUSCULAR RE-EDUCATION:** The frozen shoulder lifts up in an abnormal manner that looks strange when compared to the unaffected shoulder because of the pain that accompanies adhesive capsulitis. This coping mechanism is known as a *substitution pattern,* and it is imprinted as a movement memory (an *engram*). The shoulder is often held abnormally even after the shoulder has healed. Because of this, it is often helpful to stand in front of a mirror and point your hand up to the ceiling with your normal arm and then try to mimic that same movement with the thawed shoulder. The mirror will provide visual biofeedback, which can enable you to re-educate your shoulder, allowing it to be held normally. This may also be accomplished by the use of a biofeedback device that emits a sound when movement comes within the normal range.

- **STRETCHING:** Using a towel or wand to stretch is a very important part of shoulder maintenance. Special attention should be given to stretching the muscle group known as the *pectoralis major.* This may be done by holding the wand or towel with both hands and moving both arms in tandem through the available range of painless movement.

- **THERAPEUTIC MASSAGE:** Massage of the adjacent large muscle groups such as the trapezius, pectoralis, and latissimus dorsi can diminish protective spasm, minimize tone, and promote relaxation.

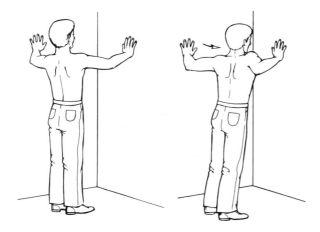

Stretching the pectoralis muscles.
Saunders HD: Evaluation, *Treatment and Prevention of Musculoskeletal Disorders*. New York: Viking Press, 1989.

■ **HOME PROGRAMS:** Motion, stretching, and strengthening as part of a home program and are essential to the successful treatment of frozen shoulder. Do not rely on getting better just from going to an office or clinic two or three times a week. Take responsibility and make your frozen shoulder your number one priority by exercising at home as often as recommended.

Conservative management is very important, especially since more radical treatments such as blind manipulation under anesthesia and surgery are fraught with so many problems. Frozen shoulder is usually manageable with appropriate therapy. Early detection, a serious willingness to get better, and adherence to a home program are all very important in healing a frozen shoulder.

29 Shoulder Separation, Disarticulation, and Dislocation

A 30-year-old female was riding her dirt bike across a mountain when the front wheel suddenly dipped into a gully and she was thrown over the top of the handlebars. She landed on the tip of her left shoulder. The immediate pain stemming from her collarbone was intense and she cradled her sagging arm with her right hand. This woman has suffered a broken collarbone.

A 44-year-old, first-time father was trying to make his 3-year-old son laugh by performing cartwheels, when he fell onto the tip of his right shoulder and felt something give away, followed by immediate pain. Now, he cannot lift his hand up over his shoulder or touch his opposite shoulder with his right hand. A large, painful bump is obvious at the tip of his right shoulder when compared to the opposite side. This man has sprained the ligaments binding his acromioclavicular (AC) joint.

The 40-year-old attendees of a birthday party split up into two teams to play touch football. Things got rough and exciting, and eventually the game became tackle football. Predictably, a twelve-man pile-up occurred, and the man on the bottom of the pile ended up lying on his side crying out in pain. Now he has a painful bump on the inner end of the left collarbone where it attaches to the breastbone. Any movement of his arm is painful and limited. This man has sprained *the ligaments of his* sternoclavicular joint.

A group of college freshman had an all-night slumber party. At one point, someone fell off the top of a bunk bed and landed on her hands. Her right shoulder immediately felt as if something was out-of-place and she yelled with pain. She could not use her right shoulder at all and cradled it protectively with the opposite arm. A lump was felt in her right armpit. This woman has suffered an anterior shoulder dislocation.

■ SPRAIN AND DISLOCATION

IN GENERAL, ligaments are not capable of stretching and are therefore able to bind the two ends of a joint securely, like taut adhesive tape. A torn ligament is called a *sprain* and results in a less stable joint. Ligament injuries occur quite often, especially in the ankle and knee joints, and they are very painful. A mild sprain (grade I sprain) involves a tear of only a few ligament fibers, while a

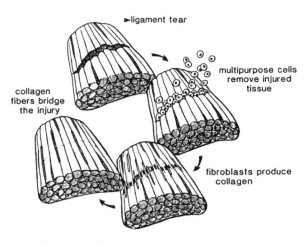

How a ligament heals.
Siegel IM: *All About Bone: An Owner's Manual*. New York: Demos, 1998.

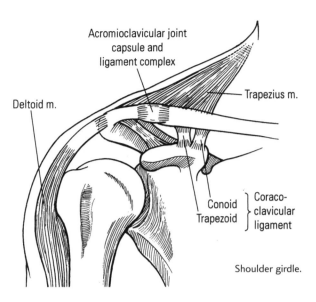

Shoulder girdle.

moderate sprain (grade II sprain) involves a tear of less than one-half of the fibers making up that ligament. A complete sprain (grade III sprain) involves a rupture of all the fibers in the ligament. In this case, the joint becomes so unstable that it may dislocate.

In addition to pain, a ligament sprain involves bleeding that causes the neighboring joint to swell after an injury and usually turn blue or purple the next day. When a ligament tear occurs, the torn space is not filled in by new ligament tissue. Instead, a poorer quality *scar tissue* fills the gap. This distributes force unevenly throughout the ligament and represents a weak site in the ligament that is prone to failure with excessive joint motion. Scar tissue is not as strong or capable as ligament and, therefore, the ligament is considered weakened and more likely to be re-injured in the future.

THE SHOULDER GIRDLE

The girdle of bones that encircles the shoulder or breast is known as either the *shoulder* or *pectoral* gir-

dle (derived from the Latin word *pectoralis*, meaning "breast"). This girdle includes the collarbone (clavicle) in the front, which spans from the inner breast to the tip of the shoulder where it connects via a joint to the shoulder blade (scapula) along the upper back. In this way, the shoulder girdle wraps around the upper part of the torso. The end of the long bone of the upper arm (the *humeral head*) is rounded and fits into a bowl-shaped depression in the shoulder blade (the *glenoid fossa*), forming a ball-and-socket joint that permits circular motion. All these bones work together in synchronous tandem every time you move your shoulder.

CLAVICLE = COLLARBONE

A collar is something that decorates the neckline. The *clavicle* (derived from the Latin word *clavis*, meaning "key") is also known as the *collarbone*. It is a unique bone that is crank-shaped when viewed from above, although it is nearly straight when looked at from the front. The human neckline is graced by the clavicle, which despite its swanlike appearance conveys strength to the shoulder girdle. Indeed, the clavicle is the only bony strut linking the trunk to the shoulder. Incredibly strong ligaments link the clavicle at either end, endowing the arm and hand with the ability to carry heavy objects.

From an engineering standpoint, the clavicle is similar to a beam supported at only one end, which is known as a *cantilever*. It is also similar to a diving springboard or a drawbridge. The clavicle is rigidly supported where it attaches to the body, enabling the side attached to the shoulder to lift weights and move relative to the stable trunk. The beauty of this arrangement is that it allows the arm to carry loads heavier than the arm itself, relying on the greater weight of the body for support.

Humans cannot typically land heavily on the arm without risking a break, unlike cats, who lack stiff ligaments. The impact absorbed by a fall onto an outstretched arm, if it does not break a bone close to the hand, will transfer up to the shoulder, pass through the clavicle, and break it at its weakest link: the middle third. A fracture may also occur from a direct fall onto the point of the shoulder. (The collarbone has been known to break in newborn babies because of the way the babies are delivered, especially during breech delivery, using forceps, and in very large babies.) When the clavicle is broken, the end at the shoulder will appear to droop lower than the opposite inner end and the arm will sag, powerless to lift anything. A clavicle fracture needs to be evaluated by a doctor to rule out any damage to blood vessels, lungs, or nerves passing just behind the collarbone.

◼ PREVENTION AND TREATMENT

Clavicle

Treatment of a fractured clavicle is accomplished by wearing a figure-eight bandage that immobilizes the collarbone in the correct position for healing, hold-

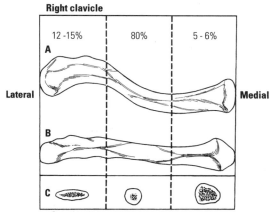

a. Superior view
b. Frontal view
c. Cross sections

When viewed from above (A) the collarbone appears crank-shaped; when viewed from the side (B), the clavicle appears straight; the cross section (C) of the inner and outer ends of the collarbone are thick and strong and therefore unlikely to break, whereas the middle part is the least stout and more likely to break during an injury. Saidoff DC, McDonough AL: *Critical Pathways in Therapeutic Intervention: Upper Extremities.* St. Louis: Mosby, 1997.

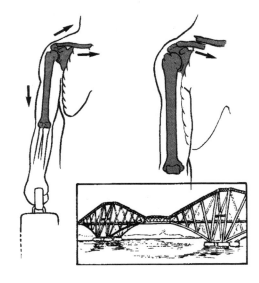

Cantilever action of the clavicle. When the clavicle is broken, the shoulder is not supported and moves downwards and inwardly. Inset: Cantilever bridge. Here, towers are built on either side and the bridge is built outward (cantilevered) from each tower to face the other tower. The weight of the suspended span in the middle is absorbed by the two towers. Dandy DJ: Essential *Orthopaedics and Trauma.* Edinburgh: Churchill Livingstone, 1989.

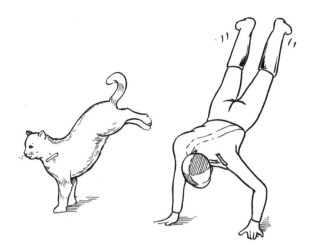

A cat is uniquely adapted to land on its forelegs because, unlike man, its clavicle does not rigidly link the sternum to the humerus. Dandy DJ: Essential *Orthopaedics and Trauma*. Edinburgh: Churchill Livingstone, 1989.

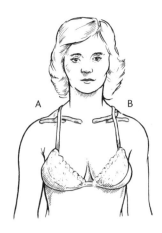

A. Bump on the collarbone at the site where healing has occurred. B. Sometimes healing may occur in such a way that the two broken ends override each other. Dandy DJ: Essential *Orthopaedics and Trauma*. Edinburgh: Churchill Livingstone, 1989.

ing the shoulder in a military-like posture. This allows the bone fragments to reattach. Reattachment often does not occur perfectly and many people have a residual bump that can be annoying. A collarbone fracture heals rather quickly. Infants heal quickly, in 2 weeks. Children heal within 3 weeks and adults take about 6 weeks to totally heal. In some cases, the bone may fail to knit together properly in what is known as "non-union," because the blood supply to the collarbone is less than ideal. Applying electrodes that deliver low doses of electricity to the skin over the fracture site, usually at night, may stimulate union and healing of the two ends of the bone fragments. Prevention of a broken collarbone is best accomplished by using protective padding when engaging in contact sports.

AC Joint

The bumpy point on the front of the shoulder is where the collarbone (in front) connects to the shoulder blade (in the back). This connection is known as the *acromioclavicular joint* (derived from the Greek word *acroma*, meaning "shoulder"). It is a very sturdy joint that is stabilized by strong ligaments. However, a fall onto the point of the shoulder can stretch, tear, or entirely disrupt these ligaments. This is an acromioclavicular joint (or AC joint) sprain, which is also called a *shoulder disarticulation*. This type of injury is quite painful. It appears as a very pronounced bump at the joint where the two bone ends have moved apart. Moving the shoulder is very painful. The bump may become permanent if left untreated and the shoulder will be weakened. Arthritis may eventually result.

Sprains may be treated in one of several ways, depending on severity. If the sprain is mild, the shoulder can be immobilized by wearing a halter that approximates the two ends of the joints, thus permitting the ligaments to heal in a shortened position. Applying ice and taking medication to ease the pain may help reduce early symptoms. If the injury is a total tear of the supporting ligaments, either a specialized sling may be used, or surgery may be performed to repair the torn ligaments. Regardless of the degree of injury, physical therapy is necessary to help get the shoulder moving normally and painlessly again.

SC Joint

The collarbone attaches on its inner end to the trunk via the *sternum*. The sternum, also known as the *breastbone*, is located at the front of the chest and protects the lung and heart. (The sternum is typically cut through during open heart surgery.) The point of attachment is known as the *sternoclavicular joint*. Strong ligaments anchor the collarbone to the sternum. However, certain types of injuries may tear these ligaments and push the collarbone inwards or outwards, causing a *sternoclavicular joint sprain* or *shoulder separation*. A hard kick aimed at the front of the chest or a head-on collision that forces the dri-

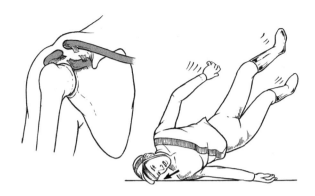

Shoulder disarticulation of the acromioclavicular (AC) joint due to spraining of its supporting ligaments.
Dandy DJ: Essential *Orthopaedics and Trauma*. Edinburgh: Churchill Livingstone, 1989.

A. Diagram of the shoulder region where the inner (medial) collarbone attaches to the breastbone (sternum)
B. A normal SC joint between the collarbone and breastbone.
C. Sprain of the supporting ligaments of the SC joint resulting in partial dislocation (subluxation) of the SC joint.
D. Backward dislocation of the inner (medial) portion of the collarbone so that it may push back upon and may even pierce the adjacent blood vessels.

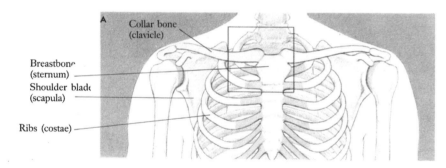

Collar bone (clavicle)
Breastbone (sternum)
Shoulder blade (scapula)
Ribs (costae)

Ligament and capsule over the joint between breastbone and collar bone

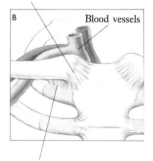
Blood vessels

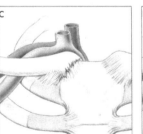

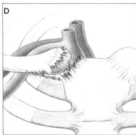

Ligament between the collar bone and the first rib

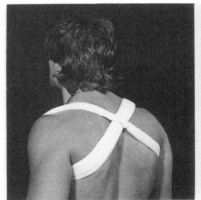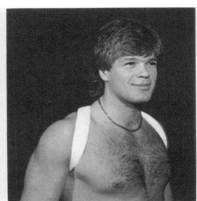

A figure-eight bandage seen from the back and front. Peterson L, Renstrom P: *Sports Injuries: Their Prevention and Treatment.* London: Martin Dunitz, Ltd., 1986.

ver's chest into the steering wheel can disrupt these ligaments and push the collarbone inward. If the guy at the bottom of a football pile-up is lying on his side, the collarbone can either sprain inwards or outward, depending on whether the shoulder is rolled backward or forward. This type of injury is very painful and may damage the lungs in severe cases. Treatment involves aligning the bones back into their original place and wearing a figure-eight strap to hold them in place. Ice and medication can

be used initially to help relieve pain. However, physical therapy is necessary during immobilization in order for the shoulder to move properly and painlessly after the strap is removed.

GH Joint

As previously discussed, the shoulder operates as a ball-and-socket joint, known as the *glenohumeral* (GH) *joint.* (See the illustration on page 246.) The rounded upper portion of the humerus is known as the *humeral head.* It rests precariously within a shallow bowl known as the *glenoid fossa.* This concave bowl is much smaller than the bulbous humeral head, but serves as a horizontal shelf for the humeral head to rest upon during most of the movements of the shoulder. This shelf becomes increasingly vertical as you raise your arm straight up to the ceiling. In fact, the humeral head would roll right off and slip downward in what is known as a *shoulder dislocation,* if not for the ligamentous thickenings of the shoulder joint capsule located beneath the shoulder joint, which tense up in order to hold the shoulder in place. However, the shoulder joint is likely to dislocate if a combination of positions and forces come to bear on it because these ligaments are pleated. In fact, the shoulder joint is the most likely joint in the body to dislocate.

Imagine your hand, elbow, and shoulder in the

Hippocratic method of reducing (relocating) a dislocated shoulder with the unbooted foot in the axilla. Dandy DJ: Essential *Orthopaedics and Trauma.* Edinburgh: Churchill Livingstone, 1989.

position in which you are taking an oath in a court of law. This is the vulnerable position. Now if someone were to grab your hand and pull it backward, the rounded humeral head might be forced through the pleated ligaments and dislocate downward and out of the joint. This can also happen during a fall. A dislocated shoulder should be immediately treated by an orthopedic surgeon who must rule out any nerve or blood vessel damage and then relocate the shoulder with a maneuver that puts the shoulder back where it belongs. It is important to avoid having a layperson try and force the displaced bone back into the socket because damage may occur to the nerves and blood vessels, as well as to the joint itself. However, once a shoulder has been dislocated and then relocated, it becomes ever more prone to dislocating in the future and may slip out-of-place from a movement as trivial as reaching behind your seat. Surgery may be necessary if the shoulder continues to dislocate in order to tighten up the shoulder ligaments and stabilize the shoulder. Microsurgery and arthroscopic techniques allow for simplified repair of dislocated shoulders by inserting a viewing tube (an arthroscope) directly into the shoulder joint. This miniature video camera allows the surgeon to manipulate tiny surgical instruments in order to make surgical repairs. Physical therapy following a medically treated dislocated shoulder may hasten recovery and help prevent recurrence by building up the muscles and stabilizing the shoulder.

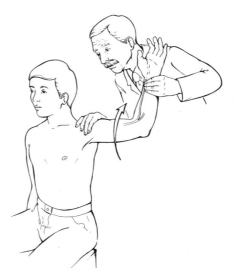

Mechanism for (anterior) shoulder dislocation. This maneuver is reproduced by the doctor to confirm (from the apprehension viewed on the patient's face during the test) that a shoulder dislocation occurred. Saunders HD: *Evaluation, Treatment and Prevention of Musculoskeletal Disorders.* Bloomington, Minnesota: Educational Opportunities (Viking Press), 1985.

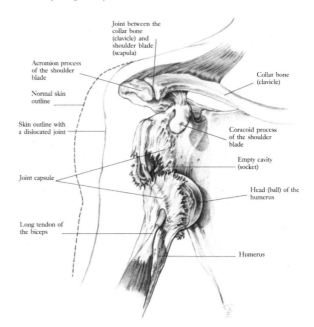

The most common form of shoulder dislocation is called *anterior shoulder dislocation.* Not only have the supporting ligaments become torn (sprained) but the entire joint is unstable and dislocates. Peterson L, Renstrom P: *Sports Injuries: Their Prevention and Treatment.* London: Martin Dunitz, Ltd., 1986.

30 Cervical Spine Disease

A 46-year-old woman complained of a sore neck and pain in her right arm after a whiplash injury several years ago, which diminished, until last week during an especially active game of tennis. The pain in her neck occurred late in the game when she quickly bent her neck back and lifted her arm in preparation for a powerful serve. The pain in her neck worsened later that day and spread to her right shoulder blade and arm. As time wore on, she noticed that she felt worse when waking up in the morning, especially on rainy days. A hot shower brings some relief. Certain movements of the neck and arm increase her symptoms. This woman has cervical spine disease due to radiculopathy, a pinched nerve in the neck.

■ CERVICAL RADICULOPATHY

APART FROM the nonspecific condition known as *neck strain, cervical radiculopathy* is probably the most common cause of neck pain. It occurs when the nerve root that exits the spinal cord is compressed (pinched) by some other structure. There are two common causes of cervical radiculopathy: a slipped disc and an arthritic spine, otherwise known as *cervical spondylosis. Spondylosis* is a Greek word meaning the "undoing of the spine." It refers to the age-related arthritic changes that occur in the cervical spine. C*ervical spondylosis* and *cervical arthritis* are both included in the category of *cervical spine disease.*

There are many possible causes of cervical radiculopathy. The most common cause in younger people is a slipped (herniated) disc, usually caused by a traumatic injury such as a whiplash. In middle-aged and older people, the most likely cause is arthritic changes in the cervical spine that affect the bones as well as the discs.

In the example at the beginning of this chapter, a previous history of whiplash injury to the neck may have predisposed the bones of this woman's neck toward injury of the emerging nerve roots. Hyper-extending (back-bending) the neck suddenly and forcefully may have caused acute pinching of a nerve root in an already sensitized area.

■ THE CERVICAL SPINE

As previously discussed, the spinal column consists of twenty-six bony segments including: twenty-four vertebrae, the sacrum, and coccyx. The spine is divided into three sections: seven cervical vertebrae (neck region), 12 thoracic vertebrae (upper back region), and five lumbar vertebrae (lower back). The twenty-four vertebrae rest upon the sacrum and coccyx at the very bottom of the spine. These vertebrae are referred to by numbers, beginning with the first vertebrae at the top of the neck being the cervical: C1 through C7; thoracic: T1 through T12; and finally, lumbar: L1 through L5.

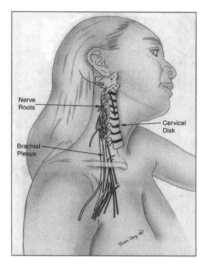

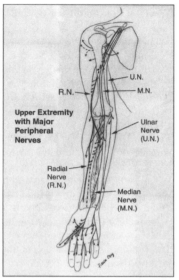

The cervical spine and discs in their normal anatomic alignment. The nerve roots exit the spine and form the nerves of the brachial plexus, then travel through the thoracic outlet to form the major nerves of the arm. Fried SM: *The Carpal Tunnel Helpbook*, Perseus Publishing, Cambridge Massachusetts, 2001.

The *cervical vertebrae* in the neck are the smallest spinal bones, and they support the head. The virtue of these multiple, small, stacked bones is that they allow us to bend our neck in different directions. They enable us to turn our head in almost 180 degrees of rotation, such as when you look over your shoulder.

The vertebrae of the spine are stacked upon one another in such a way so as to leave a small tunnel running from the spinal canal, through a ring of bone, and then outside the spine to the rest of the body. At each spinal level, two nerves exit the spinal canal (one on each side), which go to the skin (in the case of *sensory nerves*), to the muscles (in the case of *motor nerves*), or to the organs (in the case of sensory, motor, and *autonomic nerves*). Those nerves branching off the spinal cord and exiting the spinal canal are known as *nerve roots*. If the nerve roots passing through these narrow tunnels become compressed or pinched either by a disc or arthritis, the result can be severe pain and loss of normal function.

THE ARTHRITIC SPINE

The most common cause of chronic cervical neck pain due to radiculopathy, especially in those over the age of 50, is *degenerative disc disease of the spine*, also known as *cervical spondylosis*. The bones and joints of the spine may be afflicted by arthritis as we age and degenerate in the same way as the bones and joints in the hands, wrists, shoulders, and hips. Frequently, this results in local inflammation, the formation bony spicules known as *osteophytes* that overgrow the normal limits of the bone, and narrowing of the spaces between the bones. These osteophyes have an appearance similar to that of the sharp stalactites on the inside of limestone caves, and they can pinch the nerves and cause pain. Of particular concern is the narrowing of the foramen (tunnel) where the nerve roots exit the spine. This narrowing ultimately compresses the nerve root, resulting in symptoms similar to those seen with a herniated disc.

■ THE INTERVERTEBRAL DISC

Each bone of the spine consists of a very large cylindrical portion called the *vertebral body*. This portion of the vertebrae lies in the front (anterior region) of the spine and provides most of the actual structural support. Between each vertebral body lies a soft sac called an *intervertebral disc*, which together stack an extra 6 inches of height to the spinal column. The intervertebral disc was first described by the great Belgian anatomist Andreas Vesalius in 1555. These discs are almost entirely filled with fluid and provide cushioning between the vertebral bodies. Each of the twenty-three vertebral discs in the entire length of the spine allows the vertebral bodies that lie above it and below it to move against one another, permitting some degree of flexibility to the spine. Each disc consists of a soft, gelatinous center called the *nucleus pulposus* and a peripheral fibrous ring called the *annulus fibrosus*. Together they act to cushion some of the forces that are transmitted along the vertical spine. Sudden and excessive force, such as from a whiplash injury, may tear the tough outer cartilaginous envelope, allowing the gelatinous core of the disc to be squeezed out of the fibrous ring that surrounds it out like toothpaste coming out of a tube. Once the gel has escaped, it is not possible to put it back inside the disc. In medical terms, this is referred to as a *herniated nucleus pulposus (HNP),* but it is commonly called a *slipped disc.* This condition often results in severe neck, shoulder, and arm pain.

In younger people, the intervertebral discs are soft, moist, and contain a gelatinous nucleus. However, they become less moist, thinner, and a little tougher as we age, so that they are less likely to rupture when pressed. It is similar to the difference between squeezing a fresh grape versus a dried raisin.

■ SIGNS AND SYMPTOMS

As stated above, cervical radiculopathy occurs because the nerve root is pinched, most commonly due to cervical arthritis or a disc problem. The nerve root contains the sensory nerves that convey sensation from the skin. Consequently, when the sensory nerves are compressed, there will commonly be complaints of pain and/or numbness along the stretch of skin that is supplied by the affected sensory nerve. The pain is not restricted to the back alone. In fact, it may not even be felt in the back at all.

Whether the nerve root is compressed because of a disc problem or because of an arthritic problem, the symptoms are much the same and include:

- Pain in the neck that radiates to the top of the shoulders, shoulder blades, upper arms, hands, or back of the head.

- Tingling or numbness in the arms, hands, and fingers, and weaker reflexes.

- Neck stiffness, headaches, dizziness, or grating sounds with movement of the neck.

- If symptoms include leg weakness, balance complaints, or spasticity, then the condition may have progressed to cervical myelopathy, a condition wherein the spinal cord itself becomes compressed. This usually occurs in the lower cervical spine between C5 and C7. *Lhermitte's sign,* which causes tingling in all four limbs or down the back when flexing the neck, helps confirm compression of the cervical spinal cord.

Different nerves may become entrapped by a disc or arthritic bone spur and more than a single nerve root could also become pinched. Depending on the precise level of compression, there will be weakness:

- In attempting to lift the arm upward and over the head (resulting from compression at the 5th cervical level).

- In attempting to flex the bicep (upper arm muscle) as well as tingling of the thumb and forefinger (resulting from compression of the 6th cervical nerve root).

- In attempting to straighten the elbow and when bending the wrist toward the face. This is often accompanied by tingling from the forearm to the middle finger (resulting from compression of the 7th cervical nerve root).

- In attempting to use the fingers with force (resulting from compression of the 8th cervical nerve root).

The motor nerves running through the nerve root enable us to move our muscles. Consequently, there may be complaints of weakness in one arm if the motor nerves are injured. Neurological examination may show that reflexes such as jerking of the biceps or triceps are diminished or absent entirely. Motor nerve compression is much less common than sensory nerve compression, but potentially more serious.

■ Risk Factors

Risk factors for cervical arthritis include: obesity, smoking, poor posture, menopause, osteoporosis, chronic steroid use, and age. Some of these risk factors cannot be changed (age for example, although admittedly it would be nice). Other age-related changes such as arthritic outgrowths of bone are more likely to aggravate a nerve.

Risk factors for disc problems in the neck are also related to the amount of water contained within the intervertebral disc. Whereas the water content of the intervertebral disc is about 85% in preadolescents, it diminishes to approximately 70% in middle-aged adults. This happens because the chemistry within the disc alters with age. Less water means less resiliency and a diminished ability to withstand stress, making the spine more vulnerable to a disc-related injury.

■ Slipped Disc vs. Cervical Spondylosis

The two conditions of slipped disc and an arthritic spine may be differentiated from one another through a variety of clinical clues. Frequently, pain from a herniated disc is sudden in onset and follows heavy lifting or some other strenuous activity. Pain from degenerative disease of the spine is usually gradual in onset and chronic in nature. Frequently, there is no precise start time and no association with any particular activity. That being said, there are many exceptions to these rules, and there may not be a precise trigger for a herniated disc.

The surest way of determining the cause of the problem is to do radiological imaging with an MRI (magnetic resonance imaging). If an MRI cannot be done, the next best test is a *myelogram*. This procedure involves a spinal tap and the injection of a contrast agent into the fluid surrounding the spinal cord. Then, x-rays and frequently a CT scan are done in order to visualize the area of the nerve root compression. Sometimes a CT scan without the injection of the contrast agent is sufficient to visualize the problem. Keep in mind that disc herniation and degenerative disease of the spine are so common (especially in those over age 55) that they are likely to be present on the MRI or CT scan, regardless of whether they are truly responsible for the neck pain. With cervical spine disease, diagnosis is never made using imaging alone. Instead, the doctor matches the clinical symptoms to the appropriate imaging studies.

TESTS FOR CERVICAL SPINE DISEASE

There are several tests for cervical spine disease that confirm the condition by provoking symptoms, especially pain. Only medical personnel should perform these tests:

- **CERVICAL COMPRESSION/DISTRACTION:** This test refers to either pulling up or pushing down on the neck. Pulling upward may relieve symptoms because it creates more room for the nerve root; pushing downward may compress the nerve and provoke symptoms.

- **SHOULDER DEPRESSION TEST:** The already irritated nerve can be provoked by pushing down on one shoulder while side bending the head to the opposite side.

- **SPURLING MANEUVER:** This maneuver is done by rotating the head toward the painful side, bending it backward, and applying downward pressure. This will usually reproduce symptoms.

CONDITIONS TO RULE OUT

- **PERIPHERAL NERVE ENTRAPMENT:** This refers to compression of one of the many nerves that emerge from the neck and travel down the arm. One example of this is carpal tunnel syndrome. Differentiating between a compressed nerve and cervical spine disease is best done by a medical professional.

- **STINGER INJURY:** This is also known as a *burner injury*. It is caused by severe pulling on the cervical nerve roots and the meshwork they form, which is known as the *brachial plexus*. This type of injury is common in American football or during wrestling. It occurs when the shoulder is pushed down on one side while the neck is pulled to the opposite side. This will result in traction of the nerve roots or the brachial plexus. Symptoms include pain, burning, numbness, and tingling that may extend down to the hand for anywhere between several seconds to minutes. Once symptoms go away, athletic activities may be immediately resumed, taking care not to re-injure the area.

- **WRYNECK:** The disfigurement of this condition, which is also known as *torticollis*, is immortalized in the statue of Alexander the Great located in the British Museum. Approximately 3 in 10,000 people suffer from wryneck. It is a problem that can occur at any age, but it is most prevalent between the ages of 30 and 50. Women have a slightly higher incidence than men, and heredity may play a role because about 5% of those affected have a family history of the disease. Wryneck is actually classified as a mild form of torticollis in which the muscles of one side of the neck tighten or go into a spasm, causing the head to rotate to one side. Sleeping with the head bent at an unnatural angle from an uncomfortable pillow may stress the muscles in the neck. When you wake up after sleeping like this, you may find that your muscles have gone into a spasm. It can also happen from sleeping next to a window that lets in cold air over an unprotected head and neck. Taking a hot shower and/or a massage or whirlpool, and waiting a few days usually allows the muscles of the neck to get back to normal. Non-prescription medications may help. Some people may benefit from a battery-operated neck massager that can be worn like a scarf around the neck. A doctor may prescribe anti-cholinergic drugs that work by blocking certain nerve impulses in difficult cases. Alternatively, injection of tiny amounts of Botox® (a toxin produced by the organism that causes botulism) may help relax spastic neck muscles, breaking the cycle of pain and inflammation that prevents the head and neck from returning to normal.

- **ACUTE BRACHIAL NEURITIS:** This condition was very common in hospitalized soldiers during World War II, who were recovering from surgery or an upper respiratory infection. Their nerve roots somehow became inflamed. While symptoms may be confused with both cervical spine disease and peripheral entrapment, the hallmark of this condition is electrical studies of muscle that indicate both a nerve root and a peripheral nerve problem. Often, specific nerves are affected, resulting in a *winging* effect of the shoulder blade. Symptoms usually resolve of themselves, although this may take many months.

- **APEX (APICAL) LUNG TUMOR:** The top of the lung is especially vulnerable to this type of cancer in people who have a long history of smoking. Symptoms include severe and rapid weakness of all the muscles of the hand.

MANAGING CERVICAL SPINE DISEASE

For the vast majority, a combination of rest, non-steroidal anti-inflammatory drugs, and time will reduce pain and allow a complete recovery. This does not mean that the disc problem has necessarily disappeared. Rather it means that the inflammation and swelling have resolved, thereby taking pressure off of the nerve root. Conservative therapy including the following is often successful:

- **REST:** Many doctors recommend a brief period of bed rest (no more than a few days) and pre-scribe non-steroidal anti-inflammatory drugs. Some also recommend the use of muscle relaxants, but it has not been proven that they are of any significant value. It is important not to engage in activities that might provoke symptoms.

- **CERVICAL COLLAR:** A cervical collar provides some protection for the neck and serves as a reminder to take it easy. Initially, it may be worn as much as 24 hours a day for several weeks and then intermittently for the subsequent 4 to 6 weeks. The collars should not be too tight and should allow for slight bending forward of the neck.

- **MEDICATIONS:** Non-steroidal analgesics such as ibuprofen are helpful in alleviating pain and reducing inflammation. Narcotic analgesics may be used in cases of severe pain, but only for a brief period of time. Long-term narcotic use can result in physical addiction and constipation. Straining due to constipation is likely to exacerbate the underlying reason for the back pain, whatever the cause. The use of laxatives or stool softeners as recommended by a doctor may be helpful in cases where there is underlying constipation.

- **EXERCISES:** Cervical spine exercises include tilting your head towards your shoulders, moving it up and down (as when you say "yes"), and rotating it from side to side (as when you say "no"). All exercises should be done slowly and gently. Avoid those movements that cause pain. Other exercises may be added as suggested by a physical therapist or doctor.

- **TRACTION:** Spinal traction may be beneficial in dealing with neck pain. It should be performed with the neck in the slightly bent position *only* after the acute phase of pain has passed. When traction is performed correctly, it may ease the pressure against the nerve and help relieve pain.

- **MANIPULATION:** Manipulative therapy is practiced by osteopathic doctors and chiropractors. It involves a high-velocity thrust to the spine, which moves the disc away from the nerve root in order to relieve compression and pain. Physical therapists utilize a less forceful, low-velocity technique known as *joint mobilization.*

- **OTHER MODALITIES:** Cool down your painful neck by applying a commercial ice pack or package of frozen vegetable from the freezer to the painful spot for up to 15 minutes at a time, two or three times a day. Moist heat is preferred because it is more penetrating (as opposed to dry heat from an electric heating pad). Showers, baths, and whirlpools are very helpful in relieving pain and promoting relaxation once the acute phase has passed. Using TENS (transcutaneous electric nerve stimulation) has been found to help relieve pain stemming from cervical disc disease in some people.

- **MASSAGE:** Massage of the muscles of the neck, upper back, and shoulder area can be very helpful; particularly because tensing of these muscles following a pinched nerve can only irritate the nerve further. Massage may help break the cycle of pain by relaxing the muscle through which the nerves course. Other deep tissue massage techniques such as Rolfing and shiatsu may also be of help.

- **NERVE TRACT EXCURSION:** The compressed nerve root can become tethered at its point of exit from the spine. If the nerve does not move freely, scar tissue may build up and lessen its ability to move with ease as the arm moves through its normal range of motion. This makes normal movement of the neck and arm more painful and restricted. A proper nerve-sliding program is best implemented by a doctor or physical therapist.

- **INJECTIONS:** An epidural, liquid steroid injection into the area of nerve irritation, sometimes in combination with morphine, may cool down an inflamed nerve and avoid the need for surgery. The injection may be repeated once or twice, as needed.

- **NECK SCHOOL:** This approach involves 1-hour sessions over a period of several weeks in which people who suffer from neck pain learn about the anatomy of the neck, the causes of pain, and ways to prevent or lessen pain.

- **AROMATHERAPY:** Some people report relief from neck pain when lavender, marjoram, or other essential oils are massaged directly onto the skin of a painful neck and upper back. Alternately, they may be added to a hot bath.

- **RELAXATION TECHNIQUES:** Meditation and yoga are relaxation methods that may be combined with deep-breathing exercises or self-hypnosis in order to ease stress-related pain.

■ WHEN IS SURGERY NECESSARY?

If the pain fails to resolve within 4 to 6 weeks, more aggressive means of therapy may be considered. These include local injections of steroids and/or analgesics, and surgery. Many doctors will recommend surgery only if there is chronic pain that does not respond to any other option, weakness in the legs, or impairment of bowel or bladder function. Minimally invasive spinal surgery has revolutionized the management of severe cervical spine disease because there is very little post-surgical pain and a fast recovery. A ruptured disc or bony spur can be removed using *endoscopic microsurgery* through a small puncture instead of an open incision. This form of *laser surgery* involves the insertion of a tiny, thin viewing tube called an endoscope that is equipped with a laser, which painlessly vaporizes unwanted disc tissue and bony spurs.

PREVENTING NECK PAIN

The prevention of recurrent neck pain primarily involves the reduction of risk factors and firming up support for the spine. Some of these strategies include:

- **EXERCISE:** Shoulder shrugging exercises are a good way to maintain the range of motion of the neck area. Tilting the neck from side to side and rotating it in either direction is also helpful. Exercise should not be painful and should be performed slowly and deliberately in a relaxed manner.

- **STRETCHING:** Regular stretching of the muscles of the neck, upper back, and shoulder girdle are essential in maintaining optimal muscle health. A regular stretching exercise program is no less important than strengthening. It is best administered by a physical therapist, masseuse, or personal trainer.

- **MASSAGE:** Regular massage of the upper back area, shoulder area, head, and certain portions of the neck help relax the muscles through which the nerves exit the spine and course down to the arms. This is important because tight, tensed-up muscles clamp down on irritated nerves that may already be inflamed from a disc or bony spur. Massage should ideally be administered once per week or as needed by a licensed professional masseur who is state-certified. It is very important not to massage the carotid artery, especially in people older than age 35 because of the possibility of a stroke. The carotid artery is located superficially on the outer portion of the neck. This underscores the importance of utilizing a licensed masseuse.

- **POSTURAL ISSUES:** There are ways of minimizing the stress on your neck by taking care in how you perform your routine daily activities. Maintaining correct posture is one important means by which you can reduce your risk of developing neck pain. If you slouch while walking or sitting, the added curvature places greater stress on the spine. Try to walk with your shoulders back and your head up high. Slouching in a chair is a common practice because most people relax when sitting. Good posture is even more important when sitting than when standing. It is very important to sit in a chair that supports your upper back and helps you maintain a healthy posture. Placing a small pillow behind your lower back will add extra support. It is helpful to have a comfortable mattress that provides support when lying in bed. Sleep with a comfortable down pillow that provides adequate support to your head. Do not use too many pillows as this may bend your neck away from the plane of the body during sleep and strain the neck. Be sure to adjust the headrest high and forward enough when driving an automobile, to avoid placing undue stress on the muscles of the neck.

- **SMOKING:** Avoid smoking because research indicates that smoking can ruin the intervertebral discs of the spine.

31 Whiplash Injury

A 46-year-old mother was driving home from visiting her daughter when a sudden, violent thunderstorm occurred. The drenching rain created a sheet of water on the roadway. She immediately reduced her speed, but her tires began to hydroplane, which caused her to lose control of her car and slam into the median divider. She emerged from the car shaken but not hurt, and was able to walk to a telephone and call for help. She was released from a local emergency room after x-rays of her neck and spine showed no abnormality. About 6 hours after the accident, she began to experience pain in her neck and shoulders, headache, and difficulty concentrating, all of which became steadily worse. She went to her doctor, who diagnosed whiplash injury *as a result of the collision.*

■ WHIPLASH INJURY DEFINED

Whiplash injury is a nonspecific term that includes a variety of injuries to the neck and the soft tissue, as well as the bony tissues within the neck. Conceptualizing the vulnerability of the neck is easy if we imagine it to be like a tomato (the head) balanced on a soft stem (the neck). The neck can be easily damaged if too many forces are applied to the body in a particular way. Hundreds of pounds of forceful motion to the neck occurs most often during automobile accidents but may also occur dur-

ing falls, collisions involving go-carts or bumper cars, strenuous contact sports, blows to the head (boxing), or diving accidents.

■ CAUSES OF INJURY

The mechanism underlying whiplash injury is forced motion that causes the head and neck to be snapped in one direction while the body moves in the opposite direction. This can happen in one of several ways:

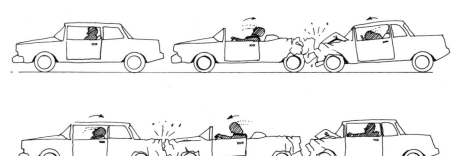

Energy in the form of force and speed can be transferred to the neck during front- and rear-end collisions.
Meals RA: *One Hundred Orthopaedic Conditions Every Doctor Should Understand*. St. Louis: Quality Medical Publishing, Inc. 1992.

- **REAR-END COLLISIONS:** The most common cause of whiplash injury involves an unaware driver in a stationary vehicle being struck from behind. This most commonly occurs in areas of high traffic density such as crowded urban areas. The collision causes the body and car to be propelled forward, while the head is thrown backward. In the absence of a head restraint, the head swiftly accelerates backward and the neck is hyperextended. The head then forcefully rebounds forward as the neck is hyperflexed and usually stops when the chin strikes the chest.

- **FRONT-END COLLISIONS:** In these types of collisions, the body and the car are pushed backward, while the head is thrown forward onto the chest.

- **SIDE COLLISIONS:** Being hit from the side causes the head and neck to accelerate to the opposite side before rebounding to the side of impact.

FACTORS DETERMINING SEVERITY OF INJURY

- **MASS AND SPEED:** These two factors represent how heavy each car is and how fast the other car was going and how fast you were moving before crashing. Both mass and speed determine how much force is imparted to the head and neck. *Acceleration*, meaning an increase in velocity over time, is mathematically defined as multiplying mass by speed, divided by time. A truck crashing into a car going 3 miles per hour is not nearly as bad as if it traveled 30 miles per hour. Similarly, a golf cart crashing into a car imparts much less force to the head and necks of the automobile occupants if it was going slowly, rather than if it was going fast.

- **HEADRESTS:** Utilizing headrests correctly by elevating them to a high position takes the punch

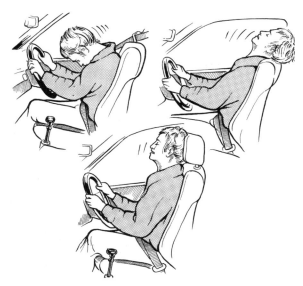

Combined flexion/extension whiplash injury of the neck. Movement of the head is limited by a head restraint.
Dandy DJ: Essential *Orthopaedics and Trauma*. Churchill Livingstone, Edinburgh, 1989.

out of potential whiplash injuries because the headrest prevents the neck from accelerating backwards.

- **AIRBAGS:** Front and side airbags that engage on impact can significantly minimize the severity of a whiplash injury.

- **AGE:** Elderly people are especially vulnerable to hyperextension injury of the neck because aging of the discs in the cervical spine as well as arthritic changes may reduce the available room for the spinal cord and emerging nerve roots. This increases the risk that the spinal cord or nerve roots will be compromised.

SIGNS AND SYMPTOMS

The signs and symptoms associated with whiplash injury may vary considerably depending on how much bodily injury occurred. The rapid stretch motion of the neck may stretch the muscles of the neck, which respond reflexively by going into painful spasm. This may cause the neck to assume an excessively rigid and upright posture. One or more of the intervertebral discs in the cervical spine may be injured. Tearing of ligaments may also occur, resulting in internal bleeding. The joints comprising the cervical spine in the neck may become dislocated or broken, injuring the nerve roots or spinal cord. The cord may become bruised from rapid bending, resulting in spinal cord contusion that manifests as tingling, numbness, or weakness of the arms and legs. The force imparted from a whiplash may be sufficient to even cause serious head injury or death.

Symptoms are often not felt until 6 or more hours after the injury. While x-rays are often normal, they may show a straight spine instead of the normally gentle curve that characterizes a healthy spine. There are often complaints of neck and shoulder pain, which may extend down to the shoulder blades. Bending the neck is painful and often not possible. The force of injury may injure the *tempomandibular joints* (*TMJ*) in the jaw. The neck can become exquisitely painful to touch, and muscle spasm may cause it to become rigid. Swelling of the soft tissues of the neck can cause problems with swallowing. The injured person may often experience irritability, dizziness, ringing in the ears, unsteady gait, headaches, poor sleep and concentration, anxiety, and depression. Other symptoms may include a racing heart, perspiration, and blurred vision. There may be muscle weakness, tingling, or numbness in the arms if the nerve roots emerging from the cervical spine are damaged. The person may experience problems with walking if the spinal cord was bruised. Confirmation of and the extent of damage to the nerves is accomplished by clinical testing and x-rays.

TREATMENT

Approximately 90% of those who suffer from whiplash injury are free of symptoms within 2 months if managed appropriately. On the other hand, the possibility of financial gain from insurance payments may play an important role in determining how soon recovery occurs. Some of the treatments involved in managing whiplash injury include:

- **REST:** A whiplash often involves sprain or strain of the soft tissues of the neck, requiring 2 to 3 weeks of rest. Bed rest is only appropriate if significant pain persists after the first day of injury. Avoid sudden or excessive bending of the neck.

- **CERVICAL COLLAR:** Cervical collars do not provide absolute stability to the cervical spine. Nevertheless, they are often worn for as much as 24 hours per day for 2 to 3 weeks and then intermittently for the next 4 to 6 weeks. The primary benefit of wearing a cervical collar is to remind the person wearing it to avoid extreme motion of the neck. The highest or widest part of the collar should be placed in the back to prevent excessive backward bending of the neck. The collar should maintain the neck and limit backward bending, while permitting some forward bending.

- **HOT AND COLD THERAPY:** Ice is usually applied within the first 48 to 72 hours following the injury in order to decrease pain and diminish swelling. After this time, heat may be applied to minimize pain and spasm and help increase local circulation.

- **MEDICATIONS:** Analgesics and muscle relaxants may be helpful in reducing pain and muscle spasm.

- **EXERCISES:** Exercising is very important because it helps restore normal muscle length to the muscles of the neck, upper back, and shoulder girdle. It is essential not to begin exercising until instructed to do so by a doctor, which is usually after the acute or subacute stage of injury has passed. It is best to begin movement from a position of minimal or absent pain. Move the neck gently through its non-painful range of motion. Motion may be increased gradually as pain subsides. Some exercises, which may be done separately or together, may include:

  - **NECK FLEXION:** This exercise stretches the muscles and joint capsules in the back of the neck. It is performed by slowly bending the chin to the chest, holding this position for five seconds in a relaxed manner, and then returning the head back to neutral.

  - **NECK EXTENSION:** This exercise stretches the muscles and joint capsules in the front of the neck. It is performed by slowly rolling the head backward so that the eyes are looking up at the ceiling. Hold this position for 5 seconds, relax, and then bring the head back to neutral.

  - **NECK SIDE BENDING:** This exercise stretches the muscles and joint capsules on the sides of the neck and upper shoulder. It is performed by bending the neck gently to one side so that the ear approximates or touches the shoulder. Hold for 5 seconds, relax, and then move the head back to neutral.

  - **SHOULDER SHRUGGING:** This exercise derives from the Feldenkreis method of exercise in which gentle up/down, back and forth, and circular shoulder-roll exercises help loosen up the muscles of the upper back, shoulder blades, neck, and shoulder.

  - **STRETCHING:** Stretching the muscles of the neck, upper back, and shoulders is helpful, although one should not push through the pain. Instead, stretch just short of experienc-

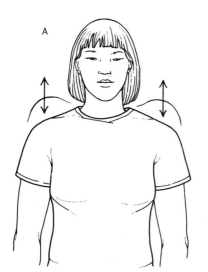

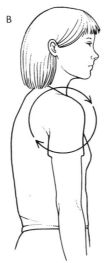

A: Lift both shoulders up to your ears and then drop them as low as they can go. Do this five times.

B: Roll your shoulders by making a circle. Lift them both shoulders and roll them forward five times, and then lift and roll them backward five times.
Allan ML, Fuerst ML: *Sports Injury Handbook: Professional Advice for Amateur Athletes.* New York: John Wiley and Sons, Inc, 1993.

ing pain. Using *cervical traction* with the head bent slightly forward may help stretch muscles and decrease spasm. Cervical traction should *only* be done after several days have elapsed since the injury

■ **EDUCATION AND PREVENTION:** It is important to adjust the headrest in your car to an adequate height as recommended by the owner's manual. In addition, it is certainly worth the expense to have a car with both front and side airbags.

32 Reflex Sympathetic Dystrophy

A 31-year-old aspiring actress with ruddy cheeks complained of a generalized burning pain in her left hand. Her hand and forearm alternately feel hot and cold, causing her loss of function. Her symptoms seem to spread up the arm toward the elbow and shoulder. Lately, her left arm appears swollen, red, and sweaty. About 2 months ago, she bruised and injured her left hand as she reached out to catch a falling toolbox. She has been seeking professional help on a weekly basis for an anxiety disorder. An x-ray of her left hand shows spotty osteoporosis of the bones of the wrist and hand. She has no other medical history. Her neurologist has diagnosed her with reflex sympathetic dystrophy.

■ WHAT'S IN A NAME?

SHAKESPEARE ONCE ASKED the question: "What's in a name?" Many would answer him: "Quite a bit!" It is a popular cultural belief that names serve as more than simple labels to hang on an object or person, but rather they sum up the essence of that something that they describe. If this is true, it would seem that *reflex sympathetic dystrophy* is poorly named because it is not necessarily *reflexive* (an illness that occurs in response to an injury); it does not necessarily involve the *sympathetic* nervous system; and it does not necessarily result in *dystrophy* of the affected body part, meaning progressive changes resulting from poor nutrition. Nevertheless, some of the early clinicians were struck by the presence of these features in many people with persistent pain in a limb following a minor trauma, so the name stuck. The large number of different names used to describe this condition, however, adds to the confusion and reflects our poor understanding of just what reflex sympathetic dystrophy is. Other commonly used names include: *causalgia of Mitchell, minor causalgia, Sudeck's Atrophy, algo-dystro-*phy, traumatic angiospasia, post-traumatic dystrophy, peripheral acute trophoneurosis, post-infarctional sclero-dactyly, shoulder-hand syndrome,* and *complex regional pain syndrome type I (CRPS-I).*

The final name on the above list, *complex regional pain syndrome type I,* is of relatively recent origin and has become widely accepted among specialists because it is more inclusive of the many different ways that reflex sympathetic dystrophy manifests. In this chapter, however, we will continue to use the classic and most familiar term: *reflex sympathetic dystrophy (RSD).*

■ REFLEX SYMPATHETIC DYSTROPHY DEFINED

The most common symptom of RSD is persistent pain, usually precipitated by some type of trauma, which need not be severe. Often the trauma may be so insignificant that it is not even remembered by the person after the appearance of the RSD. The fact that the body reacts out of proportion to the original insult is a defining hallmark of this condition. The pain may involve any body part, although most commonly any one of the extremities is usually affected first. The pain may spread to other body parts if it is not treated early. The pain may be very intense and may also involve an acute sensitivity to touch. This phenomenon is called *allodynia* or *hyperpathia* by doctors, and it results in what are normally neutral or even pleasant sensations being perceived as painful. As a result, there is loss of function of the affected area. Another feature that is commonly seen involves physical changes in the affected limb. These may include swelling, redness of the affected area, changes in sweating patterns, stiffness, warmth (in the early stages), coldness of the extremity (in later stages), and wasting away of the affected area.

▪ WHAT TO EXPECT IN EACH STAGE

RSD is a progressive disorder, which advances through several stages if it is not adequately treated early on. Although there is considerable variability from one person to the next, certain features are characteristic of each stage.

- **STAGE I:** The earliest stage typically begins with severe pain, which is limited to the site of an injury but is way out of proportion to the severity of the injury. The pain may be perceived as an intense burning sensation associated with abnormal sensitivity to touch and light pressure. At this time, physical changes may be noted in the skin. The limb may also swell. The skin usually appears red and warm, but at times it may become cold and appear blue in color. Sweating increases noticeably over the affected limb. This stage may subside spontaneously or with therapy and not progress any further, or it may go on to stage II after a few weeks.

- **STAGE II:** The pain may intensify during the intermediate stage and become more diffuse.

Skin sensitivity to what are normally innocuous sensations becomes more severe. The swelling may become more diffuse and take on a harder or tougher texture. The skin may appear shiny at this point and become more discolored. Hair is lost, and the nails may change their appearance, becoming brittle, ridged, and cracked.

- **STAGE III:** The late stage of this condition is characterized by muscle wasting, atrophy of the skin and underlying tissue, stiff joints, and demineralization (thinning) of the underlying bone (osteoporosis). These changes, once they appear, may be irreversible despite therapy. The pain also becomes intractable at this stage and highly resistant to therapy.

▪ CAUSES OF RSD

So far, the reason some people develop RSD is very poorly understood. It has long been observed that it follows some type of trauma or injury to the body. The type of injury might be very minor. For example, even a paper cut or a splinter might precipitate RSD. It has also been associated with the following:

- Major or minor trauma

- Myocardial infarctions (heart attacks)

- Surgery

- Disorders of the spine

- Repetitive motion disorders (carpal tunnel)

- Localized infections

Occasionally, the person with RSD will have no recollection of any injury at all. Most likely, the injury in such a case was too minor to have been noticed or remembered.

Some have speculated that RSD is the result of the healing process spun abnormally out-of-control. When a person sustains an injury under normal conditions, the first response of the body is to signal the presence of the injury by activating pain fibers. The sympathetic portion of the nervous system is stimulated in response to the pain, which helps organize the local reaction of the injured tissue to the injury. The small blood vessels in the area constrict and become more porous to allow *inflammatory cells* from the blood to visit the area of injury. This results in local redness and swelling. The inflammatory cells release chemicals called *cytokines* that further contribute to the redness and swelling, but also increase the sensitivity of the area to pain. The increased pain may signal the sympathetic nervous system to further increase the inflammatory response, which in turn adds to the pain. A cycle of pain and inflammatory response ensues, and some believe that if left unchecked this might lead to RSD. Ordinarily, the sympathetic nerves withdraw from this cycle after a short period of time and the cycle remains under control. For reasons that are still unclear, the cycle continues to spiral upwards in people with RSD.

Lest you get the wrong idea, it is important to emphasize that this scenario is almost certainly an oversimplification. Many people with RSD do not fit this description at all. For example, not all people with RSD appear to have significant involvement of the sympathetic nervous system. Sometimes the injury is so minor that there is no significant associated pain to initiate the cycle. Nevertheless, for many people with RSD, this framework has proven useful in understanding what is happening and has been especially useful in guiding therapy, as will be illustrated later on in this chapter.

Although the cause of RSD remains vague and elusive, studies have been convincing that there are significant physiological changes underlying the condition. For example, in one published study, eight people with RSD had their affected limbs amputated. When these limbs were studied, it was found that all of them had abnormal changes in the skeletal muscles. About half of them had loss of myelinated nerve fibers, suggesting an underlying small vessel circulatory problem called *microangiopathy*. This is the type of lesion that might be expected with abnormalities of the sympathetic nerves because they play an important role in regulating the degree of small blood vessel constriction.

People with an individual disposition toward RSD (*diathesis*) are those with increased sympathetic activity such as sweaty palms, migraine headaches, excessive flushing, or a history of fainting spells. Psychological make-up is a second type of risk factor for RSD. People who are fearful, emotionally unstable, dependent, or insecure tend to be more prone to RSD.

▓ DIAGNOSIS OF RSD

For the most part, establishing a diagnosis of RSD is based upon observing the features described above and good clinical judgment. There are no laboratory tests that can prove the existence of RSD. However, there are a few tests that may provide evidence to support the diagnosis if there is significant doubt, although their true usefulness is debated by experts.

■ **TRIPLE PHASE BONE SCAN:** In general, bone scans make use of radioactive tracers to detect areas of abnormal blood flow suggesting a fracture, an infection, or a tumor invasion. A standard bone scan is not specific enough to be useful for the diagnosis of RSD. A triple phase bone scan, however, adds an additional level of specificity that may sometimes be useful in diagnosing RSD. The first phase of this study closely follows the injection of the radionucleotide tracer and assesses the degree to which the arterial blood carrying the tracer is taken up into the bone. Increased uptake is suggestive of RSD, although it is not specific for it. The second phase of the study examines whether the blood carrying the tracer pools in the areas around certain joints in the affected extremity. If it does, this supports a diagnosis of RSD. The third stage is delayed several hours (usually 3 to 4 hours). It is suggestive of RSD if the radiologist sees diffuse asymmetric uptake of the tracer in the different joints in the affected extremity.

- **THERMOGRAPHY:** This method uses a device that measures the release of heat from different portions of the body. Abnormal patterns of heat generation may suggest the presence of RSD, but they are not in and of themselves diagnostic. In fact, neither the presence nor the absence of abnormalities in this study will prove or disprove the presence of RSD, but may be useful in supporting a questionable diagnosis. As a cautionary note, reliable thermograms are difficult to perform, and there is a great deal of variability in the outcome, depending on the skill of the examiner. It is very important, therefore, to have these tests done at an experienced and reputable facility.

- **X-RAY BONE DENSITOMETRY:** In the later stages of RSD, bone density decreases and this may be picked up by bone densitometry. Like the other tests, there is nothing specific to RSD about bone densitometry, and it is not at all sensitive to early RSD, which is when the diagnosis is most in doubt.

- **NERVE CONDUCTION STUDIES:** Nerves carry electrical messages along the length of their fibers. The ability of the nerve to carry these signals can be measured by applying electrodes over the course of the nerve and applying a small electrical current at one electrode and recording the signal from another electrode located a fixed distance away. (It feels like a small electrical shock.) By measuring the time it takes for the electrical signal to travel along the nerve from one electrode to the other, it is possible to measure the speed with which the nerve transmits signals. This is called *conduction velocity*. It is also possible to measure the height of the signal, which is also a measure of the strength of the signal. Both of these measures tell us about the health and well being of the nerve fiber itself. Nerve conduction studies are generally normal with RSD, so this test does not help us diagnose the presence of RSD, but it can be useful in ruling out the presence of other conditions that cause neuropathic pain, as discussed in the next section.

■ CONDITIONS TO RULE OUT

- **DEEP VEIN THROMBOSIS:** A clot in a vein in the leg can result in severe pain, tenderness, discoloration of the leg, and swelling. This condition looks somewhat similar to RSD. A clot may develop as the result of lying in bed for several days at a time without moving or getting out of bed (for example, after sustaining an injury) or following an infection in the leg. It is also more likely to occur in people who have a so-called *hypercoaguable state*. This means that their blood clots more quickly than it normally would. Pregnancy, for example, may lead to a hypercoaguable state. Deep vein thrombosis may be distinguished from RSD by the presence of a chord or thickened vein under the thigh and by an abnormal *venous plethysmography* or *venogram*. These are tests that measure blood flow through the veins in the leg.

- **CAUSALGIA:** This condition so closely resembles RSD that it has been named *complex regional pain* *syndrome type II* (*CRPS-II*) to distinguish it from CRPS-I, the new descriptive name for RSD. The major difference between causalgia and RSD is that there is a lesion that is destructive to the underlying nerve in causalgia, but no identifiable nerve injury with RSD. Nerve conduction studies may be helpful in differentiating the two conditions, but a careful examination by a neurologist may be equally useful.

- **NEUROPATHY:** Neuropathy includes a wide variety of conditions. Broadly it refers to any injury to a peripheral nerve. This injury might include compressive neuropathies in which the nerve is compressed (for example, in carpal tunnel syndrome; see Chapter 24). Compressive neuropathies may result in pain and tenderness in the area served by the injured nerve, but unless the condition progresses to causalgia, there is usually no swelling or discoloration. *Mononeuritis* is another type of neuropathy that affects individual nerves and their distribution, but may not be related to a direct compressive injury. Mononeuritis is often associated with other systemic diseases such as cancer and disorders of the immune system. With mononeuritis, the limb may be numb and weak, and pain may or may not be a prominent feature. Swelling and discoloration are generally not associated features.

- **CELLULITIS:** Infection of the soft tissues of a limb is referred to as *cellulitis*. Like RSD, cellulitis may include local tenderness, local warmth of the skin, discoloration, and swelling. Unlike RSD, it can be associated with fevers, elevated white blood cell counts, and generalized malaise. It is important to make the diagnosis of cellulitis quickly and treat it with the appropriate antibiotics, or run the risk of the infection spreading and becoming potentially life-threatening.

◼ TREATMENT OF RSD

The person with RSD has a painful, swollen limb that cannot be moved or used in an effective manner. The primary goal of therapy for RSD is to try to make the affected limb functional again. Treatment needs to be initiated as early as possible and needs to be focused on relieving pain and increasing mobility of the limb. A variety of different approaches are used, often simultaneously:

- **NON-MEDICINAL APPROACHES:** Aggressive physical therapy within but not beyond the limits of pain plays an important role in the early therapy of RSD. This approach makes use of techniques that train the person with this condition to keep the affected extremity mobile and avoid further injury or exacerbation. Approaches that are used include: massage, hydrotherapy, electric stimulation, intermittent limb compression, cold treatment, heat therapy using hot packs or a paraffin bath, splinting, range of motion and resistive exercises, and pool-based exercises. A valuable treatment modality utilizes stress-loading the affected limb for both pain relief and desensitization. These techniques all help avoid muscle cramps and joint contractures, and promote mobility. It is essential to begin using the affected body part as normally as possible, as soon as possible.

- **MEDICATIONS:** A number of different types of medications have been used to treat the symptoms associated with RSD. Most are directed at the pain associated with the condition. None of these drugs are particularly effective at treating the underlying condition itself. Medications used for the symptoms of RSD include:

  - **ANALGESICS:** Simple analgesics used to treat common pain syndromes associated with inflammatory states are often the first line of treatment for the relief of pain in early RSD. The drugs most commonly prescribed include non-steroidal anti-inflammatory drugs such as ibuprofen (Motrin® and Advil®), naproxen (Naprosyn®), aspirin, and indomethacin (Indocin® and Anaprox®). For people with ulcers, gastritis, or gastroesophageal reflux, newer COX-2 selective anti-inflammatory drugs such as celecoxib (Celebrex®), which are less likely to exacerbate the injury to the gastrointestinal lining, are sometimes used. When non-steroidal anti-inflammatory drugs are not effective, some doctors may prescribe stronger analgesics such as narcotics. Caution should be exercised in using narcotics for chronic conditions such as RSD because they may be addicting and have long-term side effects such as constipation.

- **ANTIDEPRESSANTS:** Tricyclic antidepressants are a class of drugs that, although traditionally used to treat depression, have been found to be useful in controlling a wide variety of chronic pain syndromes, especially pain associated with nerve injuries. These drugs include amitriptyline (Elavil®), nortriptyline (Pamelor®), and doxepin. They have a number of bothersome side effects, including: drowsiness (they should only be taken at night), dry mouth, weight gain, urinary retention, and irregular heart beats. It is therefore important that they should be used with caution and only under the careful supervision of a doctor.

- **ANTICONVULSANTS:** Several drugs that have been traditionally used to treat epilepsy have also been found to be effective at controlling the pain associated with nerve injury. These include: carbamazepine (Tegretol®), valproic acid (Depakote®), and most recently, gabapentin (Neurontin®). These drugs have not yet

been proven to be effective in relieving the pain associated with RSD.

- **SYMPATHETIC INHIBITORS:** As we will review below, one of the most effective methods of controlling symptoms of RSD is to suppress the activity of the sympathetic nervous system. This is usually accomplished with relatively invasive procedures such as sympathetic nerve block, but it may also be done on a smaller scale through the use of drugs that inhibit the normal activity of the sympathetic nerves. The most carefully studied approach to doing this is through use of a clonidine patch. Although data suggests that the clonidine patch is useful for the treatment of sympathetically maintained pain, it is not a substitute for sympathetic blockade.

- **SYMPATHETIC BLOCKADE:** *Sympathetic blocks* are useful for more than just treating RSD. For example, they may be of help in establishing the diagnosis and in determining the subtype of RSD. If a person's symptoms improve significantly following a sympathetic block (even if they are not resolved), it suggests that the condition is, in fact, RSD and that the person falls into the subgroup of those whose symptoms are related to excessive sympathetic activity. If the person does not respond to the sympathetic block, RSD is not ruled out, but it does suggest that he may have the variety of RSD that is not associated with perceptible sympathetic hyperactivity. In that case, sympathetic block or surgical *sympathectomy* is unlikely to be a useful therapeutic approach.

An anesthesiologist or some other specialist in dealing with chronic pain syndromes usually performs sympathetic blocks. It is important to be certain of the credentials of the doctor performing the procedure and to be certain that the procedure is performed in a setting where your vital signs will be monitored closely. When RSD affects the arms or some upper portion of the body, the block is performed through injection of an anesthetic to the stellate ganglion, which lies near the windpipe (the trachea). It is common to experience a change in your voice, swallowing difficulties, and drooping of the upper eyelid following the procedure. These are side effects of reduced sympathetic activity combined with inhibition of other nerves in the area. When RSD involves a leg, the injection is likely to be to the lumbar portion of the spine (lower back).

If the block is successful, the person may experience diminished pain and a warm sensation over the extremity. It is frequently necessary to perform a series of injections in order to adequately block the sympathetic nerves. Sometimes even after a successful block, it is necessary to return and repeat the block if symptoms return. It is important, however, not inject too many times because the risk of side effects increases with little additional gain in function. Rarely are more than a series of six injections necessary or useful.

■ **SYMPATHECTOMY:** When people with RSD respond transiently to sympathetic block, it is a sign that their condition is maintained by hyperactivity of the sympathetic nervous system. In that instance, they may decide, in conjunction with their doctor, that permanent inhibition of the sympathetic nerves may be warranted. Sympathectomy is a procedure in which the sympathetic nerves are permanently destroyed by either surgical transection (cutting) or by injection of a chemical such as phenol, which will destroy the nerve. The major advantage of sympathectomy is that it is probably the most effective means of controlling the symptoms associated with RSD. Disadvantages include the fact that it is also one of the most invasive means of treating RSD, and it may sometimes actually exacerbate the pain or result in new pain in a region closer to the torso than the original pain. Sympathectomy may be followed with a sympathetic block if this complication occurs.

■ **SPINAL CORD STIMULATION:** This type of treatment has been used to relieve chronic pain since 1967, but in recent years it has begun to be used to treat large numbers of people with RSD who either do not respond to sympathetic blockade or who lose their responsiveness. Studies of people with RSD report very high success rates (80% or greater) in relieving the pain associated with RSD using this procedure, especially in people with sympathetically-maintained pain for whom the beneficial effects of sympathectomy were transient. Spinal cord stimulation involves placing a temporary electrode through the epidural space (a space around the spinal cord) and advancing it until it is at the level corresponding to the area of pain. It is then tested for a period of about a week to determine whether there is a beneficial effect. If there is, then the stimulation device is permanently implanted with permanent electrodes attached. Surgical complications are common and in one study it was reported that 50% of these devices had to be removed due to complications. In most of those cases, the complications related to technical issues connected with the device itself. However, some of the cases involved infections.

Why spinal cord stimulation works is not fully understood. Some have proposed that spinal stimulation results in blockade of the sympathetic fibers in the spinal cord. Because it is also effective at relieving many types of non-sympathetically maintained pain, other mechanisms may be at work as well. For example, spinal cord stimulation might stimulate the large diameter nerve fibers that may be involved in natural pain inhibition. (See Chapter 5.)

Whole Body
Conditions

33 Arthritis

▪ ARTHRITIS DEFINED

Arthritis is defined as "an inflammation of joints due to infectious, metabolic, or constitutional causes." It is a general term for more than 100 conditions that affect about 55 million Americans and, according to a nationwide survey report by the Centers for Disease Control and Prevention, approximately one-third of all American adults suffer from some type of *joint disease*. Arthritis restricts everyday activity more often than cardiovascular disease, cancer, or diabetes, and can become so severe that it limits dressing, climbing stairs, preparing food, and getting in and out of bed. This chronic disease takes a physical, mental, emotional, and economic toll, and robs the American economy of more than 70 million workdays each year. The impaired laborer may be a nurse whose arthritic hands cannot hold a syringe steady, a pilot whose arthritic spine cannot tolerate long hours in the cockpit, or a baseball player whose arthritic shoulder silences his bat. All of this amounts to economic losses of billions of dollars per year. The Roman Emperor Diocletian understood how devastating this disease could be, so he exempted his citizens with severe arthritis from paying taxes!

People with arthritis are cared for by specialists called rheumatologists, who specialize in recognizing and treating the many forms of arthritis. Rheumatic diseases often affect those tissues surrounding the joint such as muscle, tendons, ligaments, and other parts of the body located far from joints, such as the internal organs and blood vessels.

Auguste Renoir, the famed French Impressionist continued painting for more that two decades with hands severely deformed by rheumatoid arthritis by tying a brush to his gnarled hand.

▪ RHEUMATOID ARTHRITIS

Rheumatoid arthritis (RA) is one of many forms of arthritis that are classified as *rheumatic diseases*. It is a type of inflammatory arthritis. RA is also an autoimmune disorder, which means it is a condition wherein the body attacks itself. The immune system incorrectly identifies the synovial membrane in a joint as a foreign invader, which results in inflammation that damages the cartilage and tissues in and around the joints. The surfaces of the bone are often also destroyed because the inflammation in the joints triggers the production of enzymes that slowly digest the adjacent tissue. This damaged tissue is replaced with scar tissue, which forces the space between the joints to narrow and the bones to fuse. RA causes severe pain, stiffness, fatigue, weight loss, and fever. It can strike at any age and is common in people under age 40. Approximately 2.1 million Americans have RA, and 75% of them are women. RA is often associated with stress, poor diet, and bacterial infection. It can be caused by bacterial, viral, or fungus infection in a joint. Symptoms include pain, swelling, redness, and tenderness. Often there will also be symptoms of systemic infection such as fever and chills.

OSTEOARTHRITIS

Osteoarthritis is defined as "non-inflammatory degenerative joint disease…characterized by degeneration of cartilage, bone, and changes in the synovial membrane…accompanied by pain and stiffness, particularly after prolonged activity." Osteoarthritis is the most common type of bone and joint disease. It is also known as *wear and tear* or *degenerative joint disease*. This form of arthritis affects as many as 21 million people in the United States, and this number is expected to reach 40 million by the year 2020. Osteoarthritis can begin as early as the second decade of life and is responsible for about 7 million doctor visits per year. According to the National Institutes of Health, workdays lost due to osteoarthritis total about 68 million per year. There is no cure for osteoarthritis and, by age 60, almost all Americans will have some degree of osteoarthritis.

Doctors once believed that osteoarthritis was a disease of old age. In fact, osteoarthritis is not only a disease of older people. This disease, which breaks down the cartilage lining inside your joints, begins its relentless, initially painless course as early as age 20. However, you do not even begin to feel the tell-tale twinges of symptoms until middle age. By then, the damage has been done and even the best treatment cannot do more than ease symptoms and try to maintain the status quo of progressively degenerating joints.

While many people in their 30s and 40s have it, about 16 million Americans with osteoarthritis are over 65 years of age. Women are affected more than men. By the fifth decade of life, 90% of all Americans will have some visible arthritic changes in their cartilage, and one in five will have moderate to severe osteoarthritis.

WEAR AND TEAR ON JOINTS

Whether you live on land or in the sea, if you have bones and joints, osteoarthritis is a fact of life. Nearly all vertebrates suffer from osteoarthritis, including dolphins and whales, who are buoyed up by water. There is evidence that long-extinct terrestrial animals such as dinosaurs had osteoarthritis. Only sharks do not have osteoarthritis, because they have an internal skeleton entirely made up of cartilage.

Wear happens in a pencil eraser when it is used to erase lead writing from paper. Even human teeth, which are stronger than bone, can wear out over time. Just about everything wears out given enough time. For example, the relatively low-lying Catskill Mountains in New York were once as high as the Himalayas, but they were eventually worn down by the effects of wind, rain, and erosion. Osteoarthritis develops when the cartilage covering the long ends of bones wears out and the bones rubs against each other.

This wear and tear leads to a process of cartilage

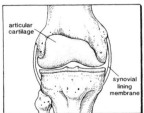

A Healthy Knee Joint

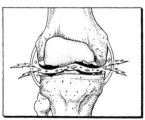

Osteoarthritis–articular cartilage degenerates and fragments

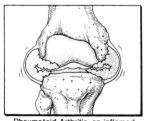

Rheumatoid Arthritis–an inflamed synovial membrane erodes the joint

The sequence of joint degeneration in arthritis.
Siegel IM: *All About Bone: An Owner's Manual.* New York: Demos, 1998.

breakdown known as *degeneration*, which is common is people over age 65, but it may appear decades earlier. This process is accelerated in the Baby Boom generation, which is currently heading into middle age, because of the cumulative affect of decades of high-impact aerobics, jogging, and running with less than perfect alignment of the joints of the hip, knee, and ankle. This is a sure recipe for osteoarthritis, especially when coupled with being overweight.

◼ NATURAL JOINT PROTECTION

The human body has incorporated a number of strategies into its evolution in order to reduce the effect of impact loading on joints, which are lined with a special *synovial membrane* that produces lubricating fluid. This lubrication is known as *synovial fluid,* and it is largely responsible for limiting the wear and tear on joints. Joints that have this type of lubricating system are known as *synovial joints.* In joints with menisci, their elastic nature also helps bear the brunt of weight-bearing forces because they act like a soft cushion to protect cartilage. The soft, elastic nature of fat within the joint also acts as a cartilage cushion. Ligaments surround and support the joints, connecting the bones to each other and preventing excessive movement. Muscles surround the ligaments and provide an additional layer of protection because their active contraction acts to splint and protect the cartilage within the joint.

◼ THE BENEFITS OF CARTILAGE

Cartilage is the remarkable material that caps the ends of our long bones and enables our skeleton to bear weight without pulverizing our bones into mush. Like the air cushions in good tennis shoes, cartilage prevents joint grinding by acting as a shock absorber. Cartilage is an elastic tissue that is full of water.

Everyday, the joints of our bodies take incredible abuse from merely moving around, whether we are running, jogging, or simply walking. Each time we take a step forward, the downward force of our body weight is conveyed through our spines, hips, knees, and ankle joints. Imagine banging a baseball bat repeatedly against a concrete floor. Sooner or later the bat will simply fall apart. We are fortunate in that, unlike the dead wooden baseball bat, we have the ability to regenerate and recover from the damage inflicted on our bodies throughout our lives.

◼ DAMAGED CARTILAGE IS UNABLE TO HEAL

Joint cartilage is also referred to as *hyaline cartilage* because its pearly white appearance is similar to frosted glass (in Greek, *hyalos* means "glass"). Because of its elastic nature, joint cartilage may compress down to as much as 40% of its height during weight bearing and then quickly recover its shape when the stress is removed. Because cartilage deforms so readily, it cannot contain any blood vessels or nerves because they would not tolerate being crunched with each step. Unfortunately, cartilage cannot heal once it becomes damaged because it lacks a direct blood supply. The inability of cartilage to regenerate means that anything that mars its polished surface will eventually cause osteoarthritis.

◼ OIL FOR THE TIN MAN

Wear and tear is caused by friction, which is not always a bad thing. Constant friction is needed in automobile brakes so that you can stop your car. However, a low level of friction is good in some instances—for example, the internal mechanism of a watch. Lubrication cuts down on friction, and the natural lubricant of the synovial joint reduces friction so well that it can be compared to two pieces of wet ice rubbing against each other. Synovial fluid is made up primarily of *hyaluronic acid*, which is a gel-like liquid similar to mucus. Its primary purpose is to reduce friction and wear and tear on cartilage. Synovial fluid is normally a viscous, pale yellow, clear fluid resembling raw egg white (the *-ovial* in synovial comes from the Latin *ovum*, meaning egg). The lubrication ability of the synovial joint is about ten times superior to the best mechanical lubrication systems known to modern engineering!

A thin layer of synovial fluid known as *boundary lubrication* separates the thigh and shinbones at the knee. This layer of synovial fluid slides on the boundaries of the bone ends and prevents the two ends of cartilage from touching during slow movements. When weight bearing forces increase during fast movements, the cartilage ends minimally contact each other, but they are prevented from grinding against each other by means of a mechanism which may be compared to hydroplaning. In this instance, the synovial fluid acts in a manner similar to rainwater on wet asphalt, wherein the rainwater will prevent the tire and road from contacting each other. This can cause an automobile to hydroplane.

AGING CARTILAGE

The cartilage of young, healthy people is about 85% water, whereas the cartilage of older people contains as little as 60%. Water is an incompressible fluid that is essential to the stress- absorbing role of articular cartilage. Articular cartilage loves water, which is another way of saying it is *hydrophilic*. This is due to the presence of certain large molecules that have the unique ability to attract water into cartilage. These molecules are known as *chondroitin sulfate* and *keratin sulfate*. Chondroitin sulfate is more common in young people and is the better attractor

of water, which allows cartilage to be a better cushion. The problem is that as you grow older, keratin sulfate replaces chondroitin sulfate, leaving the cartilage worse off and less capable of acting as a cushion. This downhill process begins in the 30s. Because of this, the joint cartilage of older people is more susceptible to wearing down.

IT STARTS WITH CARTILAGE WEAR

The type of damage that occurs to joint cartilage during the development of osteoarthritis follows a sequence of progressive destruction of the joint. Early on, the hyaline cartilage gets shredded and its surface becomes frayed and cracked. The small fragments of cartilage get swept inside the joint during joint motion and irritate the synovial lining of the joint, causing the lining to become inflamed. Over time, the cartilage softens and develops fissures and pits, similar to a shaggy carpet. Soon, the normally blue-white, smooth, and glistening appearance of healthy cartilage becomes yellow, dull, and grainy looking. Eventually, all of the cartilage on the two ends of bone is worn away, causing the bones to rub painfully against each other. The joint compensates for thinning cartilage by having the bone along either side of the cartilage growth thicker. It is as if the bone attempts to limit motion and reduce friction by growing sharp spurs of bone along the sides of the joint. This helps to stabilize the joint and more broadly distribute the loading forces. The joint is now shorter than it was, and the ligaments surrounding it are placed on slack so that they now offer less protection to the joint. In response to pain, the muscles around the joint may go into spasm and may fatigue over time. This high level of muscle contraction is an attempt to splint the painful area, but it also results in diminished motion. If this situation continues, the joint will continue to be held tightly. Over time, the joint may lose its ability to move freely and its natural shape due to contracture.

RISK FACTORS

Why do some joints wear out more readily than others? Why is it that women with healthy, strong bones that are not susceptible to the brittleness of osteoporosis are at greater risk for developing osteoarthritis? No one really knows the answer to these questions. However, some people are clearly more likely to develop osteoarthritis because of *risk factors*, which may include:

- **AGE:** Osteoarthritis more frequently occurs in males before the age of 45, whereas after age 55, it more commonly occurs in females. Osteoarthritis is not exclusively a disease of the elderly, and Baby Boomers are at risk for this chronic condition.

- **GENDER:** Both men and woman are affected by osteoarthritis, but where in the body the disease strikes is different for each sex. Woman are more likely to have osteoarthritis of the fingers, wrists, hands, and knees, while men more often suffer from wear and tear of the spine, hips, and knees. Osteoarthritis of the knee is twice as common in women as in men and females are more likely to have both knees affected, although this may be related to wearing high-heeled shoes. The gender differences may be related to the traditionally different lifestyles of men and women, although a dominant sex-influenced gene is thought to be responsible for arthritic finger nodes in females.

- **OBESITY:** Six out of ten Americans are overweight; of these, one in four is obese. Obesity is defined as being 20% over the ideal weight.

Being overweight is certainly a risk factor in the wear and tear of weight-bearing joints because of the increased loading and consequent pressure on the joints. About 4 to 8 times your body weight presses on your knees when jumping or climbing stairs. Every extra pound of fat increases the pressure to the hips and knees by 4 to 8 pounds. This factor may affect women more than it does men.

- **ETHNICITY:** Caucasians have a much greater risk than Asians in developing osteoarthritis of the hip, although Asians have a higher risk of wear and tear of the knee than Caucasians. Both Caucasians and Asians have an equal risk of developing osteoarthritis of the spine. Black women are twice as likely as Caucasian women to have osteoarthritis of the knees.

- **OCCUPATION:** Heavy physical labor has been correlated to wear and tear at the knee joint in farmers, firefighters, and construction workers. Miners, who are predominantly male and whose occupations involve heavy lifting, typically get osteoarthritis of the hips and knees much more so than those in white-collar occupations. Miners and dockworkers often develop osteoarthritis in their knees, while riveters report the condition in their elbows. Women employed in weaving jobs often develop osteoarthritis in the favored hand. Computer work can also lead to the development of osteoarthritis of the hand, wrist, and shoulder joints.

- **SPORTS:** Gymnastics, figure skating, and diving often involve movements such as doing a split with one leg straight out in front and the other leg pointing backward. These positions place extreme stresses on the body joints and ligaments, causing premature osteoarthritis as early as the late 20s. Dorothy Hamill, the American figure skater and winner of the figure skating Gold

Medal in the 1976 Winter Olympics, is a victim of osteoarthritis. For similar reasons, ballet dancers are often stricken by osteoarthritis in their hips, ankles, and feet. Despite their excellent flexibility, muscle strength, and cardiovascular conditioning, ballet dancers are quite vulnerable to developing osteoarthritis due to the constant and unnatural distribution of weight, and the stress on impact of landing with their full weight on one foot. Low-impact aerobics are preferable to high-impact aerobics for this reason. Similarly, violent sports such as American football exert excessive force through the joints. Joe Namath, the great New York quarterback, had an osteoarthritic condition of the knee that resulted from the repeated injuries he suffered while playing football.

- **HYPERMOBILITY:** People who are hypermobile, such as kids who show off to friends by bending their thumbs back to touch their forearms, or who bend their ankles around their necks, can also push their joints beyond the limits for which they were intended, causing injury.

- **GENETICS:** There appears to be a greater coincidence of arthritis between parents and children or between siblings, than between husbands and wives. This suggests that osteoarthritis might be inherited.

- **CLIMATE:** Eskimos and other people who live in cold environments have less osteoarthritis than people who live in warm climates.

- **MARITAL STATUS:** Bachelors are twice as likely to have arthritis of the knee as married men.

- **MUSCLE WEAKNESS:** Normal muscles contract and, thus, they help absorb the injurious forces that pass through a joint. Someone with weak-ened or thinning muscles will have less muscle tissue to bear the brunt of joint force, causing the joint cartilage to absorb more pressure and impact.

- **LACK OF NORMAL MOTION:** Sometimes, a mildly arthritic hip or knee that never had any symptoms will become moderately or severely osteoarthritic after being in a cast for several weeks. This is because joint cartilage needs motion in order to stay healthy and nourished. Lack of normal motion may unmask a barely noticeable osteoarthritis and turn it into a painful problem.

- **JOINT CONTRACTURE:** When the muscles and other soft tissues around a joint become shortened so that the joint cannot move normally, it causes forces to pass through the joint in an abnormal way. This results in injury to the joint cartilage.

- **TRAUMA:** Trauma to a joint might occur from an external source such as being hit by car or baseball bat, or undergoing surgery. An internal source of trauma might be bleeding within the joint, a meniscus, or other loose body marring the articular surface, or from joint infection. Blood within a joint has the effect of rapidly destroying the smooth cartilage that makes up the joint surface.

- **ANATOMIC MALALIGNMENT:** The hip and knee are designed to absorb and transmit weight in such a way that they avoid injury. However, some people may have a deformity of a joint, thigh, or shinbone, such as bow legs or knock knees, or have one leg longer than the other. These anatomic variations cause the weight of the body to be distributed unevenly on the hips and knees, and may result in premature wear and tear of these joints. Also, if the foot is too flat or has an excessively high arch, forces will be unevenly distributed at the knee and hips joints, predisposing the person toward osteoarthritis.

TYPES OF OSTEOARTHRITIS

There are two types of osteoarthritis: primary and secondary. *Primary osteoarthritis*, which is also known as *idiopathic arthritis*, occurs for no reason in particular and usually shows up in middle age or later. It most commonly involves women during their fifth and sixth decades and affects multiple joints. It usually only affects one hip joint when it affects men. This form of arthritis seems to be an accelerated aging of cartilage, similar to premature graying of the hair.

Secondary osteoarthritis occurs because of an underlying insult or injury to cartilage such as joint infection, trauma from an injury or surgery, bleeding into a joint from an injury or in someone with hemophilia (whose blood has living cells that will literally eat away at a joint surface), a loose meniscus or bone flake, or from uneven weight-bearing because one leg is bowed or shortened. Accumulated microtrauma from occupational stress such as that generated by the vibrations of a pneumatic drill are particularly damaging to joints.

WHERE DOES OSTEOARTHRITIS USUALLY DEVELOP?

Osteoarthritis is not a systemic disease, which means that it does not spread throughout the entire body. Rather, it concentrates in one or several joints. Unlike rheumatoid arthritis, osteoarthritis does not affect symmetrical parts of the body. Osteoarthritis affects the hips, knees, spine, hands, and fingers. Although the ankles bear the same heavy loads as the hips and knees, for some reason, osteoarthritis does not usually happen in the ankles in the general population, with the exception of ballet dancers. Osteoarthritis is likely to develop in:

- The main weight-bearing joints are those that are nearest the ground: the hips and knees. These joints are the most susceptible to arthritis because they absorb the downward forces from the weight of the body and the equal, opposite forces moving up the body from the ground (Newton's Third Law). Osteoarthritis of the hips and knees occurs more frequently in men and may be due to the heavy manual labor performed more often by men. Wear and tear of the hip joints is very common in the United States, but the risk is lower in Asia and some Middle Eastern countries.

- Each level of the spine can become affected by osteoarthritis. In addition to slow deterioration of the discs, the bony spurs that grow out of the spine may compress on a spinal nerve, causing pain and disability.

- Osteoarthritis of the hand most commonly occurs in females during their fourth decade of life, typically at the base of the thumb. Often, knobby spurs of cartilage and bone develop in the joints of the fingers, causing pain, tenderness, and stiffness. They are known as *Bouchard nodes* when they occur in the middle finger joints and *Heberden's nodes* when they occur at the ends of the finger. Once they grow to full size, they stop hurting, although they give the fingers a gnarled appearance. These nodes occur ten times more commonly in woman than in men and tend to run in families. It is not true that just because you have nodal osteoarthritis of the fingers in middle age that you will experience worsened arthritis during your 60s; there is no correlation between the two.

■ Signs and Symptoms

The vast majority of people develop arthritis as they get older, but only about a fourth get worse in terms of increased pain, deformity, and decreased function. Osteoarthritis can be deceptive because it does not make you feel sick with a fever. People with osteoarthritis often feel good one day and miserable the next. It may go into remission with little or no symptoms for weeks at a time. Some people with osteoarthritis experience muscle weakness, tenderness to the touch, and joint *crepitus*, a condition in which a squeaking, creaking, or grating sound is heard during motion. People with osteoarthritis of the leg may limp from pain. People with many of these symptoms also experience a loss of function, meaning that they can no longer perform simple activities like opening a jar or putting on their socks. There are several particularly common signs and symptoms that include:

■ **Pain:** This is often the earliest symptom of arthritis. It may be sharp when you move the affected joint, particularly if you have been inactive for a while and overdo it. Most often the pain is a constant, dull, nagging, ache that worsens with activity, especially early on. Sometimes the pain from arthritis of the hip is felt at the knee. This is known as *referred pain*. Arthritis of the knee most commonly develops at the inner side of the knee, and there will be pain when the front of the leg, just below the kneecap on the inner side of the knee, is pressed. Each individual has a different threshold and tolerance for pain, which is often affected by emotional and physical factors. The ache may be present at nighttime and may disrupt sleep, causing the person with arthritis to wake up feeling tired.

■ **Stiffness:** It is common for the joints to be stiff, especially after a night's sleep or resting for some time. This stiffness often goes away in the morning after moving around, especially after a nice, hot shower.

■ **Diminished Motion:** The joint will have a diminished ability to move through the normal available range of motion, particularly fully bending or straightening.

■ **Inflammation:** The synovial membrane may become inflamed because of osteoarthritis, secondary to the destruction of cartilage. This inflammation will heighten the sense of pain and result in swelling and warmth of the joint.

■ Your Own Internal Barometer

Believe it or not, people with osteoarthritis can sometimes predict the weather based on how their joints feel. When rain and snowstorms approach, the humidity rises and the barometric pressure drops, causing an increase in the pain in arthritic joints; this is how people with arthritis know inclement weather is on the way. On the other hand, low humidity and higher air pressure generally signal better weather, and the person with arthritis can often tell when a storm is passing. Why is this so?

Subchondral bone is the bone beneath the cartilage. Changes occur in the subchondral bone when all the cartilage has worn away. Normally, bone is full of fluid that ebbs and flows within the bone through minute channels known as *canniculi*. Osteoarthritic changes in bone cause many of these fluid-filled channels to become closed off from each other. A chamber filled with fluid is basically a barometer because the fluid within the chamber will expand and contract with changes in air pressure. The rapid expansion or contraction of fluid within bone causes pain to be felt. People with osteoarthritis will often complain of pain on the day before the storm because changes in barometric pressure usually happen the day before a storm. The pain in their bones lets them know a storm is coming. Arthritic pain also decreases as the temperature rises, which is why many sufferers of arthritis move to climatically hot, dry areas such as Arizona.

DIAGNOSES OF OSTEOARTHRITIS

Osteoarthritis may be visible on x-rays because there is a loss of the normal space between bones, causing the joint space to appear narrowed, but cartilage itself will not show up on x-ray because it does not have any calcium salts. However, a diagnosis of osteoarthritis is made by the presence of signs and symptoms. Laboratory tests for osteoarthritis are not useful except to rule out other conditions. A diagnosis of osteoarthritis based only on x-rays may be inaccurate because two-thirds of all people may appear to have joint wear and tear on their x-rays, even though there may be no pain or stiffness. Other conditions can masquerade as osteoarthritis. Some of these include rheumatoid arthritis, gout, lupus, gout, psoriatic arthritis, ankylosing spondylitis, and scleroderma. Diagnosis is made by a rheumatologist.

PREVENTION AND TREATMENT

There is no sure way to prevent osteoarthritis or slow its progression, but some changes in lifestyle may reduce or delay symptoms:

- **WEIGHT LOSS:** Excessive body weight places excessive stress on the weight bearing joints and makes arthritis much worse. One study showed that loss of only 10 to 15 pounds by women of medium height decreased their risk of developing osteoarthritis of the knee by one-half. A diet for weight control should go hand in hand with an exercise program, so that calorie intake is limited at the same time that excess weight (especially around the chest, thighs, and waist) is slowly burned off. It is important to eat a varied diet that emphasizes low-fat, high-fiber foods. If osteoarthritis has affected one knee or one hip, losing weight will diminish the likelihood of getting it in the other hip or knee. Most of all do not over do it. For example, arthritis may develop in the thumb joints because of excessive videogame playing. Moderation is *always* the maxim.

- **REST:** While it is important to keep arthritic joints moving, excessive activity will exacerbate pain and inflammation. The proper amount of activity depends on the severity of symptoms at any given time. More activity and less rest are needed during times when active inflammation eases up, and the opposite is true during flare-ups. It is very important for those with arthritis to get enough sleep, even if it means taking short, daytime naps.

- **EXERCISE:** The idea behind exercise in the treatment of osteoarthritis is that strengthening the muscle around a joint in osteoarthritic stress can help interrupt the cycle of degeneration because the bulk of the muscle will help absorb the forces delivered through the joint. Applicable exercises include range of motion, strengthening, and stretching. These activities increase stamina, help maintain a positive self-image, and enable the person with arthritis to hold onto their sense of control and accomplishment. Moderate weight-bearing exercises help protect joints by strengthening the supporting muscles and tendons surrounding a joint. Plan on exercising twice a day for the rest of your life. It is important to start at a comfortable level and gradually increase the amount of exercise. Choose a time and place for your daily workout, and stick to it. Exercise during that part of the day when you have the least pain, stiffness, and fatigue.

- **RANGE OF MOTION EXERCISES:** Normally, joints require motion to stay healthy. Range of motion (ROM) refers to the normal ability to move a joint in all directions allowed. Daily activities of living such as dressing, cleaning, lifting, bathing, and cooking exercise a joint through its full range of motion. Aside from these activities, it is important to move your joints through their full range of motion every day in order to reduce stiffness and maintain flexibility. Range of motion exercises should even be performed on bad days when joints are very painful and swollen, although at such times exercise should be done more slowly and gently. Do not forgo your range of motion exercises just because you are having a flare-up. If necessary, only do part of your exercise routine.

- **STRENGTHENING:** Muscle strength is especially important in the prevention and treatment of arthritis because strong muscles support and protect the joint more efficiently and possibly decrease joint pain. *Isometric strengthening*, in which you tighten your muscles without moving the joint, is best reserved for those times when there is a flare-up because this type of exercise stresses the joint the least. *Isotonic exercises* involve contracting your muscles by moving the joint. Follow the guidelines of a physical therapist in the use of this type of exercise. Strengthening the legs by using a stationary bicycle is a good idea because it allows muscle strengthening without the stress of weight bearing that accompanies running, jogging, or aerobics. A recumbent bicycle takes the pressure off sensitive joints such as the hips and knees by allowing exercising in the recumbent position. Raise the seat in order to

decrease the resistance and reduce stress to the knee joint. Also, remember to avoid sudden changes in the intensity of exercise.

- **STRETCHING:** It is important to stretch muscles on either side of a joint in order to maintain flexibility and optimal motion of that joint. Follow the guidelines of a physical therapist in stretching exercises.

- **JOINT PROTECTION:** A variety of assistive devices such as a cane or splints may aid in protecting a joint. Every 5 pounds of pressure that is applied to a cane relieves the supporting leg of 25 pounds. Hold the cane in the hand opposite the hip or knee that is painful in order for it to be the most effective. Splinting a joint with an orthoses helps rest the joint and holds it in an ideal position, which will help keep the muscles and ligaments around it limber. Using a cane or walker is helpful in relieving pain in the joints of the leg during walking. The correct length for a walker or cane is best determined by a physical therapist. There are many assistive devices for opening car and kitchen doors, and cans and bottles. Using a viscoelastic arch support or wearing shoes with an air pocket in the heel may help diminish stress to the joints of the leg and spine.

- **ESTROGEN:** Studies show that hormone replacement therapy that includes estrogen significantly reduces the risk of osteoarthritis in post-menopausal women.

- **NUTRITIONAL SUPPLEMENTS:** *Chondroitin sulfate* and *glucosamine* are two nutritional supplements that are naturally used by the body to build cartilage. Some believe that synthetic versions may help slow, stop, or even reverse osteoarthritis. While there has been circumstantial evidence of pain relief, there is only preliminary evidence that these oral supplements can help maintain existing cartilage and stimulate new cartilage to grow. S-adenosyl-methionine (SAMe) has been used for many years in Europe to manage arthritis and depression. It is available as a nonprescription supplement in the United States. SAMe may relieve osteoarthritic pain in a manner similar to non-steroidal anti-inflammatory drugs, but with fewer side effects. However, there is no evidence that it helps regenerate cartilage. Cerasomal-cis-9-cetylmyristoleate and cetyl myristoleate (brand names: CMO®, CM Pure®, CMPlus®, CM Protocol®, and Arthro-Balance®) are two popular animal substances touted as cures for arthritis without the backing of scientific studies. Vitamins A, E, and C, and soybean and avocado oils are currently being studied as possible treatments for arthritis. Some research suggests that omega-3 fatty acids from coldwater fish such as salmon, mackerel, and herring may offer modest, temporary relief from inflammation.

- **ELIMINATION DIETS:** According to the Arthritis Foundation, food sensitivities may play a role in arthritis. Elimination diets require that people with arthritis stop eating the foods that may irritate the joints. The problem is that scientists cannot agree on exactly which foods cause problems or whether all people with arthritis are food sensitive. Consult your doctor before altering your diet.

▉ ARTHRITIS MANAGEMENT

Although the search continues, there is no known cure for arthritis. Arthritis can lead to a vicious cycle of pain, depression, and stress. However, remember that is possible to have arthritis and still have a life. Many of the prevention strategies may also be used in the management of osteoarthritis. No single approach works for everyone, and so an eclectic approach is recommended.

- **ANALGESICS:** For those osteoarthritis sufferers who do not experience inflammation, analgesics are often all that is needed to control their symptoms. Analgesics containing acetaminophen, commonly known as Tylenol® or Panadol®, do not have anti-inflammatory properties, although these nonprescription painkillers are the first line of defense for mild pain, especially because they may relieve discomfort without harming the digestive tract. Early-stage osteoarthritis has a minor inflammatory component and so these nonprescription medications are effective because of their pain-fighting properties. Acetaminophen is less likely to irritate the stomach than non-steroidal anti-inflammatory medications. However, acetaminophen tends to lose its effectiveness with continued usage. *Capsaicin cream* is a nonprescription drug derived from the pepper plant, which provides pain relief by inhibiting pain transmission.

- **NON-STEROIDAL ANTI-INFLAMMATORY DRUGS (NSAIDs):** This classification of drugs includes: aspirin and ibuprofen (Motrin®, Advil®, and Nuprin®), indomethacin (Indocin®), naproxen (Naprosyn®), naporxen sodium (Aleve®), and piroxicam (Feldene®), and others. These drugs were first introduced in the early part of the twentieth century and have an analgesic effect in reducing pain. However, their main emphasis is on reducing inflammation. Aspirin was first discovered by Bayer in 1889, and soon after became available without a prescription. One good thing about aspirin, including Bayer's Aspirin®, Excedrin®, and Anacin®, is that you do not become resistant to it. It will work just as well in 10 years as it does the first time. Aspirin should never be taken with either alcohol or vitamin C because this combination may seriously irritate the digestive tract. About 2 to 4 percent of all people who take high doses of NSAIDs develop ulcers or other digestive tract problems, which is a major drawback. To prevent irritation of the stomach lining and even internal bleeding, aspirin (also known as salicylic acid) may be taken with meals. Alternately, aspirin may be enteric-coated, meaning that it is covered with a substance that dissolves so slowly that it prevents stomach irritation. It is best not to take aspirin with milk because milk interferes with its dissolution. Various herbs such as cumin, cinnamon, ginger, dandelion, celery seed, and evening primrose are also believed to have anti-inflammatory properties.

- **Cox-2 Inhibitors:** Drugs such as Celebrex®, Vioxx®, and Mobic® relieve pain without side effects on the stomach lining. They work by inhibiting the enzyme cyclo-oxygenase (*cox*). This enzyme is responsible for the production of prostaglandins, the principal directors of pain and inflammation. These drugs are very helpful because they lower the production of prostaglandins, thereby helping reduce both pain and inflammation. There are two different types of cox enzymes. The cox-1 molecule is found in most of the tissues of the body. It directs the formation of a lining in your stomach that protects against acid damage. In the presence of inflammation, however, different messengers are formed, cox-2 enzymes, which, in large quantities, promote the inflammation and pain of arthritis. The problem with most NSAIDs is that when they inhibit the cox-2 enzymes in order to ease joint symptoms, they also inhibit the cox-1 enzymes, leaving the stomach lining exposed to the possible development of bleeding ulcers. The cox-2 inhibitors relieve pain by targeting only the cox-2 enzymes, leaving the stomach lining uninjured. They offer relief from pain and inflamma-

tion without the downside of gastrointestinal distress. Cox-2 inhibitors are expensive, however, and recent studies have linked their usage to an increase in heart-related problems.

- **Injections:** Corticosteroids are synthetic versions of the hormone cortisone. They are the most potent anti-inflammatory medications available. Steroids may be injected directly into a painful joint that does not respond to other forms of treatment. This is occasionally helpful, but should not be performed more than two to three times because of the potential for damage to the joint. In addition, if the injection is not done very carefully, infection may be introduced into the joint. Oral steroids should not be prescribed for osteoarthritis because of their serious side effects.

- **Hyaluronic Acid:** Hyaluronic acid is a lubricant normally found within the synovial fluid of the healthy knee. This substance is depleted in the osteoarthritic knee. Synvisc® and Hyalgan® are trade names for hyaluronic acid, which is obtained from chicken combs (the fleshy crest over the head of the fowl). These substances may be injected into the mild to moderately osteoarthritic knee in order to function as a substitute for *hyaluronic acid* in those who cannot get relief from pain medication, exercise, or physical therapy. Five or six injections are given at weekly intervals. These injections have the additional advantage of not causing the side effects associated with oral pain medications. These treatments are given as a series of several injections by a rheumatologist or orthopedic surgeon. They may provide relief for up to 6 to 12 months at a time.

- **Cloning:** New advances in the science of cloning involve the removal from a person with arthritis of a few healthy cartilage cells that are then cloned to grow new cartilage in a laboratory. These genetically identical cartilage cells are then surgically introduced into the diseased joint without concern for autoimmune rejection. This form of cartilage replacement appears to work best in people below the age of 40 who have experienced cartilage damage due to sports-related activities.

■ **TETRACYCLINE:** This antibiotic is chemically designed to kill bacteria, but it seems to also slow the erosion of cartilage.

■ **APPLYING COLD:** Cold is best applied during the acute stages of osteoarthritis when the joint painful, tender, and swollen. Cold should not be applied for more than 15 minutes at a time. A good way to apply cold is to place ice in a plastic bag, wrap it in a towel, and apply it to the painful joint. This can also be done using a bag of frozen vegetables from the freezer.

■ **APPLYING HEAT:** It is best to reserve the application of heat for when the osteoarthritic joint is not acutely painful. Heat is best applied as a moist hot pack wrapped in towels and placed around a painful joint. Heat can ease stiffness and spasm. When applying heat, it is important to use enough towels to prevent a burn. A hot paraffin bath is also very helpful in easing the pain of arthritic hands and feet.

■ **ELECTRIC STIMULATION:** Transcutaneous electric nerve stimulation (TENS) directs mild electrical impulses to nerve endings in order to block pain signals to the brain. TENS has been used by people with arthritis with very limited success.

■ **POOL EXERCISES:** Regular, moderate exercise is a key element in keeping the pain of arthritis in check. It is important that you enjoy exercise and not exacerbate the pain. Pool exercises are especially helpful for arthritic joints because they allow movement and minimize the concussive effects of weight bearing. The buoyancy of water cancels the effect of gravity's weight bearing pressure. Swimming in a pool may also help relieve pain because of the comforting, gentle pressure by the water on the body. A water temperature of around 86 degrees Fahrenheit is recommended.

■ **EDUCATION:** Learning to avoid activities and positions that may exacerbate arthritis is very important. For example, avoid deep knee bends. It is essential that people with osteoarthritis of the hip and spine sit on relatively high chairs and elevated toilet seats. An elastic knee brace may be helpful by providing support to the knee during weight bearing activities. In the kitchen, use lightweight pots and pans and electric appliances when possible. Use baking pans with nonstick coating to reduce scrubbing. Sit on a chair with good back and foot support for good posture in the office.

■ **HERBAL REMEDIES AND SUPPLEMENTS:** The National Center of Complementary and Alternative Medicine, an arm of the National Institutes of Health, received $89.1 million dollars in federal funds last year to explore alternative and complementary treatments. This money is to be used to fund studies that will determine the efficacy of these types of treatments. Many human studies from Europe show that internal use of chondroitin sulfate (1,200 mg. per day, divided into two doses), a component of human cartilage derived from the windpipes of cattle, relieves symptoms of osteoarthritis with little or no side effects. There have been reports of diminished pain and stiffness, although relief is slow acting, and it may take up to 2 months to be effective. Glucosamine naturally occurs in the body, and internally ingested supplements made from chitin in the shells of shrimp, crab, and lobster (1,500 mg. taken in two doses per day) are believed to ease pain and stiffness and contribute to cartilage repair. Relief of symptoms has been confirmed by many European studies. It is important not to take large doses of these remedies and always tell your doctor that you are taking them.

WHEN IS SURGERY NECESSARY?

Surgery is the only option available to people with severe osteoarthritis of the hips and knees. In the past, wear and tear would progress to the point of causing depression due to immobility. The avoidance of pain leads to weakness due to lack of activity. *Arthroscopy* is a procedure used in some joints to remove bone fragments and damaged cartilage by means of a tiny camera and instruments that are inserted through small incisions. Joint replacement surgery, which was developed in the 1960s, is known as total joint *arthroplasty*. This procedure has offered hundreds of thousands of people a chance to set the clock back and face their future with a new lease on life. All the major joints of the body, including the hip, shoulder, elbow, knee, and thumb may be replaced, although artificial hips and knees have been the most successful. Each year, doctors in the United States perform about 270,000 knee replacements and 170,000 hip replacements. Orthopedic surgeons are doctors who specialize in bone surgery, and they perform these types of operations. The Chicago Bears' Hall of Fame tight end Mike Ditka has had both hips replaced.

REMEDIES YOU DO NOT NEED

Henry VII's doctor treated Henry's swollen joints by applying baked ox dung wrapped in cabbage leaves. Chronic pain can make people feel desperate enough to believe shamans who claim to have the cure for arthritis. Americans spend as much as $6 billion a year on useless "miracle cures," and about 94% of those with arthritis will try one of these unproven remedies at least once.

Some of these "get better quick" cures can be downright dangerous. For example, some "alternative cures" include radioactive uranium mittens or bracelets, sitting in abandoned uranium mines at 175 times the federally accepted standard for radiation levels for up to several hours a day, self-administered steroids and injections of bee, ant, or snake venom, and injections of turtle blood. Some equally bizarre but less dangerous "treatments" include standing naked under the full moon, WD-40 lubricant sprayed on joints, seaweed or copper bracelets, eating shark or baby chick cartilage or New Zealand green-lipped mussels, lying in vibrating beds or sitting in vibrating chairs, and covering the body with cow manure twice per day. Mega doses of fat-soluble vitamins like vitamin A can accumulate in the body to toxic levels. Joint manipulation in the treatment of osteoarthritis is practiced by some chiropractors without any evidence that manipulation can cure arthritis, although some people may anecdotally report circumstantial evidence of pain relief. Direct manipulation of the osteoarthritic joint may relax the tissues surround the joints, thereby improving their mobility and circulation.

Many of these or other bogus treatments may offer temporary relief simply because you think they will. This is called the *placebo effect*, and it shows how truly powerful the mind is when it comes to hoping for a cure. As many as 40% of those who try a new treatment will experience a reduction of pain due to the placebo effect. In fact, many of the so-called "arthritis clinics" are often located in beautiful settings and warm climates located far away from the stress of everyday life. Just being in this kind of environment would probably help most people feel better, regardless of what was troubling them. The moral of all this is: Do not fall for the dubious promises and smooth talk of testimonial advertising that promises "secret" cures. If in doubt, research these so-called cures by contacting the National Arthritis Foundation to find out how legitimate they really are before wasting your precious time and resources.

34 Osteoporosis

OSTEOPOROSIS DEFINED

OSTEOPOROSIS is a painless condition in which the bones become thinner and more porous as calcium is progressively lost; the word "osteoporosis" means "porous bone." It occurs so insidiously that it is often not noticed. About 7 to 8 million people in the United States have some degree of osteoporosis and approximately 20 million people are at high risk because of low bone density. This slow process of bone thinning and weakening becomes painful when the bone weakens to the point of breaking from its own weight. This is known as a bone fracture. More than 1.5 million fractures occur in mostly older American women each year, usually in the spine, hip, and wrist. Osteoporosis is second only to osteoarthritis as the most common skeletal disorder, and the costs are staggering. Osteoporosis-related problems cost an estimated $14 billion each year. As many as one in every three women older than 65 years old can expect to break a bone due to osteoporosis. Osteoporosis is preventable to some extent, essentially through education, diet, and exercise.

ELEMENTS OF BONE

Bone carries the body and it is as strong as steel-reinforced concrete. The thighbone, for example, is so strong that it is able to bear the weight of a compact car. The strength of bone is based upon the idea that a tube is stronger than a rod. Bone is made of protein and minerals, making it similar to other two-phase materials such as steel-reinforced concrete, bamboo, or fiberglass. The internal structure of bone is made of a tough protein fiber known as collagen, which is organized like a scaffold for strength.

The scaffolding within bone is arranged as a lattice of flat crystals organized like cross-braced struts. From an engineering point of view, this organization endows bone with maximal strength using a minimum of material. It allows bone to withstand compressive forces as intense as 30,000 pounds per square inch!

Within this latticework are salts including calcium, magnesium, phosphorus, and other minerals, which form like a pearl within an oyster and make bone as hard as rock. Bone is far from being just an inert framework; it is a dynamic living tissue that is constantly being remodeled by specialized bone cells called *osteoblasts* and *osteoclasts*. Osteoblasts create bone and osteoclasts absorb bone. Together they work to remodel bone.

These specialized bone cells play a tug-of-war with calcium in the body, resulting in constant bone remodeling. This continuous remodeling causes us to lose calcium each day through urination. To offset this constant calcium drain, sufficient dietary intake of calcium must occur daily for us to stay healthy. This daily loss and replenishment of calcium causes us to have completely replaced all of the calcium in our bodies by age 25. This cycle of replenishment continues throughout our lives, once every 7 years.

■ HORMONES - THE CONTROL CENTER

The hormone glands in the neck known as the thyroid and parathyroid glands control bone growth and loss in healthy bone. Bones basically hoard calcium, and like bankers who carefully control currency deposits and withdrawals, they selectively release mineral crystals into the bloodstream according to the amount needed by the body. Minerals such as calcium are needed for more than simply hardening bones. They are also needed for the heart and other muscles to contract, for blood to clot, and for nerves to transmit impulses. Too much calcium can cause kidney stones or blood poisoning, and too little calcium might cause the heart and nerves to stop working! Therefore, calcium must be very carefully released into circulation. Only 1/40th of an ounce of calcium should be in the blood at any given time in order to maintain this delicate balance. In this way, calcium is either given out or taken back according to the body's changing needs.

■ THE FORCES EXERTED ON BONES

Astronauts on the Gemini and Apollo space missions suffered bone loss while floating around weightless in space, and when they came back to Earth their relatively young bones were thin and brittle similar to people who have osteoporosis or who have been sick in bed for a long time. Bones need to experience gravity in order to be healthy. This is why a broken leg needs to have weight placed on it in order to fully heal. Simply keeping it in a cast will not completely heal a bone fracture. Bearing the weight of one's own body is essential in preserving healthy bones. Gravity is a force, and bones are kept healthy by having force applied to them. They will become wider and stronger when used—for example, professional tennis players may have forearm bones in their racquet arm that are wider and stronger than their other hand. This is known as Wolff's law. In the same way, cavalrymen will develop larger and occasionally altogether new bones in the buttocks and thighs as a result of heavy horse riding.

■ IT'S DOWNHILL AFTER AGE THIRTY-FIVE

Normally, minerals such as calcium constantly move in and out of the bones. There is also continual remodeling throughout a lifelong process of bone deposition and resorption. In the healthy child and young adult, bone growth is greater than bone loss until age 35, at which time the skeleton reaches its peak mass because deposition (an increase in bone) dominates resorption (diminishment) of bone. Bones are dense and strong enough to bear pressure of up to 24,000 pounds per square inch during their peak strength and size! Unfortunately, after the middle 30s, this process reverses itself and bone loss progressively outpaces bone growth. Men and women over the age of 35 lose about 1 to 3 percent of their bone mass each year. This is because our body still needs the same amount of calcium released into the bloodstream for essential life functions, and it draws upon the calcium reserves within the bones, at the cost of weakening the skeleton. This is a great price to pay.

Calcium loss is the precursor of osteoporosis. It occurs when there is more bone loss than resorption. There are several reasons for why we lose calcium as we get older. We absorb it less efficiently from the food passing through our gut as we get older, which results in calcium deficiency. Osteoporosis also affects men. The male hormone testosterone is the equivalent of estrogen in females, and because the levels of this hormone are lessened with aging, the bones become weaker and more porous. However, calcium loss usually affects woman more than men because males start out with more overall bone mass than females, due to having larger and heavier skeletons. As a result, men are less likely to get broken bones secondary to osteoporosis. Women also lose calcium if they have had children. This is because they actually build the baby's skeleton from the calcium within their own bodies. They may lose as much as 300 to 400 mg of calcium per day if they breastfeed, leading to a serious condition known as osteomalacia in which the bones becomes so leached of calcium that they actually turn soft. (A high occurrence of osteomalacia occurs in Bedouin Arab women who nurse their children longer than in other countries. This problem is also compounded by a lack of vitamin D, which is caused by the wearing of modest clothing that does not allow any more than their eyes to be exposed to sunlight.) The ovaries shut down at menopause, causing the mineral drain to accelerate, dramatically hastening the process of osteoporosis. Having fragile bones means that a bump or fall that once resulted in a mere a bruise now causes bones to easily break.

As many as one in every four women over the age of 65 years may develop a broken bone due to osteoporosis. The bones that break most often are the vertebrae in the spine, a wrist, a rib, or the neck of the thighbone in the hip. Bone can tolerate compression and tensile forces rather well, but it is vulnerable to breaking from torsion forces in which opposite rotating forces are applied. This is especially so in bone made brittle by osteoporosis, which can become as fragile as fine china. Hips may break from a blow following a fall, but they often break from torsion force. This can occur when suddenly twisting instead of turning in a circle, so that the bone breaks before the person falls and hits the ground! The annual number of hip fractures is projected to rise by more than 500,000 per year by the year 2030 because of the nation's aging population. Wrists often break when attempting to break a forward fall, because people react by spreading out

their hands to catch themselves. Interestingly, women who have broken their wrists during middle life are more likely to break their hips in later years.

The spinal vertebrae often break because suddenly bending over or lifting a heavy object can cause a painful crush fracture. This can even happen from something as trivial as sneezing violently or turning around in bed at night in a susceptible person. Such fractures cause loss of height, especially when they happen over and over. Shrinking from these spontaneous vertebral fractures is often accompanied by a protruding hump or gibbous at the site of the collapsed vertebra. The posture takes on a hunched over appearance when this involves multiple spinal vertebrae.

■ RISK FACTORS

There are factors that predispose some people to developing osteoporosis. Interestingly, although being obese increases your risk for osteoarthritis, it is also a protective factor against osteoporosis. Advanced age, loss of estrogen, and immobility are all high risk factors for many people because they result in low bone-mineral density (BMD). Other risk factors that contribute to BMD include menopause, being underweight, lactose intolerance, living a sedentary lifestyle, and having lots of kids or a small body frame, and breastfeeding. Estrogen is a magical hormone, and it acts to ward off brittle bone disease in women. However, this benefit may be lost in females who cease menstruating before age 45 because of premature ovarian failure, undergo ovary removal or hysterectomy, experience scant or infrequent periods, have three to six missed menstrual cycles, long menstrual cycles, or enter menopause because of excessive athletic activity. Older men also develop osteoporosis and should take preventative measures such as getting regular exercise and ensuring that their diets include an adequate supply of calcium and vitamin D, which is necessary for the proper absorption of calcium. The Caucasian and Asian races are thought to be particularly vulnerable to developing osteoporosis, as are people who have freckles or blond or red hair. People of African descent are less likely than other ethnicities to develop osteoporosis. A diet poor in calcium and vitamins D and C will also result in weakened bones. This is especially so in older people whose upper digestive tract becomes less efficient in absorbing calcium and vitamin D. Some people have an impaired ability to absorb calcium from food because they have had part of their stomach or bowel removed. The most common cause of osteoporosis in young men is alcoholism because alcohol depresses bone growth and alcoholics typically have poor nutrition. Anorexia nervosa is a psychiatric condition common in adolescent girls who refuse to eat because of their distorted body image. This illness can become very serious, even leading to death from starvation. Obviously, it results in poor nutrition and calcium-poor bones. Smoking breaks down estrogen in the body, leading to bone loss in females. Caffeine increases both urinary and intestinal loss of calcium. A diet high in sodium increases urinary loss of calcium. Long-term use of steroid medications such as prednisone, which is used for asthma or rheumatoid arthritis, also causes calcium to leach out of the bones. A diet that is high in fat or salt increases the risk for osteoporosis. Taking medications such as thyroid medications, anticoagulants, and antacids containing aluminum (Mylanta® and Maalox®) have a negative effect on bone. Be careful about drinking too many carbonated drinks if you have a family history of osteoporosis. The phosphorus in carbonated beverages may more than double your risk of osteoporosis because it leaches the calcium out of the bones.

YOU ARE WHAT YOU EAT

Simply saying that osteoporosis stems from a deficiency of calcium is being oversimplistic. Osteoporosis is common in Western, industrialized countries and stems from a lifetime of poor dietary and exercise habits that prevent the buildup of sufficient bone mass. Eating the right food is one of the easiest and most effective ways to help prevent osteoporosis, and the best time to start good eating habits is in childhood when adequate dietary intake of calcium will make sure that bones get off to a good, strong start in life.

THE COUCH POTATO

In the United States, where the automobile is such an important part of the American dream and life can be so fast-paced, people would rather drive down the block or around the corner than take the time and trouble to walk. The human body was not designed for this unnatural lack of exercise, although driving may be useful in saving time for our other pursuits. A typical white-collar employee has their dinner after a long day at the office and then turns into a couch potato in front of the television for an hour or two each night. Lack of proper exercise causes demineralization, a condition in which the minerals that strengthen the bones slowly leak out of the skeletal system, leaving the skeleton weaker and more vulnerable to damage. Watching television would be so much healthier if you disciplined yourself to walk on a treadmill at the same time you watched it. It pays to change your lifestyle from sedentary to active because, in general, the fact that active people live longer is borne out by statistics.

Bone can be quite deceptive. It has the appearance of a hard, inert scaffold that is used to hang your organs, muscles, skin, and latest fashions on. In fact, bone is a living organ that continually under-goes a process called remodeling. Just like someone may try on many different outfits according to the season, occasion, or mood, bone must also model itself according to the amount of pH (acid or alka-line levels) in the bloodstream. A swing in the direc-tion of too much acid can cause serious problems. Bone avoids these problems by being vigilant in keeping the blood-calcium levels in a steady state known as *homeostasis*. Bone maintains the balance of pH by continuously changing the amount of cal-cium released into the blood according to the needs of the body.

The human body is very sensitive to changes in pH and functions best in a more alkaline than acid state. The problem with the standard American diet, which is high in animal protein, processed foods, and baking soda, is that it tends to maintain the body in an acid state. In order to neutralize acid-ity, calcium, magnesium, and potassium must be released by the bones into the bloodstream. In addi-tion, although meat is an important staple of the American diet, it is a poor source of calcium. Over a lifetime, this slow loss of minerals from the bones leaves the skeleton weaker and more vulnerable to fracture.

■ SUGAR, TOBACCO, COFFEE, AND ALCOHOL

Americans seem to crave sugar, and just about every-thing available in the stores has some sugar in it, but too much sugar is especially problematic for bone health. Even some varieties of salt have sugar in them in the form of dextrose that helps boost fla-vor! Sugar causes bone loss in more ways than one. Eating excessive sugar limits calcium absorption and increases urine output of valuable minerals such as calcium, magnesium, chromium, copper, zinc, and sodium. Sugar also increases the produc-tion of hydrochloric acid in the stomach, which

adds to the overall acidic condition of the body. The morale: enjoy sugar in your coffee, but only in mod-eration.

Type II diabetes is a disease of sugar metabolism that is on the rise worldwide at a frightening rate. Diabetes is a group of diseases characterized by high blood sugar levels that result from defects in the body's ability to produce and/or use insulin. Dia-betes is the sixth leading cause of death by disease in the United States. It may lead to severely debili-tating complications such as heart disease, blind-ness, kidney disease, or amputation. At present, an estimated 124 million people have this form of dia-betes, and this number is expected to increase to 221 million by the year 2010. Type II diabetes usu-ally occurs because of insulin resistance, wherein the body fails to use insulin properly. Type II dia-betes is also known as adult onset diabetes or mid-dle age onset diabetes because it usually occurs in adults over 40 who are overweight; it is also known as non-insulin dependent diabetes. In addition, according to the American Diabetes Association, an increasing number of children and teenagers are developing the juvenile form of diabetes. About 60% of the adults in this country are overweight or obese, and nearly 13% of children are also. The cur-rent increase in diabetes in the general population is thought to be strongly linked to sedentary lifestyle and the easy availability of processed foods. The Surgeon General recently warned that diabetes may soon overtake tobacco as the chief cause of pre-ventable death in the United States.

About 90% of all people with diabetes have type II. Excessive sugar in the blood leads to atheroscle-rosis of the arteries in the brain, heart, and limbs, and increases the risk for stroke. According to the American Diabetes Association, type II diabetes can be prevented by changing eating and exercise habits. Lifestyle modifications can reduce the inci-dence of type II diabetes by almost 60% in people who are at high risk for the disease. Modest weight loss of less than 10 pounds combined with a healthy diet and regular, moderate exercise can mean the difference between health and disease.

Americans drink the most coffee. It has been our national drink since it became downright unpatriotic to drink tea after Samuel Adams led raiders to the Boston docks and dumped the tea into the ocean during the Boston Tea Party. Smoking tobacco has also become very popular since American plantations began growing tobacco on a massive scale. Americans also drink more than 500 million gallons of pure alcohol a year, about 2½ gallons per person. Excessive alcohol, caffeine, nicotine, and sugar all rob the bones of minerals, thereby preventing them from being strong and healthy.

■ SIGNS AND SYMPTOMS

Screening for osteoporosis does not need to be part of your regular health checkups unless you are at risk. Younger women do not benefit from screening unless they have hormone disorders, premature menopause, anorexia, ovarian removal, or unexplained bone fractures. Osteoporosis may be detected on x-rays, but bone density testing is more accurate. Bone density tests can be expensive and may need to be repeated. The most common accurate bone density test is a painless test similar to taking an x-ray known as dual energy x-ray absorptiometry (DEXA).

■ YOU ARE WHAT YOU EAT

This old adage rings especially true with regard to keeping bones strong and healthy. It is important to maintain a high dietary intake of calcium: at least 800 mg. every day. Dairy products are the best source. A full 1000 mg are recommended for men and premenopausal woman. As much as 1,500 mg

of calcium, the equivalent of six glasses of vitamin D fortified milk, is recommended for postmenopausal women who are not taking estrogen. It is recommended that women who breastfeed take 2,000 m. per day of calcium.

The key to beating the inescapable fact of gradual calcium loss after age 35 is to increase your intake of calcium and exercise during the childhood and early adulthood when calcium deposition dominates resorption. By achieving peak bone density during the time that the bones are being built (until about age 25), you will be insured against the loss of too much bone after age 35.

Milk and milk products such as yogurt and low-fat cheese are excellent sources of calcium, although 2% milk is recommended because it contains less cholesterol than whole milk, which contains 4% fat. Green leafy vegetables contain considerable calcium, but their high fiber content may cut down on the amount of calcium absorbed. Vegetables high in calcium include broccoli, soybeans, turnip greens, kidney beans, collards, and Chinese cabbage (bok choy). Sunflower and sesame seeds, dried figs, and tofu are good sources of calcium. Eggs and bread are also good sources of calcium. Fruit, while tasty, is not a particularly good source of calcium. Try to get at least 15 minutes of sunlight daily in order to increase the amount of vitamin D in the body. There are only a few food sources of vitamin D, including salmon, mackerel and other fatty fish. Cod liver oil (Ugh!) is also a good source of vitamin D. Be careful not to take excessive vitamin D, however, because too much of it may be toxic. Rely on advice from your doctor.

Meat is generally a poor source of calcium, although using vinegar to marinate meat that contains a bone is a good idea because it helps move the calcium from the bone and into the meat. Hard water that contains a high degree of minerals is preferable for drinking because it contains more calcium than soft water. Try to avoid high-protein diets because protein consumption removes calcium from the body. Try to eat foods containing calcium and foods containing high amounts of fiber at separate times because the fiber may decrease the amount of calcium absorbed. Limiting alcohol intake to no more than two drinks a day is a good idea because alcohol robs bones of minerals and prevents the buildup of strong bone.

The following supplements are believed to be helpful in preventing osteoporosis when taken on a daily basis:

    1,200 to 1,500 mg of magnesium

    1,000 to 2,000 mg of vitamin C

    20 mg of manganese

    25 to 30 mg of zinc

    1 to 2 mg of boron.

■ USE IT OR LOSE IT

Regular exercise, particularly weight-bearing exercise, is essential in combating the effects of calcium loss. Exercise is vital to maintaining healthy bones. It strengthens the muscles, and strong muscles result in strong bones. Sedentary elderly people who exercise with weights can increase their muscle mass by 15 to 20 percent and their muscle strength by almost 22% in just 10 weeks. In order to maintain healthy bones, it is more important to exercise regularly than to exercise vigorously, which makes walking the dog every day is better than an active game of tennis once a week.

Aerobic exercise such as walking at least 30 minutes per day, jogging, playing tennis, or aerobic dancing increases the total amount of calcium in the upper body and upper thighs, the areas most at risk for osteoporotic fractures. Walking or jogging 1 to 2 miles per day and playing tennis or cross-country skiing for at least 30 minutes at a time at least three times per week is ideal. Stair climbing is an excellent exercise for the lower limbs as well as a good way to get an aerobic workout. These exercises can be performed with cuff weights attached to the ankles or wrist, which can further increase bone density. Generally, the longer and more frequently you exercise, the stronger your bones will become.

Although swimming is a great exercise for the heart, lungs, and muscles, it is less than ideal in combating osteoporosis because of the buoyant effect of water. Water exercises should not be considered a substitute for calcium supplementation and medication, but they are of great assistance in stopping and even reversing osteoporosis in some cases.

Activities that twist the back, such as bowling and tennis, are discouraged in people who have already developed significant osteoporosis because of the danger of breaking one of the spinal vertebrae. For the same reason, low-impact aerobics are preferred to high-impact aerobics. People with osteoporosis should regularly perform the type of extension exercises of the back where they bend backward. It is especially important to regularly stretch all of the major muscles, particularly the pectoralis major, which are the muscles under the breasts. These large muscles often become tight, causing increased bending forces on the thoracic spine, which is that part of the mid-spine most vulnerable to osteoporotic compression fracture. This is especially true when bending forward. A stretching program suited to your needs may be learned from a physical therapist.

■ PREVENTION IS THE BEST CURE!

- **BE CONSCIOUS AND CAREFUL:** People who have moderate to severe osteoporosis should play it safe and take commonsense precautions. All telephone lines, throw rugs, and extension cords should be placed away from walkways where they might cause a fall. Non-skid rubber pads should be placed under all area rugs, and linoleum floors should be regularly polished with non-skid floor wax. Using a non-skid shower and bath mat is a must. Beware of wearing only socks or smooth-soled slippers on waxed floors. Women should not wear shoes with high or spiked heels. Nightlights should be used in hallways, bedrooms, and bathrooms. Light switches should be installed at the top and bottom of stairways. If the house has a second floor, sturdy handrails may be installed on both sides of the stairwell and the first and last step may be marked with bright tape. In the bathroom, grab bars should be installed near the toilet and in the shower. In the kitchen, commonly used items should be placed within easy reach in order to avoid excessive bending or stooping. Using a shopping cart to transport groceries is preferable to carrying them, especially if the bag weighs more than 5 to 10 pounds. Using an assistive device such as a cane or walker may be appropriate for people who feel dizzy or lose their balance, even if it is only when trying to get up and go to the bathroom at night. A person at risk for osteoporosis should not use ladders, chairs, or stools to reach high places. Vision and hearing tests should occur regularly because both vision and hearing can affect the ability the sense of balance. It is wise to bend over at the knees or hips rather than bending the back.

- **QUIT SMOKING:** Tobacco not only increases the likelihood of early menopause, but it has been shown to interfere with normal bone metabolism. Tobacco also lowers estrogen production. Some studies suggest that women become more easily addicted to nicotine than men. Therefore, women should consider taking medication that blocks nicotine cravings in order to quit smoking, if necessary.

- **LIMIT INTAKE OF BONE DEPLETING FOODS:** Limit your caffeine intake to no more 2 to 3 cups of coffee per day; avoid beverages that contain phosphorus—this includes all carbonated sodas; limit alcohol intake to no more than 2 ounces per day; and cut back on salt intake.

- **AVOID HARMFUL ANTACIDS:** If you must use antacids, take calcium carbonate, which helps build bone, rather than those containing aluminum salts, which promote bone loss.

SUPPLEMENTS AND MEDICATION

- **CALCIUM SUPPLEMENTS:** There are several types of calcium supplements on the market. Calcium carbonate is often derived from oyster shells. It is the least expensive, readily absorbed form of calcium, but it may cause bloating from gas, nausea, and constipation. This can be avoided by taking it with meals. Calcium gluconate is a better choice, but this form of calcium requires taking numerous tablets daily. Calcium citrate is the most easily absorbed, but it is more expensive than other forms of calcium supplements. Because some organic supplies of calcium have undesirably high levels of lead, a safe source is the Tums® brand antacid tablet, which is pure calcium carbonate. To prevent excessive calcium supplementation from causing joint problems, it is best to take calcium with magnesium. It is usually recommended that calcium and magnesium supplements be taken as two-thirds calcium and one-third magnesium. Supplements are best taken with meals so that they can be better digested. Taking calcium supplements is most effective when taken in sufficient quantities before age 35. Regardless of the drugs taken for osteoporosis, all patients should take calcium, magnesium, and vitamin D daily. Because taking calcium supplements increases the risk of kidney stones, an upper limit of 2,500 mg per day is recommended. No more than 500 to 600 mg should be taken at any given time, but rather the supplements should be taken throughout the day. There is no evidence that calcium intake above the recommended daily dietary allowance is beneficial in preventing or treating osteoporosis.

- **VITAMIN D:** This vitamin is necessary for the absorption of calcium. African, African-American, Asian, and Caucasian people have the capacity to produce vitamin D from sun exposure. Exposing an area of skin the size of your face to sunshine for an hour each day allows the skin to metabolize the necessary amount of vitamin D. (One of the first diseases caused by industrial pollution occurred in the smoke-filled foggy coal mining villages of Wales and England in the nineteenth century when rickets due to vitamin D deficiency secondary to inadequate exposure to sunshine became more prevalent.) Africans, African-Americans and Asians require more time in the sun to produce the same amount of vitamin D as Caucasians. If you live in a northern city such as Boston, New York, or Minneapolis, studies suggest you can sit in the sun for 4 to 5 hours a day between November and March without yours skin producing significant amounts of vitamin D because of the low sunlight intensity in those latitudes. The skin's ability to manufacture vitamin D from sunlight also decreases with age. Unless you spend 15 to 20 minutes per day in bright sunshine, supplementation of vitamin D is essential. Good dietary sources of vitamin D include fortified milk, sardines, herring, salmon, tuna, liver, dairy products, and egg yolks. The recommended amount of vitamin D per day is 400 IU, and as much as 600 IU per day if you are over age 61. No one should take more than 1,200 IU per day because vitamin D is toxic in high doses.

- **ESTROGEN SUPPLEMENTATION:** Whether or not to take prescribed estrogen is an individual choice. Estrogen may be used to relieve the symptoms of menopause regardless of age, although it is less potent in those who begin using it after age 70. The powerful effect of this female sex hormone results in the slowing down of bone loss by as much as 50%. Many of the benefits of ingested calcium are lost because it is flushed out of the system when it is not taken with estrogen. Estrogen replacement therapy is most helpful if taken soon after menopause begins and continued for 15 years or longer. Whether taken by pill, patch, cream, or implant, estrogen has the additional advantage of reducing the risk of developing heart disease and stroke. On the down side, taking estrogen quadruples the risk of uterine cancer and increases the risk of blood clot formation. It may also increase the risk of breast cancer. The increased risk for developing uterine cancer is minimized by also taking progestin for women who still have their uterus. The menstrual period and breast soreness may resume during treatment because estrogen stimulates the uterus. Estrogen treatment may cost between $15 and $30 per month, depending upon the type prescribed.

- **ISOFLAVINS:** Recent studies suggest that plant chemicals known as isoflavins are structurally similar to estrogen and may help prevent osteoporosis. Good sources include soy products such as tofu and the various plant-based supplements available in health food stores.

- **CALCITONIN:** Salmon calcitonin (Miacalcin®) is a synthetic form of thyroid hormone that helps slow bone loss by controlling the breakdown of bone by osteoclasts. Calcitonin is very safe, but it is expensive (about $60 per month) and it requires daily injections. It should be taken with calcium and may work for men who cannot take estrogen. Because of unpleasant side effects such as facial flushing and possibly rash or nausea from self-injection, calcitonin nasal spray is a better tolerated method for taking this prescription medication. The use of parathyroid hormone (PTH) is also being investigated for its promising ability to increase bone mass.

■ **FLUORIDE:** Fluoride treatment for osteoporosis is widely used in Europe, and breakage of the narrow neck of the upper thigh bone is less common in populations drinking fluoridated water. Fluoride actually stimulates new bone growth in cancellous bone, but not cortical bone. Sodium fluoride is helpful because it incorporates fluoride into the mineral crystals of the bones, rendering the crystalline structure more stable. However, fluoride treatment can weaken bone unless calcium and vitamin D supplements are also taken. Fluoride treatment is especially good for treating men with osteoporosis of the spine who cannot take estrogen. An enteric coating will help prevent stomach upset. The monoflurophosphate form of fluoride has fewer side effects than sodium fluoride.

■ **BISPHOSPHONATES:** This class of medications includes alendronate sodium (Fosamax®), which is the only one of this class approved for the treatment of osteoporosis. Other similar medications include risedronate sodium (Actonel®) and raloxifene (Evista®). Actonel® is also used to treat Paget's disease, a bone disorder. California researchers found that osteoporotic women who received this drug experienced a 40% reduction in spinal fractures and a 5% rise in bone density. Daily use of these medications for 3 years increases bone mineral density and reduces bone loss in a manner similar to estrogen. Fosamax® has few side effects and reduces the chance of having a spinal or hip fracture, but it does not increase the likelihood of breast or uterine cancer. Fosamax® is also a good alternative for people who are unable to take estrogen. This drug must be taken on an empty stomach, and it requires the taker to remain in the upright position for one-half hour after it is taken in order to prevent backflow into the esophagus.

35 Fibromyalgia

A 47-year-old bank manager has been complaining of diffuse aching pain in her shoulders, hips, and low back for about a year and a half. Her symptoms have gotten worse recently, and she also complains of increasing stiffness. She often wakes from a night's sleep feeling exhausted and often experiences episodes of diarrhea. She has multiple sites of tenderness over the skin on her neck and her upper and lower back. She has little time to relax and has not been on a vacation in 3 years. After visiting her doctor and receiving negative results on all her medical tests, she was diagnosed with fibromyalgia.

■ FIBROMYALGIA DEFINED

Fibromyalgia is a painful, chronic, non-transmittable, debilitating condition that may affect as many as 2% of all Americans. The prefix *fibro* refers to fibrous tissues such as muscle, tendon or ligament, and the suffix *algia* means pain in the fibrous tissue. There is usually no accompanying inflammation. Fibromyalgia occurs in muscles, tendons, and ligaments, but not joints. It is the second most commonly diagnosed musculoskeletal disorder. For many years, skeptical doctors wrote off the symptoms of fibromyalgia as psychological because medical tests were negative and the presenting complaints were accompanied by depression and anxiety. Prior to the endorsement of the term *fibromyalgia* by the American College of Rheumatology in 1990, the condition was referred to by other names, including fibrosistis, tension myalgias, chronic muscle pain syndrome, and psychogenic rheumatism.

■ WHO IS MOST LIKELY TO HAVE FIBROMYALGIA?

Fibromyalgia affects 3.5% of women and .5% of males, and costs the U.S. economy more than $10 billion annually. Not only are two-thirds of all those with fibromyalgia women, but the symptoms are generally more severe in females. Fibromyalgia is most commonly diagnosed between 35 and 55 years of age. Fibromyalgia is prevalent in the thirty-something age range, but it is relatively uncommon in people older than 65 years of age. Because it is so difficult to define, fibromyalgia is called a *syndrome* —a collection of signs and symptoms—rather than a specific disease.

The cause of fibromyalgia is unknown, although various factors such as stress, emotional or physical trauma, overexertion, immune system challenges, weather changes, or simply being out of shape may trigger the condition. People with fibromyalgia tend to have low levels of the neurotransmitter *serotonin* and its precursor, an amino acid called *tryptophan*. Low levels of these essential chemicals are associated with the symptoms of fibromyalgia, including depression, anxiety, migraine headaches, and

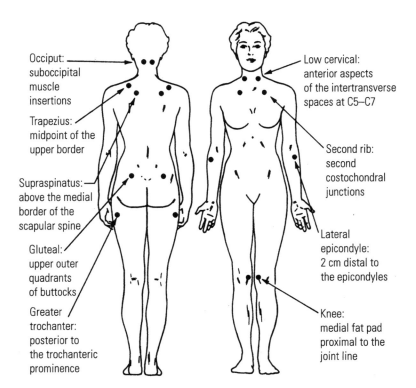

Occiput:
suboccipital
muscle
insertions

Trapezius:
midpoint of the
upper border

Suprasinatus:
above the medial
border of the
scapular spine

Gluteal:
upper outer
quadrants
of buttocks

Greater
trochanter:
posterior to
the trochanteric
prominence

Low cervical:
anterior aspects
of the intertransverse
spaces at C5–C7

Second rib:
second
costochondral
junctions

Lateral
epicondyle:
2 cm distal to
the epicondyles

Knee:
medial fat pad
proximal to the
joint line

Location of many of the typical sites of deep tenderness in fibromyalgia.
Bulletin on the Rheumatic Diseases; Rodan GP, Schumacher HR: *Primer on Rheumatic Diseases*, 8th Edition. Atlanta: The Arthritis Foundation, 1983.

gastrointestinal distress. Fibromyalgia is thought to have an autoimmune etiology similar to illnesses such as rheumatoid arthritis and systemic lupus erythematosus. Interestingly, many people with posttraumatic stress disorder experience fibromyalgia syndrome.

■ DIAGNOSIS OF FIBROMYALGIA

Because no specific test can rule out or confirm the condition, fibromyalgia can be difficult to diagnose. The diagnosis of fibromyalgia, therefore, is one of exclusion—meaning that it is diagnosed when tests for other conditions come back negative and the person still complains of pain. Tests usually include laboratory tests, x-rays, muscle strength, reflexes, and joint range-of-motion, and neurological examination for sensation. According to the American

College of Rheumatology, a person must meet two criteria to be diagnosed with fibromyalgia. They must have widespread pain above and below the waist that has existed for at least 3 months. Additionally, they must verbally complain of intense pain when light pressure is applied to 11 out of 18 possible tender points in the body.

■ SIGNS AND SYMPTOMS

The primary symptom of fibromyalgia is an aching feeling all over the body that is accompanied by marked limb stiffness, although the joints are not affected. Diffuse pain may be accompanied by swelling in soft tissue as well as muscle spasms. People with fibromyalgia often have *tender points* (also known as *trigger points*) that cluster in regions around the neck and shoulders, the upper chest wall, and the lower back. Trigger points are localized spots within muscle that elicit radiating pain in response to pressure. Painful trigger points are thought to arise because of buildup of a waste product known as *lactic acid* in muscles that are overworked, preventing waste removal that would normally occur when a muscle is at rest. Many of the muscles involved early on are muscles of the neck and upper back. These muscles may tense up during times of increased emotional stress and inadequate rest and relaxation. This, in turn, may cause decreased blood supply (*ischemia*) and metabolic malfunction of muscles. Pain typically radiates in characteristic patterns known as *referral zones*. President John F. Kennedy suffered from painful trigger points in his back that were treated by his personal doctor Dr. Janet Travell. She prescribed daily sessions of sitting in a rocking chair as part of his treatment program.

Other symptoms of fibromyalgia include morning and daytime fatigue, nonrestorative sleep, chronic tension, migraine headache, bowel and bladder irritability, bowel cramping, alternating diarrhea and constipation, chest pains, anxiety, and depression. Typically, discomfort is experienced on awakening and worsens throughout the day. The genesis of fibromyalgia suggests interplay between both psychological and biologic factors because many of these symptoms are associated with psychological and physical stress.

CONDITIONS TO RULE OUT

Fibromyalgia was not very widely known or respected as a genuine physical condition until very recently, and a certain amount of stigma was attached to it. In 1987, the American Medical Association recognized the syndrome as an illness and major cause of disability, thereby negating the notion that fibromyalgia was purely a psychological phenomenon. Once diagnosed, many people experience a significant reduction in anxiety and feel validated because they now know their symptoms are caused by an actual illness. Some of the conditions to rule out in making a diagnosis include:

- **CHRONIC FATIGUE SYNDROME:** This condition manifests as persistent fatigue lasting 6 or more consecutive months. Chronic fatigue syndrome has symptoms similar to fibromyalgia. The difference between the two conditions is that pain is the most prominent feature of fibromyalgia, and unremitting fatigue is the prominent feature of chronic fatigue syndrome. The cause of both these conditions is unknown. Chronic fatigue syndrome affects approximately 5 to 10 of every 100,000 thousand American adults. Over 75% of all cases occur in white females, with an average age of onset of 30 years.

- **LYME DISEASE:** This condition is an infectious bacterial disease transmitted by deer ticks. It is named for Lyme, Connecticut, where it was first identified in 1975. Because the bite of the tick is painless, the tiny tick may go unnoticed. After the initial phase, which may or may not include a circular smooth rash, flu-like symptoms accompanied by muscle soreness, neck stiffness, fatigue, fever, and joint pain may occur several weeks after the initial infection. Arthritis may set in if Lyme disease goes undetected and is not treated with antibiotics. Eventually, chronic problems affecting the heart and nervous system may develop. Differentiating Lyme disease from fibromyalgia is done by a doctor.

- **POLYMYALGIA RHEUMATICA:** This condition is most common in women over age 50. It manifests as severe pain and stiffness in those parts of the arms and legs closer to the trunk. People with this condition often have a high fever and symptoms similar to fibromyalgia. This condition is identified by blood tests. The cause of polymyalgia rheumatica is unknown, although it responds well to steroid treatment under the care of a doctor.

■ TREATMENT

Fibromyalgia can be mild or disabling; the condition is neither progressive nor fatal; and remission may occur in people who participate in a program of rehabilitation. No single treatment will cure this syndrome, but a multifaceted approach to symptomatic control is often helpful, especially when accompanied by a healthy lifestyle. Eating and sleeping correctly, and regular involvement in a stress reduction program can help minimize symptoms or, when coupled with other treatments, may cause symptoms to disappear altogether. Management of symptoms allows people with fibromyalgia to lead more productive lives. The following measures can make living with fibromyalgia easier:

- **REST:** Allowing enough time to rest each day and foregoing the opportunity to work even harder at personal and professional projects will help reduce stress. We live in a society that measures success by how productive we are, making it easy to lose sight of the importance of finding time when our minds and bodies are free to relax and not be accountable to pressures from others or our own internally generated pressure to be productive.

- **EXERCISE:** Physical exercise is thought to be the most effective intervention for long-term management of fibromyalgia because deconditioned muscles use energy poorly and are more susceptible to fatigue, microtrauma, and pain. It is important to start exercising lightly and as gently as possible. Performing a very low level of exercise such as weight-lifting for 5 minutes per day and then increasing the duration of activity by 1 minute per session every few days is a good approach. While this may be painful at first it is important to continue. The pain of fibromyalgia usually gets worse before it gets better. Eventually, you can gradually build up to 30 or 40 minutes of exercise 3 or 4 times per week. Aquatic exercises can be very helpful because of the relaxing benefits of buoyancy. Aerobic exercises such as swimming, walking, or biking are excellent choices for exercise.

- **STRETCHING:** Stretching is very important because it helps restore muscle flexibility. Improved extensibility is essential to relieving pain in muscles. Stretching should be done slowly and gently, and without increasing the level of pain. Consulting a physical therapist or personal trainer as to a stretching regimen is an essential step in relieving the symptoms associated with fibromyalgia.

- **MASSAGE:** Gentle massage may promote muscle relaxation, and deep friction massage across the trigger point may help diminish the long-term sensitivity of the trigger point.

- **STRESS REDUCTION:** Cognitive-behavioral therapeutic techniques such as meditation, hypnosis, yoga, deep-breathing exercises, biofeedback, acupressure, acupuncture, and tai chi may be helpful to people with fibromyalgia. Psychological or psychiatric counseling may also be helpful in teaching people with this syndrome to cope with the stressors in their lives and negotiate disappointments due to unfulfilled expectations.

- **ADEQUATE SLEEP:** It is important to develop regular sleep habits with an emphasis on getting adequate rest each night because fatigue makes the symptoms of fibromyalgia worse. People with fibromyalgia should moderate their use of caffeine, alcohol, and nicotine to increase restorative sleep patterns.

■ **SPRAY AND STRETCH:** This pain-reduction technique utilizes a vapor coolant that is sprayed over painful muscles, thereby diminishing pain and allowing a therapist to stretch the muscle adequately.

■ **TRIGGER POINT INJECTIONS:** This form of treatment is performed by a doctor. It is reportedly effective in reducing pain and tenderness in some people with fibromyalgia. The injection of steroids and/or analgesics causes intense, temporary pain in the trigger point, followed by significant relief later on, thus allowing for an enhanced ability to stretch the muscle. Several injections may be required.

■ **MEDICATIONS:** Nonprescription non-steroidal analgesics in modest doses may help relieve some of the pain and stiffness associated with fibromyalgia. Some doctors may also prescribe muscle relaxants. Antidepressant medications may be prescribed to help promote deep sleep. Your doctor can prescribe a variety of different drugs that may relieve your pain and allow you to sleep better.

■ **MODALITY USE:** Using moist hot packs, heating pads, whirlpools, warm baths or showers to increase blood flow and decrease muscle spasm and tension may be helpful. Using cold modalities such as ice massage, cool baths, or ice packs may be helpful in anesthetizing the painful tender points and breaking the cycle of pain.

■ **EDUCATION:** It is important that people with fibromyalgia understand the necessity of adhering to an adequate home exercise program and not rely entirely on therapists to provide relief. Understanding fibromyalgia allows many people to maintain control over their lives. Knowledge is power and it can help people with fibromyalgia cope with their condition. Attending support groups may also be helpful. Weight control and a well-balanced diet are also advised.

36 Remedies for Pain Relief

THIS CHAPTER discusses some of the different types of treatment for pain that are available, when they should be used, and when to exercise caution. It is a guide to some of the management strategies available to help resolve the symptoms of common pain syndromes and athletic injuries, but not a comprehensive discussion.

■ REST

"Take it easy." "Take a load off." "Chill out." "Relax." These are just some of the terms commonly used to describe "rest." The human mind is stronger than the body in the sense that it can push the body beyond its physical limits, but the human body needs an adequate amount of rest. Sure, there are times when you want to push yourself as if you were running a marathon. At times, that approach is appropriate, but often it is not. This level of intensity is not always good for the body in the long run, although in the short run it may be useful. Unfortunately, many people convince themselves that every day is a mini-crisis. They push so hard that they reach the point of causing themselves harm. This is true for the athlete and stockbroker alike. Listen to your body. If it hurts, avoid the activity that causes pain rather than tolerate or embrace it. Take some time off and rest.

Rest plays an important role in providing relief from pain. Pain is the product of the inflammation that accompanies injury. (See Chapter 4.) Inflam-

mation helps us heal in many ways. Cells involved in the inflammatory process break down injured and dead tissue, clearing the way for new tissue to regenerate. Cells also release proteins that play a role in recruiting the cells that participate in the rebuilding process. The process of restoring damaged tissue is a complex one and demands the full focus of the body parts involved. Inflammation causes the pain that lets us know it is time to slow down, rest, and give the body time to heal.

Rest does not always have to mean sleep, or even absolute rest. Sometimes rest can be accomplished by reducing the level of your activity so that healing and restoration may occur. Rest can also be accomplished by cross-training, wherein you train your muscles to work in a different way by engaging in activities other than your usual routine. If the cross-training activity is well chosen, you may be able to rest the muscles that need it and engage in a rigorous exercise routine using different muscles at the same time. Many people return to harmful activities too soon, only to re-injure themselves. Rest allows you to heal before irreparable damage occurs.

■ COLD AND HEAT

The first recorded use of cold as a remedy for pain was by the Greek physician Hippocrates, who applied snow and ice to soft tissue injuries. Cold is very helpful when experiencing the hot, sharp, or aching pain that comes on right after an injury such as a sprained ankle. It is also helpful when applied to a hot, swollen joint after an arthritic flare-up. The intense pain felt during a flare-up or immediately after an injury is called *acute* pain. Applying a cold compress for 15 to 20 minutes to the site of an acute injury may help numb the area and relieve inflammatory pain. You can use a package of vegetables from your freezer, a frozen cup of ice, or crushed ice and water in a zipper lock bag. Alternatively, placing the injured part in a bucket filled with ice slush, applying a gel-refrigerant or chemical pack, or using a coolant spray may also be effective. Applying cold for more than 20 minutes is not advisable because it may damage the skin.

Heat provides great relief of chronic pain and it is also helpful in reducing muscle spasm. A hot bath has been used since time immemorial to relieve the pain of aching joints or the back. For this reason, naturally hot mineral springs are very popular. Alternately, applying heat in the form of an electric pad can provide relief, although it is best to leave the setting on low, in the event you fall asleep with the hot pad in place. Be sure to place as many as 6 to 8 layers of towel between the hot pack and your skin when using a moist hot pack to protect yourself from a burn. While this may seem excessive, it is not. Initially, you may not feel the heat, but as the heat seeps through the towels, you will most certainly feel it.

A paraffin bath is another example of applied heat for the relief of pain. With this treatment, a smaller body joint such as those found in the hand, foot, or elbow is momentarily (for a few seconds only) placed in a tub containing liquefied paraffin and mineral wintergreen oil mixed in a 6:1 ratio that has been heated to 131 degrees Fahrenheit—do not worry; you will not be burned. The melted paraffin quickly turns hard at room temperature after the limb is removed from the container. It acts like a glove to hold in the warmth. The body part is then wrapped in wax paper or plastic to make certain that the heat is not lost and then further insu-

lated with a thick towel. After 20 minutes the glove may be peeled off.

Fluidotherapy involves circulation of heated cellulose or silicon particles that creates the sensation of a dry whirlpool. Typically, these units are located in physical therapy offices. The limb is placed in a sleeve, which is then placed inside the whirlpool for the treatment.

TENS

Electric current has been used to treat ailments since early Roman times in the form of electric eels, rays, and torpedo fish. The child who has a scrape learns early on that holding and rubbing the injured area brings relief. Why is this so? The pain signals may be modified many times by interactions with other parts of the nervous system between the stimulated pain receptor and the cortex of the brain. Modification of the signal begins even in the peripheral nervous system. In the early 1960s, it was noticed that stimulation of large-diameter peripheral sensory nerve fibers, not thought to be directly involved in pain sensation, decreased the responsiveness of spinal cord neurons to signals coming from pain receptors. Spinal cord neurons will respond more intensely to pain signals coming from pain receptors if the activity of these other sensory neurons is blocked. This led Patrick Wall and Ronald Melzack to propose the "Gate Control Theory of Pain Perception." This theory maintains that pain perception may depend upon a balance between the activity of the pain-sensitive nociceptor neurons and the other, larger-diameter, better-insulated sensory neurons. Pain sensation is heightened when activity is high in the pain-receptor neurons and low in the large-fiber neurons. When the opposite is true, pain sensation is diminished.

The practical outcome of this theory is that it supplies a rationale for other non-medicinal approaches to pain management. For example, the Gate Control Theory may explain why vigorous rubbing of the skin at the site of a minor painful injury often helps relieve the pain. Rubbing the skin stimulates the large-diameter sensory fibers. It also explains the rationale underlying a popular non-medicinal method of pain control called *transcutaneous electrical nerve stimulation* (TENS). This method involves the use of a battery-powered electrical device that stimulates the large-diameter sensory fibers. This is believed to have the effect of suppressing the transmission of pain signals. The weak TENS current is applied through electrodes placed on the skin over the painful area. TENS is particularly helpful in relieving chronic pain from osteoarthritis and bursitis. It is also sometimes used to treat neuropathic pain.

ULTRASOUND

Ultrasound is a form of energy with a frequency that is higher or beyond that detectable by the human ear. These frequencies are generated when electricity is passed though special, naturally occurring crystals that vibrate at ultrasonic frequencies. Dogs can hear ultrasound, which is why dog whistles can not be heard by people but are heard well by dogs. Dolphins and whales communicate via ultrasound; submarines use ultrasound waves to navigate through dark waters and avoid bumping into objects; and bats use it to fly successfully in the dark. Using a similar principle, ultrasound is used in diagnostic medicine to visualize a baby within its mother and to detect how much blood is ejected out of the heart valves in a damaged heart. Ultrasound waves penetrate deep into tissue and transfer their energy as heat, thereby healing the tissues and easing the pain associated with chronic conditions. This method of treatment should not be done during the acute stage of injury because the heat generated may exacerbate the pain from the acute inflammatory process. Ultrasound applied in the pulsed mode (*phonophoresis*) may deliver pain-relieving medications to problem areas. Diagnostic or therapeutic ultrasound should only be administered by a health professional because improper use may cause injury.

WHIRLPOOL

Hydrotherapy in a whirlpool relieves pain, relaxes muscles, and is useful in the treatment of joint stiffness and arthritis. Archimedes the Greek mathematician was the first to discover that water has the property of buoyancy. His story is interesting and worth mentioning. The king suspected that a crown presented to him by the local goldsmith was alloyed with silver, and he commissioned Archimedes to figure out whether the goldsmith had hoodwinked the royal treasury. Determining whether the crown was alloyed with silver without injuring the crown was a daunting prospect. Archimedes pondered the matter while lowering himself into the water at the public bathhouse. Understanding the principle of buoyancy in a flash of sudden insight caused Archimedes, in his excitement, to run naked out of the bathhouse and into the street yelling Eureka! Eureka! (meaning, "I have discovered it"). The crown proved to be alloyed, and we can only speculate about the fate of the unlucky goldsmith.

You feel lighter in water because of buoyancy. Minimizing the constant tug of gravity provides rest to your muscles and allows inflammation to subside somewhat. Whether the water is hot, tepid, or cool, whirlpool water is usually agitated by a turbine that adds air to the water in a process known as *aeration.* This turbulence can be very relaxing and provides additional relief to sore, injured areas.

▪ CONTRAST BATHS

Contrast baths involve alternating between placing the injured area in hot and cold tanks or a whirlpool bath. The hot water should be about 102 to 105 degrees Fahrenheit, and the cold water should be between 50 and 60 degrees Fahrenheit. Begin with hot water first for 5 to 10 minutes, then the cold water for 1 to 2 minutes, for a hot to cold ratio of 3:1 or 4:1. Contrast baths stimulate circulation by alternating between vasoconstriction (cold) and vasodilatation (heat) of the superficial blood vessels. This maximizes blood flow to the painful area. The entire treatment lasts 30 minutes and is always concluded with the cold bath in order to reduce swelling. Improved circulation promotes healing and may reduce pain over time, although it provides little immediate pain relief.

▪ MOBILIZATION

Mobilization of body joints refers to a technique often employed by physical therapists to restore normal motion to a joint. The idea behind mobilization is that certain injuries cause stiffness at the joint from wearing a cast or brace. The joint may have trouble moving normally after removal of the immobilizing device because the joint capsule surrounding it may have become tightened in an unnatural position. Mobilization involves wiggling the joint through small, gentle, oscillations with the intention of stretching the tight ligaments and capsule. The joint will be able to move through its normal range of motion once it has been stretching in this manner.

▪ MASSAGE

Ancient Chinese and Egyptian manuscripts make mention of massage as a method of treatment for pain. Hippocrates advocated its use, and one of the Roman emperors' physicians, Galen, wrote many books relating to massage. Massage has a wonderful effect on the person being massaged, and the direct benefits include improved circulation, muscle relaxation, and stimulation of the lymphatic system. Today, the most popular style of massage that is being used is Swedish massage. It can be beneficial in alleviating stress, improving some types of low back and neck pain, and relaxing tight muscle groups. Massage involves stroking, kneading, squeezing, pounding, and striking, or applying friction to the skin or tissues below the skin. A state-licensed massage therapist or physical therapist is preferred.

▪ ACUPUNCTURE

The Chinese have practiced acupuncture as a method of healing and pain relief for centuries. Acupuncture gained notoriety in the West when Western observers documented surgery performed in China without conventional anesthesia; only acupuncture was used to block pain. No one really knows how acupuncture works, although it has been hypothesized that local needling excites the endorphin system of pain control, providing pain relief for hours or days. Proponents of acupuncture see the body as a bioelectric system with energy pathways known as meridians that run throughout the body. Along these meridians are as many as 365 acupuncture points. When energy is disrupted along the meridians, pain and illness may result. Energy disruption is corrected by using needles to stimulate energy flow along these pathways and, thus, the flow of energy is brought back into balance and health is restored. It is very important to choose a well-trained acupuncturist who is either state- or county-certified. Acupressure operates along these same principles but uses applied pressure that is focused at certain body areas instead of using needles. Electro-acupuncture utilizes needles that are electrically stimulated.

A frequently asked question is whether there is any objective scientific evidence that acupuncture is effective in relieving pain. This is a more difficult question to answer than might be thought. A review of the medical literature reveals a plethora of contradictory studies, some of which support the efficacy of acupuncture and others that suggest it is no better than a placebo. Some of the variability may be related to the different types of pain studied in each trial. There are suggestions in the literature that acupuncture may be effective in relieving some types of pain, but not all types. Reviews of large numbers of studies suggest that many were done improperly without an adequate number of participants or proper study design. After all this time since acupuncture was introduced to Western medicine, it still appears that no large, adequately designed, unassailable study has been conducted to provide a definitive answer to this question.

▪ CREATIVE VISUALIZATION

Imagining or visualizing yourself in better health has been advocated by some people and may reduce pain and pain-related anxiety. Focusing on positive imagery in which the body is seen as free from pain and injury may make pain less prominent. Tapping into the power of suggestion may positively affect pain through a psychoimmunologic mechanism.

▪ MEDICATION

Despite the non-medicinal approaches to pain control briefly discussed above, medication remains the major approach to pain control in use today. There are several different categories of drugs that are commonly used. They differ from one another in their pharmacological properties, their mechanisms of action, the types of pain they treat, and their potential side effects. Each class of drug is discussed individually below, with the caveat that in any given situation you should rely on the specific recommendations of your doctor.

▪ NON-STEROIDAL ANTI-INFLAMMATORY DRUGS (NSAIDS)

Oral non-steroidal anti-inflammatory drugs (NSAIDS) are probably the most commonly used pain medications. They include drugs like aspirin and ibuprofen (Motrin® and Advil®), naprosyn (Naproxen® and Anaprox®), indomethacin (Indocin®), clinoril, and others. NSAIDs are very helpful in controlling the pain and inflammation associated with acute and chronic musculoskeletal conditions. They have both anti-inflammatory and analgesic properties and, in that respect, not only do they provide pain relief, they also address the underlying cause of the pain to some degree. As an additional bonus, they are also effective in suppressing fever. Although most of the NSAIDs are similar in structure and mechanism of action, there is a surprising amount of variability in how individuals respond to the different drugs. For example, one person may respond beautifully to ibuprofen but not at all to naprosyn. Another may have the opposite response, or respond better to a third drug. No one fully understands why this is the case or why any given individual will respond to any particular drug. However, the significance of this observation is that if one NSAID does not work, that does not mean you should give up on NSAIDs. However, if two or three do not work, then you may want to consider some other alternative.

Many NSAIDs are now available in nonprescription strength, but they are not completely benign.

Excessive use of NSAIDs can lead to gastritis, ulcers, hearing loss, bleeding disorders, and kidney damage. Everyone should limit the number of NSAIDs they take and the length of time they take them. Individuals with a medical history of any of the problems listed above should consult their doctor before taking NSAIDs at all. Even if there is no such medical history, elderly people, in particular, should be especially careful about taking large doses of NSAIDs. There are newer varieties of NSAIDs such as the Cox-2 inhibitors Vioxx® and Celebrex® that may have a lower risk for some of these side effects. These are effective NSAIDs and they have become increasingly popular. Keep in mind, however, that although the risk of complications is lower with Cox-2 inhibitors, excessive use can still be dangerous.

ACETAMINOPHEN

In addition to the NSAIDs, there are other medications that are highly effective in relieving pain. The most important one in common use is acetaminophen, better known by the brand name Tylenol®. Acetaminophen is similar to many of the NSAIDs in that it is effective in both relieving pain and reducing fever. It is a weak anti-inflammatory drug, however, and appears to work through a mechanism of action different from that of NSAIDs. Just how it works is still not fully understood. Acetaminophen has been shown to be effective in treating many different types of pain, although it may be less effective in treating moderate to severe pain than the classic NSAIDs.

The major advantage of acetaminophen over the typical NSAIDs is that it is safe when taken as directed. Acetaminophen will not cause ulcers, gastritis, or esophageal reflux. This does not mean that acetaminophen is safe in any quantity. High doses of acetaminophen can result in severe, even life-threatening liver failure. It is therefore important to try to stay within the manufacturers' recommended dosing guidelines, which for the average adult is a cumulative maximum of 4,000 mg a day.

OPIOID ANALGESICS

Opioid analgesics—so named because they are all derived or structurally related to opium—are the most potent analgesics available. They are also referred to as narcotics. Some varieties of opioids, such as heroin and codeine, are illegal in the United States. Opioids are chemicals that bind to three types of receptors that are found naturally in the body. Although opioids themselves are not found naturally in the body, small peptides called *endorphins* are found naturally. Endorphins mediate analgesic functions at the opioid receptors. (See Chapter 4 for a more complete discussion of endogenous opioids.)

The opioids that are most effective in relieving pain all bind to the *mu* opioid receptor. Most of these are derivatives of and structurally related to morphine. Although the entire class of mu receptor opioids is similar in structure, they differ from one another in potency. This means that smaller quantities of a potent opioid may give you the same analgesic benefit as a much greater quantity of a less potent opioid. Unlike NSAIDs, however, there does not appear to be much difference between opioids in terms of individual response. If you took sufficient quantities of codeine (a relatively weak opioid) so that it would be equal to a given quantity of hydromorphone (a very potent opioid) there would likely be little difference in the degree of pain relief. There are differences among the opioids in the degree to which they bind to other types of opioid receptors and, therefore, there may be differences between them in some of their other effects.

Opioids are very powerful analgesics, and they have become the drugs of choice for severe acute pain. There are downsides to opioid use, however. Opioids are highly addictive and can cause physical dependency. Although these two terms are frequently used interchangeably, they do not mean the same thing. Physical dependence suggests that if someone stops taking the drug, they will experience physical symptoms of withdrawal. These include restlessness, sleepiness, insomnia, irritability, shaking, tremors, nasal congestion, diarrhea, and other symptoms. Addiction implies that the person's behavior has changed in an antisocial way in order to obtain narcotics. For example, stealing, doctor-shopping, and prescription fraud are all signs of addiction. Some people may become addicted to and physically dependent upon prescription opioids such as morphine, just as they would illegal opioids such as heroin.

Opioids also have other potentially serious side effects as well. They frequently cause nausea, vomiting, constipation, sleepiness, hallucinations, impaired judgment, and abnormal thinking. At high doses they may cause coma, respiratory suppression (difficulty breathing), and death. In addition, people on longstanding therapy with opioids frequently develop tolerance to their analgesic effects. This means that over time they require larger and larger doses of the opioid to get the same analgesic effect.

Many doctors prefer to prescribe opioids only for acute pain of limited duration (often no more than 1 to 2 weeks). Doctors are likely to be more liberal in prescribing higher doses of opioids for longer periods of time in cases where there is malignant pain from cancer. There is currently a great deal of debate among doctors as to whether it is appropriate to prescribe opioids for chronic, non-malignant pain when other pain medications have failed. Several leading medical organizations have published recommendations suggesting situations where it is appropriate to do so. The issue is far from settled. Some drug companies are currently working at formulating new types of opioid drugs that will be less dangerous and less likely to cause physical dependence or addiction. So far, few are currently on the market.

STEROID INJECTIONS

Steroids are natural substances made by glands within the body. Many hormones, including the sex hormones, have structures similar to steroids. One of the most important properties of a group of steroids called glucocorticoids is that they reduce inflammation. Although they have no analgesic properties per se, their ability to reduce inflammation enables them to inhibit the major cause of pain following a tissue injury. This makes steroids highly effective in reducing the pain associated with most types of stress injuries and chronic pain syndromes.

Steroids may be administered by mouth, inhaler, systemic injection (to the whole body), or by local injection directly at the site of injury. Local injections are the most effective route of applying steroids because they result in a high concentration of steroid right where you need it. In addition, using local injections avoids the side effects of systemic injections, which include weight gain, swelling, osteoporosis, abnormal hair growth and distorted features, gastric irritation, abnormally high blood sugar, and suppression of the immune system, which may lead to opportunistic infections.

One problem with local injections is that steroids are so powerful that they weaken the tissue into which they are injected. No more than two or three steroid injections should ever be administered to a single area. Too many injections, for example, into a painful tendon may cause the tendon to become weakened to the point of being unable to handle stress, and it will eventually rupture. Another problem with steroids is that because they often cause a dramatic decrease in symptoms, people often feel that they are cured and apply themselves vigorously to the same activity that caused the pain and inflammation in the first place. This catches up with them sooner or later and they typically exacerbate the injury that caused their original symptoms. The bottom line is that when used judiciously, steroid injections can be very useful in controlling pain and aiding the healing process, but when used carelessly or cavalierly, steroids can make a bad situation much worse.

MEDICATIONS FOR CHRONIC PAIN

Often, the drugs that are usually effective in relieving the pain associated with an acute injury become less effective when the pain becomes chronic. Alternatively, a doctor may have good reasons not to prescribe one of the treatments for acute pain over a prolonged period of time. This may be because of the associated risks such as addiction, gastroesophageal injury, or other complications. There are drugs available that are specifically useful in dealing with chronic or chronic/recurrent pain. They may be taken on a daily basis for long periods of time with limited adverse effects and significant long-term efficacy. These drugs are not able to eliminate acute pain. However, they are effective in improving longstanding chronic pain. Although a wide variety of drugs has been tested and prescribed over the years for this purpose, the most successful and popularly prescribed drugs for chronic pain are the tricyclic antidepressants and the anticonvulsants. As you may have noticed from their names, neither class of drug was originally developed for the purpose of treating chronic pain.

TRICYCLIC ANTIDEPRESSANTS

As the name implies, tricyclic antidepressants were developed for the treatment of depression. They are still popularly used for that purpose, although with the introduction of so many other classes of antide-pressant drugs they are used less commonly to treat depression than they once were. In addition to treating depression, tricyclics were discovered early on to be effective in treating chronic pain of various sorts. Why they are effective in this way is not completely understood, although many researchers believe that it may have to do with the fact that tricyclics serve to increase the effects of serotonin (a chemical transmitter in the brain) by preventing its removal from the site of activity. Serotonin is believed to play an important role in modulating chronic and recurrent pain, although precisely how is not understood.

Tricyclics are not analgesics, and they are ineffective in relieving acute pain or primary inflammatory pain. They have been reported to be effective in treating neuropathic pain (pain related to nerve injury) and many types of headache. There are many agents available in this class of drugs. Some of the more popular ones are: amitriptyline (Elavil®), nortriptyline (Pamelor®), doxepin (Sinequan®), and imipramine (Tofranil®), to name a few. They are similar in their actions, but there is some individual variation in their efficacy and the associated side effects.

The tricyclics have a number of side effects, which some people have difficulty tolerating, including daytime sleepiness, dry mouth, increased appetite, weight gain, fluid retention, bizarre dreams, and rarely, hallucinations. More serious side effects include urinary retention, abnormal heart rhythms, and acute closed-angle glaucoma. It is recommended that these drugs be used with special care in the elderly and people with cardiac histories, enlarged prostates, or a history of glaucoma or elevated ocular pressures.

ANTICONVULSANTS

Anticonvulsants are drugs that are generally used for the treatment of seizures in people with epilepsy.

They work by a variety of different mechanisms, but they share in common the fact that they inhibit the propagation of electrical signals in the nervous system. It is through this mechanism that they interfere with seizures in the brain, and it is likely that this mechanism also interferes with the chronic pain associated with peripheral nerve injury.

There are many different kinds of anticonvulsant drugs in common use today, but only a few have been shown to be effective in the treatment of chronic pain. The earliest anticonvulsant to be used for this purpose was carbamazepine (Tegretol®). It is still popularly used for this purpose as well as for the treatment of specific acute painful syndromes such as *trigeminal neuralgia.* Valproic acid (Depakote®) has also proven useful for the treatment of chronic neuropathic pain. Gabapentin (Neurontin®) is a relative newcomer, but it is a drug that is quickly becoming very popular for the treatment of neuropathic pain. The anticonvulsants may be better tolerated than the tricyclics by some, but they also have side effects, and care should be taken with their use. Sleepiness, clouded thinking, dizziness, nausea, vomiting, and double vision are sometimes experienced. Carbamazepine may cause a severe form of bone marrow suppression in rare instances, so your doctor may elect to follow your blood count for a while when first starting this particular medication.

37 Staying in Shape

■ FITNESS: THE BEST FORM OF PREVENTION

THE OLD ADAGE "active life, long life" runs true—the two are practically synonymous. Americans have been increasingly preoccupied with greater fitness over the past several decades. People everywhere are swimming, running, cycling, walking, playing tennis, and engaging in numerous sport-related activities. Studies have shown that the more you walk, the longer you will live. In addition to providing a healthy and more attractive appearance, exercise reduces anxiety and promotes self-confidence, greater levels of energy, more restful sleep, and sharper concentration. In addition, exercise—in conjunction with diet—can halt the progression of osteoporosis. It also protects the heart. The bottom line: The fit live longer and healthier lives.

■ MR. AND MRS. FIX IT

Some people do not like to exercise by participating in sports-related activities. However, fitness can also be accomplished by other activities such as gardening, which involves weeding, hoeing, and digging. Gardening can burn as much as 400 to 450 calories per hour. Find an activity or project around the house that you have been putting off for a while and get to it! Performing household chores such as carpentry, cleaning windows, painting, mowing the lawn, scrubbing floors, shoveling snow, chopping and stacking wood, and washing and polishing the car are just some of the activities that can be done around the house to increase fitness. These activities can accomplish as much as exercises done at a gym when they performed vigorously for more than half an hour every day.

■ THE COUCH POTATO

Many people believe in the myth that they are still physically fit during middle age because they were athletic and played lots of basketball or some other sport when they were young. In addition, simply being in your 30s or 40s is no guarantee that you are physically fit. In fact, a 65-year-old man who exercises three times per week for an hour may be in better shape than a 25-year-old couch potato! Generally, sedentary people lose about 10% of their lean muscle mass each decade after age 30. Because of this, it is extremely important to avoid getting out-of-shape. Statistically, people with more education tend to be more physically active. So, get off that couch and start exercising!

■ THE BIG MISCONCEPTION

Some people think that being strong is all there is to it; they think that all they need to do is pump up for a few years during their 20s and then they can just coast through life with their "pumped iron" physic. They could not be more wrong. Exercise is a constant daily requirement that must be followed throughout life. It is important to think of exercise in the same manner as we think of the activities we consider mandatory, such as taking a regular bath or shower, using deodorant, shaving, and brushing and flossing our teeth—you just have to do it. The great thing about exercise is that it does not have to be boring. Exercise can be done while watching TV, listening to music, or reading the paper. Exercise can also be a social activity, such as when you play tennis or take a power walk with a friend. Remember to enjoy yourself when you exercise.

THE BENEFITS OF EXERCISE

Virtually every body system is enhanced by the effects of exercise. The muscles burn more fat; the liver produces glycogen more efficiently; more oxygen is delivered by the lungs; the heart pumps stronger; the circulatory system builds more capillaries; and glucose and insulin are better regulated by the pancreas. Additionally, the mitochondria—the principal sites of energy generation within the cells of the body—enlarge and increase in response to exercise. Moreover, bones respond by becoming denser, the "good" cholesterol increases, and the "bad" cholesterol decreases. Blood pressure drops within 24 to 48 hours of exercising and will stay down with continued exercise. The likelihood of developing blood clots also diminishes with regular exercise. Vigorous exercise increases lean muscle mass by consuming fat for energy, thereby helping you maintain a healthy weight. Regular exercise will help you sleep better and will increase your amount of endorphins—the body's natural opiates that make you less sensitive to pain and bring on a feeling of wellness. Exercise also elevates mood by releasing an abundance of the neurotransmitter serotonin, which works to elevate mood. Exercise will leave you feeling relaxed, with more energy, and looking better, too! Perhaps this was what inspired

the great American naturalist and philosopher Henry David Thoreau to claim, "Methinks that the moment my legs begin to move, my thoughts begin to flow."

STRETCHING FOR FLEXIBILITY

Another big misconception that many people share is that all you have to do in order to maintain fitness is strengthen your body. This could not be further from the truth. Muscles benefit greatly from contracting, but they must also elongate or stretch. Many of the muscles in the body are paired on either side of a bone so that when one contracts, the opposite muscle elongates. The problem is that certain muscles normally have a higher resting tone than other muscles, causing your body to favor certain positions when you are at rest. For example, you will tend to curl up with your legs in the fetal position when you are sleeping because the hamstring and calf muscles have greater tone than the quadriceps muscles, and they tend to pull the knee joint into the flexed, bent position. Consequently, these muscles are typically tight in many people and become even tighter as the years go by. Because of this, stretching is just as important, if not more important than strengthening. Stretching improves joint mobility and muscle extensibility. Everyone's body is different, which is why it is important to be guided by a professional such as a physical therapist or athletic trainer regarding the stretches that would be best for you.

BUILDING MUSCLE STRENGTH

You are never too old to build muscle strength. Studies have shown that men in their 60s and 70s were able to increase their muscle size by greater than 10% and their strength by a staggering 170%

after adhering to a weight-training program for just 12 weeks! Resistance-training does more than just build muscle. It also stimulates and strengthens bones.

However, always exercise with conscious regard for your body. Resistive exercises such as pumping iron may increase the muscle mass of people in their 30s and 40s, but if it is done to excess, it can enlarge the heart at the expense of decreasing the volume of the heart's chambers in a way that is indistinguishable from elderly people who develop pathologic enlargement of the heart. Even younger people in their 20s should be cautioned about not pumping an increasingly heavier bench press. This type of exercise is good in the short run, but it builds up the pectoralis muscles, which have a tendency to revert to fat a decade or so after the exercise is stopped. This may have the long-term effect of giving the male chest a flabby look. It is best to seek the guidance of a physical therapist or athletic trainer in choosing the right strengthening program for you.

■ STAMINA FOR ENDURANCE

Stamina, staying-power, aerobic power, and endurance are all synonyms describing the ability of the heart and lungs to work together in order to bring oxygen and nutrients to the far reaches of the body and remove waste products in an efficient manner. A good way to understand this concept is to understand the difference between cold- and warm-blooded creatures. Cold-blooded creatures do not have cold blood; rather the word "cold" in this instance refers to the fact that they are unable to generate enough energy to move around very quickly, or very often for that manner. This is because the heart and lungs of cold-blooded animals are relatively small. Thus, it is easier to stand still and rest on a sunny, warm rock if you are a tur-

tle because your metabolism does not burn enough fuel to provide heat. On the other hand, warm-blooded animals have relatively larger hearts and lungs than their cold-blooded counterparts, thus they are able to luxuriate in the warmth created by their own more efficient cardiopulmonary systems. This also makes them capable of quick movements.

Human beings are warm-blooded mammals, which makes them prone to developing poor endurance with the onset of modern living. Our bodies were originally designed for running, hunting, and protecting ourselves from predators. Now, fast forward to the Industrial Revolution, fast foods, television (and the couch that goes with it), and working at desk jobs. This spells trouble for the human cardiopulmonary system. The health of this system is measured by our endurance and stamina, and how easily we get out of shape as we huff and puff through activities like snow shoveling that we hardly gave a second thought to during our 20s. It is never too late to reverse these changes if you notice this in yourself. A study of over 3,000 men conducted at the University of North Carolina at Chapel Hill discovered that aerobic exercise offers more protection to the heart than pushing back the clock 19 years!

This is why endurance exercise is ranked as the most important component of any fitness program. It keeps your heart and lungs in top working order. Aerobics, for example, is a high-endurance exercise that results in high fat loss, high flexibility, and moderate strength-building. Basketball, biking, jogging, running, rowing, skating, cross-country skiing, swimming, and a brisk game of tennis, can all improve your aerobic power. Here is the rub—weight-lifting has low endurance. So does baseball, golf, downhill skiing, and doubles tennis. It is far more important to perform aerobic exercise, even as early as the 30s and 40s, than it is to pump iron. While the latter may make you look better, aerobic exercise addresses the body's need for strength, flexibility, fat loss, and most important of all—cardiopul-monary function. Consult your doctor and seek the advice of a physical therapist, exercise kinesiologist, or athletic trainer before beginning an endurance program.

EXERCISE IN MODERATION

While most people do not exercise enough, others are so overzealous that they may harm themselves. Exercise is not advocated as a cure-all for the difficulties of modern life. It should be performed in moderation and enjoyed because it is one of the most important things we can do in order to live healthy, well-balanced lives.

You know you are overdoing it if you leave an exercise session thinking about the next session with loathing. Excessive exercise will result in many problems:

- Less energy to enjoy the other things in your life

- Trouble sleeping

- No appetite at all or an appetite that is out-of-control

- New aches and pains

- A high morning pulse rate

- You may need to wear a knee or other brace, and

- You may need to ice parts of your body or pay for massage just to be able to keep up your routine.

If you have been overdoing it—beware! Stop and re-evaluate your reasons for exercise and slow down. Relax by reading a good book, talking with a friend, spending time with your family, or learning how to take care or yourself in some other constructive way.

SOME HELPFUL HINTS

The credo of some coaches and athletes known as "no pain, no gain," is best reserved for young, professional athletes. Most people who strengthen, stretch, or perform endurance exercises past the point of pain are well advised to take heed and avoid pain. The goal of exercise for most people is to stay healthy and feel good. Have a good experience exercising so that you will enjoy it and want to come back and participate again. Here are some helpful hints regarding fitness:

- **START SLOWLY:** A key concept is *gradual* conditioning. Do not rush right into exercise at breakneck speed. Ease into an exercise regimen calmly and at a relaxed pace. Increase your activity over time, but stop short of pain. For example, if you are working on your aerobic conditioning and your muscles start to hurt after 2 miles of running, then stop short of 2 miles the next time. Do not improve your endurance at the price of sore muscles.

- **WARM UP:** Not warming up prior to exercise is like turning on your car engine on a cold day and driving off without allowing the engine to properly warm up. Your body must warm up before taking off. Warm muscles are more elastic and, therefore, less vulnerable to injury. Also, the ability of muscles to utilize oxygen and fuel more efficiently increases with an increase in temperature.

  Walk before you jog, and jog before you run. A good way to warm up is by slowly stretching the hamstring, quadriceps, and calf muscles, and the muscles of the arms and shoulder girdle, such as the pectoralis major; gentle back stretching is also helpful. You are less likely to injure yourself when exercising if you have warmed up first.

■ **HOLD YOUR STRETCH:** Each stretch should be held for anywhere between 30 and 40 seconds. Count: 1,000, 1,001, 1,002, 1,003, etc., while you hold the stretch in order to ensure that you do not speed up too quickly. Holding a stretch helps preserve any extensibility gained from the stretch. Also, stretch both before and after exercise and remember, stretching should not hurt; at most, you should feel a gentle pull.

■ **BOUNCING:** Bouncing into a stretch should never be done because it can cause microtrauma within muscle tissue, which is then filled in with scar tissue. This weakens the muscle and predisposes it to further injury.

■ **STRENGTHENING:** Begin with a weight that you can lift comfortably eight times. Research indicates that performing a single set of twelve repetitions with the proper weight can build muscle just as efficiently as three sets of four repetitions of the same exercise. This is good news for busy people who are not able to spend 90 minutes each day in the weight room. Instead, simply spending 20 to 25 minutes several times per week can build strength. Always avoid jerky movements when handling weights.

■ **TRAIN IN CYCLES:** If you participate in several sports, rest for a few days between them, because you may not always be able to exercise at your peak level of activity. It is best to rest one full day between exercising each specific muscle group in order to allow that group to recover. Cross-training helps maintain fitness, especially if your muscles have gotten sore from a particular exercise.

■ **COOL DOWN:** Do not stop activities such as stretching, strengthening, or aerobic exercise abruptly. Instead, slow down gradually. For example, if you have been jogging or running, walk for 3 to 5 minutes afterwards to allow your circulatory system to slow down gradually.

■ **AEROBIC EXERCISE:** Aerobic and strengthening exercises require a minimum of 20 to 25 minutes at least three times per week in order to have a significant physiologic impact. Riding a bike, walking, or any other activity that can be done with a partner will help keep you both motivated. If you can hold a normal conversation without getting out of breath while you are walking, you are walking at the right pace.

■ **KNOW YOUR LIMITS:** Pace yourself. When first beginning an exercise program, do a little bit the first day, a little more the next, and then more the following day. Gradually increasing your level of activity will allow your body to reap the benefits of exercise in a safe manner. Back off for a day or two if a muscle starts to get sore and resume exercise when the soreness has eased up. Also, remember not to exercise when you are sick with a cold or the flu, because your body is already challenged enough without being overloaded with challenging exercise.

■ **BE REALISTIC:** Remember not to expect miracles right away, especially if you have neglected your body and are beginning to exercise after many years. You are likely to become discouraged and discontinue exercising before giving your body a reasonable chance to get back into shape if you expect immediate and dramatic improvement. It is reasonable to allow 6 to 8 weeks before you notice an improvement.

■ **USE THE RIGHT EQUIPMENT:** Wearing the correct shoes and using the correct sports equipment can go a long way in preserving safety and avoiding injury.

■ **ASK QUESTIONS:** If you are unsure about something—however trivial you think it may be—be sure to ask an athletic trainer or physical therapist.

WALKING IS THE BEST FORM OF EXERCISE

According to the Centers for Disease Control and Prevention (CDC), approximately two-thirds of the U.S. population fails to get 30 minutes of daily exercise. In fact, a full one-third of all people live a life officially defined as sedentary. Recently, the National Academy of Sciences reported that 30 minutes per day of exercise may not be enough. Upping the ante to 60 minutes of moderately intense activity per day is preferable. Unfortunately, only 3% of Americans exercise 60 minutes per day.

One of the best ways to exercise moderately is by walking. Walking is free, pleasant, safe, easy to accomplish, and hard to do wrong. A growing body of evidence suggests that the benefits of walking include a lowered risk for heart attack, diabetes, stroke, osteoporosis, and breast and colon cancer. Walking also helps reduce weight, cholesterol levels, constipation, age-related dementia, impotence, and depression. It also increases muscle mass, flattens the belly, and helps reshape the thighs.

Because a majority of Americans are overweight and, hence, carry around more poundage than they ideally should, walking is a much safer choice than jogging, running, or aerobics. The plain and simple reason is that with each step taken, walkers land with only one-fifth of the force that a jogger or person performing aerobic exercise does. Attempting to reach a goal of 10,000 steps a day (about 5 miles) was the ideal put forth by the former Surgeon General C. Everett Koop in an attempt to help Americans become fitter and leaner; this program was called "Shape Up America." A person who works in an office typically walks an average of 2,500 to 5,000 steps per day. It might be worth purchasing a pedometer and clipping it to your waist from morning until bedtime for inspiration!

Index